Comprehensive
Anatomy for Martial Arts

Comprehensive Anatomy for Martial Arts

A Systems Approach to Anatomy and Biomechanics

for Sports, Martial Arts, & Modern-Day Warriors

Barry A. Broughton, PhD

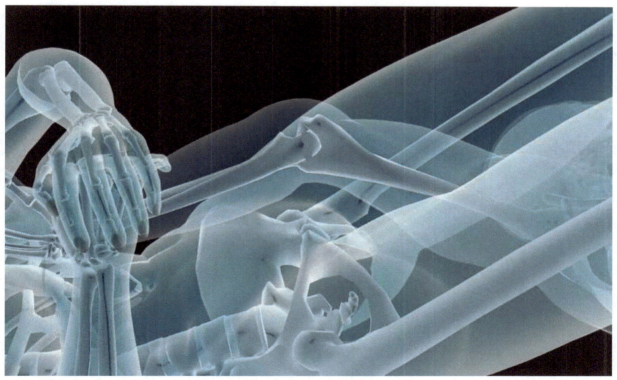

Fig. 0.1 Skeletal Armbar. Image Credit: FatalHolds, 2010. Used with artist's written permission. Not for reuse.

Comprehensive Anatomy for Martial Arts

A Systems Approach to Anatomy and Biomechanics

for Sports, Martial Arts, & Modern-Day Warriors

Disclaimer: This book is intended for educational purposes only. The medical information in this text is provided as a resource only and is not to be used or relied upon for any diagnostic or treatment purposes. The information contained herein is intended for academic use only, and does not create a doctor-patient relationship, and should not be used as a substitute for professional diagnosis and treatment. By purchasing or reading this text you agree to the foregoing terms and conditions. The author and publisher of this book are not responsible in any manner whatsoever for any adverse effects or injuries that arrive directly or indirectly from the material presented in this text.

Published by Rustic Studio Publishing

ISBN 978-1-939263-94-0

Library of Congress Number: TX 9-263-673

Copyright © 2022 Barry A. Broughton

All rights reserved. No part of this publication may be reproduced or utilized in any form or by any means, electronic or mechanical, including recording, photocopying, or by any information storage or retrieval system, including any future means not yet known or created without the prior express written consent of the author.

Dedication

This book is dedicated to all the AKT Combatives-Jujitsu practitioners, martial art students, college self-defense students, and Black Belt students who have allowed me to turn nearly every class for over four decades into an anatomy lesson. Your patience and continual thirst for knowledge are a true motivator in the writing of this reference text.

Contents

About the Author xiii
Preface xv
Introduction xvii

SECTION ONE: *BIOMECHANICS* 1

Chapter 1 1
Principles of Biomechanics 1
Newton's Laws of Motion 2
Force 5
Moment, Moment Arm, and Torque 6
Base and Balance 11
Martial Arts Relevance: 12
    Throws and Takedowns 12
    The Science of Punching (and Striking) Power 14
Levers 17
Motion 20

SECTION TWO: TERMINOLOGY 27

Chapter 2 25
Martial Arts Relevance: Talking The Language 25
The Anatomical Position 26
Anatomical Terms of Movement 28
Anatomical Terms of Location 32
Body Cavities 35

SECTION THREE: Introduction to the Human Body 37

Chapter 3 — The Integumentary System 41
Layers of Skin 41
Clinical Significance and Martial Arts Relevance 46
    Scalp Lacerations and Facial Lacerations 46
Appendages of the Integumentary System 47
Clinical Significance and Martial Arts Relevance: 49
    Skin Infections 49

Chapter 4 — The Skeletal System 55
Structure of Bone Tissue 56
Classification of Bones 59
Classification of Joints 61
Accessory Structures of a Synovial Joint 66
Clinical Significance and Martial Arts Relevance: 67
    Bursitis 67
    Post-traumatic Osteoarthritis 67
The Human Skeleton 68
Skeletal Terms 71

Axial Skeleton (80 bones) 76
Clinical Significance and Martial Arts Relevance: 77
    Fractures of the Pterion 77
    Fracture of the Cribriform Plate 78
    Facial Fractures 80
Clinical Significance and Martial Arts Relevance: 82
    Fracture of the Hyoid Bone 82
Vertebral Column 83
▪ Cervical Spine 84
Clinical Significance and Martial Arts Relevance: 86
    Injuries to the Cervical Spine 86
▪ Thoracic Spine 92
▪ Lumbar Spine 93
Clinical Significance and Martial Arts Relevance: 94
    Fractured Coccyx 94
The Thoracic Cage 94
Clinical Significance and Martial Arts Relevance: 101
    Rib Fractures 101
Appendicular Skeleton (126 bones) 103
Shoulder Girdle 103
Clinical Significance and Martial Arts Relevance: 106
    Acromioclavicular Dislocation 106
    Clavicle Fracture 107
    Two major types of SC joint dislocation: 108
Upper Extremity 109
Arm 110
Humerus 110
Glenohumeral Joint 111
Clinical Significance and Martial Arts Relevance: 113
    Dislocation of the Shoulder Joint 113
Elbow Joint 115
Clinical Significance and Martial Arts Relevance: 117
    Injuries to the Elbow Joint 117
    Straight Armbar 119
Forearm 125
Clinical Significance and Martial Arts Relevance: 131
    Common Fractures of the Radius 131
    Mid Shaft Ulna Fracture 132
Wrist 134
Clinical Significance and Martial Arts Relevance: 137
    Scaphoid Fracture 137
    Anterior Dislocation of the Lunate 138
    Triangular Fibrocartilage Complex Tear 138
    Wrist Locks 139
Hand 140
Clinical Significance and Martial Arts Relevance: 141
    Boxer's Fracture 141

- Knuckles 143
- Fight Bite 143
- Arthritis of the Hand... 143
- Finger Injuries 145
- Pelvic Girdle.. 148
- Clinical Significance and Martial Arts Relevance:.................................. 149
  - Pubic Symphysis Injury 149
  - Pubic Rami Fractures... 149
  - Acetabulum Fractures 150
- Lower Extremity 151
- Thigh... 152
- Acetabulofemoral Joint 154
- Knee Joint 155
- Clinical Significance and Martial Arts Relevance:.................................. 158
  - Patellar Dislocation 158
  - Patellar Fracture... 158
  - Medial Collateral Ligament Tear... 159
  - Anterior Cruciate Ligament Tear... 160
  - Meniscus Tear.. 161
  - Attacks to the Knee: Low Kicks, Kneebars, Reaps, Heel Hooks.... 162
- Leg 164
- Clinical Significance and Martial Arts Relevance:.................................. 169
  - Fractures of the Tibia... 169
  - Fractures of the Distal Fibula 170
- Ankle Joint 171
- Clinical Significance and Martial Arts Relevance:.................................. 174
  - Ankle Movement and Stability 174
  - Ankle Locks 175
  - Ankle Sprains 178
  - Avulsion Fractures 178
- Foot 179
- Clinical Significance and Martial Arts Relevance:.................................. 183
  - Fractures of the Talus and Calcaneus... 183
  - Fractures of the Metatarsal Bones.. 184
  - Plantar Fasciitis 185

Chapter 5 — The Muscular System 189

- Types of Muscle Tissue... 190
- Understanding Muscle Names 193
- Muscles of the Head and Neck.. 195
- Muscles of the Torso 196
- Clinical Significance and Martial Arts Relevance:.................................. 199
  - Abdomen vs Stomach 199
- Muscles of the Upper Extremity.. 207
- Clinical Significance and Martial Arts Relevance:.................................. 212
  - Rotator Cuff Tendonitis and Rotator Cuff Tear 212
  - Bent Armbar 213
  - Rupture of the Biceps Tendon 216

  Epicondylitis 221
  Making a Proper Fist 221
  Mallet Finger 228
  A Boutonniere Deformity 229
  Jersey Finger 229
 Muscles of the Lower Extremity 236
 Clinical Significance and Martial Arts Relevance: 248
  Osteitis Pubis 248
  Injury to the Adductor Muscles - "Pulled Groin" 249
  Myositis ossificans 249
  Hamstring Injury: Muscle Strain 254
  Avulsion Fracture of the Ischial Tuberosity 254
  Baker's Cyst 264
 Skeletal Muscles: Their Origins, Insertions, and Actions 266

Chapter 6 — The Nervous System 285
 How Does the Human Body Create Electricity? 286
 Nerve Tissue 287
 Organization of the Nervous System 290
 Central Nervous System Overview 291
 Clinical Significance and Martial Arts Relevance: 293
  Extradural and Subdural Hematomas 293
  Concussion 297
 The Peripheral Nervous System 302
 Autonomic Nervous System 310
 Clinical Significance and Martial Arts Relevance: 312
  Solar Plexus 312
 The Somatic Nervous System 313

Chapter 7 — Special Sensory Organs 319
 The Ears 319
 Clinical Significance and Martial Arts Relevance: 321
  Auricular Hematoma and Cauliflower Ear 321
  Perforation of the Tympanic Membrane 324
  Mechanisms of Equilibrium 336
 The Eyes 339
 Clinical Significance and Martial Arts Relevance: 345
  Hyphema 345

Chapter 8 — The Respiratory System 347
 Mechanics of Ventilation 348
 Clinical Significance and Martial Arts Relevance: 350
  Compression of the Chest 350
 Respiratory Passages 351
 Clinical Significance and Martial Arts Relevance: 353
  Nasal Fracture 353
  Epistaxis 353
  Airway Chokes 357
 Bronchi, Bronchial Tree, & Lungs 359

Chapter 9 — The Cardiovascular System 361
- Heart...362
- Cardiac Conduction System...366
- Blood 367
- Blood Vessels...367
- Clinical Significance and Martial Arts Relevance:...............................371
  - *Carotid Triangle*..371
  - *Vascular Neck Restraints*..372
  - *Injury to the External Jugular Vein* 373

Chapter 10 — The Lymphatic System.............................377
- Components of the Lymphatic System 380
- Clinical Significance and Martial Arts Relevance:...............................385
  - *Rupture of the Spleen*..385

Chapter 11 — The Digestive System 387
- Organs of the Digestive System 389
- Clinical Significance and Martial Arts Relevance:...............................393
  - *Liver Shot*..393

Chapter 12 — The Genitourinary System 395
- Components of the Urinary System 396
- Components of the Reproductive System..399
- Clinical Significance and Martial Arts Relevance:...............................402
  - *Injuries to the Genitalia*...402

Chapter 13 — The Endocrine System 407
- Endocrine Glands & Their Hormones..409
- Clinical Significance and Martial Arts Relevance:...............................413
  - *Fight, Flight, or Freeze*...413

SECTION FOUR: *PHYSIOLOGY* 419

Chapter 14 — The Physiology of Specific Techniques 421
- Vascular Neck Restraints 421
- Airway Chokes 424
- Physiology of the Liver Shot 426

SECTION FIVE: *PSEUDOSCIENCE* 429

Chapter 15..431
- Pseudoscience In Martial Arts..431

Bibliography... 441

Glossary 447

ABOUT THE AUTHOR

Barry A. Broughton, PhD has applied his years of experience in orthopedics and sports medicine to his extensive training in the martial arts to create and found AKT Combatives-Jujitsu, a comprehensive reality-based martial arts system.

Dr. Broughton served on active duty in the US Army for nine years, initially as a Combat Medic and then as a Battalion Medical Officer. As an Orthopedic Specialist, he holds a Bachelor of Science as a Physician Associate, completed a 2-year Orthopedic Surgery PA Residency Program, and holds a PhD in Health and Human Services. Having been board certified in both primary care and surgery he has completed hundreds of hours of Continuing Medical Education (CME), and certified in Pediatric Advanced Life Support, Advanced Cardiac Life Support, Advanced Trauma Life Support, and has also completed the USA Boxing Ringside Physician Course sponsored by the American College of Sports Medicine.

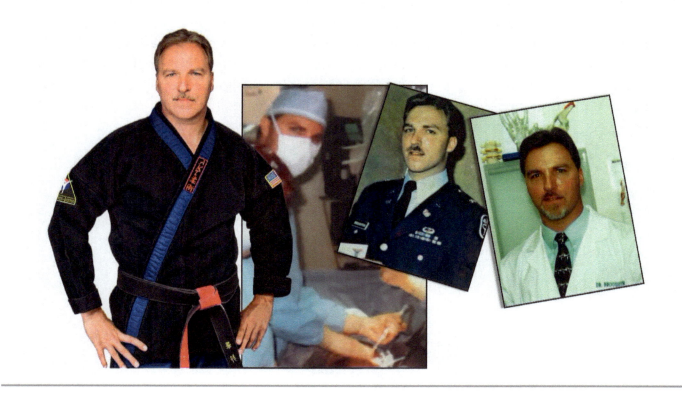

Broughton has earned Black Belts in several martial art styles and has been inducted into multiple Martial Arts Halls of Fame, and the Bare Knuckle Boxing Hall of Fame. He has served on the Board of Directors of several martial arts organizations and is the North Atlantic Regional Director for the American Sport Jujitsu League at the time of this publication. Due to his numerous accomplishments, he has been featured in *The Martial Directory: International*

Instructors Edition; Who's Who in the Martial Arts; Black Belt Power; US Veterans Magazine, and more.

Broughton is the head coach of Team AKT Sport Jujitsu team and was on the coaching staff of the 2017 and 2019 Gold Medal US National Jujitsu Teams. As a competitor he has won numerous tournaments culminating his competition career with Silver and Gold Medals at the World Jujitsu Championships. He has taught Emergency Medical Technician (EMT) and Paramedic courses for City Colleges of Chicago; Self-Defense, MMA, and the AKT Combatives-Jujitsu curriculum as Physical Education credit courses for State University of New York (SUNY) — Jamestown Community College; was the Martial Arts Club Advisor at Saint Bonaventure University; and teaches Police Defensive Tactics, Personal Protection, and Jujitsu related seminars both nationally and internationally.

He is the bestselling author of *Beyond Self-Defense: AKT Combatives Reality-Based Personal Protection* that is used as a textbook for college self-defense classes and is the contributing author to several bestselling martial arts compilation works as well.

Drawing on his multi-faceted experience, Dr. Broughton has created this comprehensive reference text to aid martial artists in improving their understanding of human anatomy and biomechanics. This text is also intended to raise the level of professionalism amongst martial arts instructors by assisting them in teaching relevant human anatomy more accurately while dispelling many antiquated misconceptions related to biomechanics and martial arts. This book is intended to be used as a reference text to aid in the understanding and teaching of human anatomy as it relates to martial arts training but can also be a valuable resource for other sports.

For more information about the author and AKT Combatives-Jujitsu, or to schedule a seminar with Dr. Broughton in your area, visit www.AKTcombatives.com.

PREFACE

▪ Motivation

I have treated thousands of broken bones, knife wounds, gunshot wounds, and other self-defense, martial arts, and combat sports related injuries over the course of my career in orthopedics and sports medicine. In addition to those acute trauma related injuries, I have also treated countless chronic overuse (and degenerative) injuries. Most injuries occur purely by accident, yet too often they occur due to poor training and a lack of preparation. Unfortunately, there is a subset of injuries (both acute and chronic) that occur inadvertently because of a misunderstanding of the biomechanics and human anatomy involved in executing certain techniques.

As a martial arts instructor, it is my responsibility to minimize the potential for injury to my students while training, in competition, or during real-life/real-world self-defense situations. The pursuit of martial arts prowess is fraught with the potential for injury, some of which can be career-ending. Therefore, to extend the longevity of our training- and survival, we must attempt to diminish the potential for injury of those under our charge. If needed, techniques must be modified to be more practical, and yet have maximum effect on an assailant while using the most efficient and safest means possible. However, that cannot be achieved without a comprehensive understanding of human anatomy and the biomechanics involved with the execution of self-defense related techniques. Let me explain…

The first time I dissected a human shoulder during my anatomy cadaver lab in college, it was not at all what I had envisioned! With my gloved fingers inside of the joint capsule, I pushed the humeral head forward. I focused deep beyond the formaldehyde-soaked muscles of the rotator cuff. *Stabilize the scapula. Rotate the humerus. Apply the pressure.* POP! *Success!* I'd dislocated the shoulder! While I *should* have been observing the mechanics of the ball-and-socket joint as an eager student of medicine, I found myself exploring human anatomy through the lens of a martial artist trying to determine the most efficient and effective way to dislocate the shoulder joint.

Again, early in my orthopedic surgery training, while performing a surgical procedure on a patient with chronic recurrent anterior shoulder dislocations, I examined the range of motion of the surgically exposed shoulder (glenohumeral) joint. This intimate view allowed me to examine the limitations of the joint. I could see in which directions the humeral head was *not* supposed to go, and why. I immediately thought — although I never told my patient this! — *that's why a bent armbar doesn't always work!* I realized that a *bent armbar* would be much more effective if I made some subtle changes to the way in which I positioned the arm while executing the technique.

Beyond studying in just the classroom, I was able to gain a deeper appreciation of human anatomy in the cadaver lab, which was reinforced via fresh autopsies during my clinical training, and then "re-learned" in the operating room with live patients. Having the opportunity to evaluate x-rays, CT scans, and MRIs, and *then* compare those finding to actual living anatomy in the operating room provided an invaluable foundation for a detailed understanding of human anatomy. Similarly, reducing (putting back into place) innumerable displaced broken bones and joint dislocations, provided an in-depth grasp of which way joints should and should not move. I understand that not everyone has these same opportunities. Fortunately, however, everyone does not need to take that same journey to reap the benefits. I am honored to be able pass this knowledge along to others with this work: *Comprehensive Anatomy for Martial Arts*.

▪ Purpose

Because we live in a three-dimensional world, our bodies move in more than just a one-dimensional plane. Therefore, one cannot gain a full appreciation of human anatomy and biomechanics by just memorizing a two-dimensional basic anatomy chart hanging on a dojo wall. Doing so only provides a superficial understanding of anatomical locations at best. Conversely, understanding the nuances of human anatomy and the biomechanics involved in kinesiology quickly shortens the learning curve, increases the efficiency and efficacy of applying techniques, and in the process, elevates the skill level of martial artists and perhaps could save someone's life in a real self-defense situation.

In this text, I strive to change the way in which martial artists comprehend and apply their knowledge of human anatomy as it relates to the learning and teaching of martial arts techniques. My hope is to raise the level of proficiency surrounding accurate and relevant human anatomy and biomechanics within the martial arts community. In addition to personal use, I also envision this reference text being incorporated into the curriculum of martial arts styles, academies, and instructor certification courses.

~Barry A. Broughton, PhD

INTRODUCTION

▪ What This Book Is... and is Not!

Not understanding anatomy in martial endeavors is like blasting birdshot at a target with a shotgun. In a physical altercation, you can throw a bunch of punches and kicks, and splatter the target with potentially non-lethal strikes — a lot of wasted effort without a very good return on your investment — or you can attack anatomic vulnerabilities with the precision of a sniper rifle. Snipers are martial scientists. Their every shot is calculated as they judge the distance, the geography, wind conditions, and the position of their target, as well as their own skill level. For a martial artist, understanding anatomy allows one the precision laser-like target acquisition of a sniper, while avoiding haphazard techniques that expose your own vulnerabilities.

As with most books of a science related nature, *Comprehensive Anatomy for Martial Arts* is meant to be used as a reference text; to be read, studied, and re-read as needed. Although it may be read straight through, cover-to-cover; it will likely be most useful by reading the sections that are most pertinent, or of most interest, at any given time. However, for those who do not have a background in medicine, healthcare, or the sciences it is advised to read Section One (Biomechanics) and Section Two (Terminology) before reading the chapters in Section Three (Introduction to the Human Body, and specific organ systems). Doing so will provide a better understanding of the anatomical descriptions discussed throughout most of this reference text. Please refer to the Terminology section or use the Glossary at the end of the book if you are not familiar with the usage of a certain word or phrase.

Even though this book is written at a college graduate school level, it is presented in a descriptive format with copious images and illustrations that makes is accessible to most readers. The use of medical and scientific descriptive terminology is used throughout this book because it allows for more precise and accurate explanations of human anatomy and their interactions with other structures. In using these terms, martial artists will not only become more familiar with the scientific vernacular but will be better able to provide accurate descriptions and instructions while teaching martial arts techniques.

This book is designed to be a *systems* approach to human anatomy, presenting each organ system individually. However, as discussed later in this text all organ systems must work together to achieve any given task. With that in mind, there will be some discussions in certain sections of this book that will overlap.

Because the physical nature of martial arts is related to human movement, the vast majority of injuries sustained during training, competition, and real-world self-defense are musculoskeletal related. Therefore, the chapters related to musculoskeletal anatomy will be presented in greater detail than other organ systems.

This reference text is not just a picture book with labeled diagrams and is not intended to be an instructional book on how to execute certain techniques. However, specific anatomical structures that can be injured during certain techniques, or how a specific technique may be executed more effectively will be presented.

To aid in the application of the material presented in this text, there are sections titled *Clinical Significance and Martial Arts Relevance* disbursed throughout each chapter. These sections will provide more insight and detail related to the anatomical structures being discussed as they relate to martial arts techniques and injuries. An often-overlooked concept in martial arts training is that most techniques are designed to inflict harm and injury to the assailant. These sections will aid in understanding how that occurs, or how to possibly prevent it from happening.

Because this reference text is written from a modern scientific physical anatomy perspective; mysticism, meridians, and chi will not be presented as quantifiable or relevant entities. The ideas of meridians and chi (qi or ki) are only addressed in the last chapter on Pseudoscience in the Martial Arts.

Academia in the Martial Arts

▪ Professional Warriors

"The only true wisdom is in knowing you know nothing." ~ Socrates

"Knowing that you don't know is the first step to true wisdom"
~ *The third tenet from the AKT Student Creed*.

Anyone who has studied martial arts for any length of time knows that the ancient samurai of Japan were not only proficient on the battlefield but were also well versed in the arts and philosophy. In addition to military tactics, archery, swordsmanship, and unarmed combat, samurai also pursued the development of intellectual virtues.

Being samurai was not just about the physical aspect of the *martial spirit*. In fact, samurai were expected to be just as skilled in the literary arts as they were with a sword. As the essential nobility of their era, members of the samurai class were far more than mere warriors. Most samurai were well-educated. At a time when very few Europeans could read, the level of samurai literacy was extremely high. Participating in numerous cultural and artistic endeavors, samurai studied poetry, monochrome ink paintings, and calligraphy, as well as literature and history.

The dedication to the arts, sciences, and literature among warriors was not isolated to Japan or Asian cultures. Throughout history, warriors in many cultures nurtured their personal and intellectual development in addition to their physical martial arts training. True growth in the martial arts is only possible if we cultivate ourselves both mentally and physically.

Direct physical combat experience can indeed perpetuate a military that can fight and win *battles*; but it is *education* that provides the intellectual depth and breadth that allows soldiers to understand and succeed in *war*. Lieutenant General Sir William Francis Butler was a British Army officer and prolific writer in the late 19th-century.

"The nation that will insist on drawing a broad line of demarcation between the fighting man and the thinking man is liable to find its fighting done by fools and its thinking done by cowards." ~ Sir William Francis Butler

Butler's conclusion that academic rigors are requisite for soldiers goes beyond that of a nation's military and its leaders. Individuals concerned with their own personal-protection, and that of their family and loved ones, would also benefit in pursuing a similar balance.

Even modern professional career military soldiers are required additional training and education beyond the physical skills required of combat. Career commissioned officers, warrant officers, and non-commissioned officers of today's military must seek continuing education in order to get promoted and remain on active-duty status. "Leaders are readers" is a popular adage in today's business and political arenas, but the phrase is even more relevant within the military. In a military combat setting, leaders who do not read must learn by experience — the hard way! The consequence of their ignorance comes at the expense and lives of young soldiers. Most people are not aware that the primary educational focus of the United States Military Academy at *West Point*, perhaps the most revered military institution in history, is not on the study of military science, but on mathematics, engineering, and the hard sciences. It was not until General Douglas MacArthur served as the Academy's Superintendent from 1919 to 1922 that the educational focus shifted towards *liberal arts* and the *humanities*. Graduates from the Military Academy have a well-rounded education in the humanities, technology, and sciences to stimulate critical thinking and problem-solving.

▪ Missing *Martial:* Why is This Relevant Now?

Prevalent in today's "light-to-no contact" era of competitions, and training with only compliant partners who never give resistance, are practitioners of flawed theories who have never pressure-tested their techniques or concepts in an arena (test lab) of non-compliance and reality.

Having never done so, either via aggressive competition with heavy contact and full resistance, or by the pressure-testing of techniques against a non-compliant assailant, a false sense of confidence and security ensues. Stephen Hawking is noted as saying "The greatest enemy of knowledge is not ignorance; it is the illusion of knowledge." Psychologists refer to this *cognitive bias* as the Dunning-Kruger Effect. It is a condition in which incompetent people suffer from *illusory superiority* and mistakenly tend to believe they are competent; while competent people tend to believe that they are less competent than they actually are.

It is typically those people who know a great deal about a certain topic who remain attentive and teachable. This is usually because those who are truly competent understand there is always more to be learned even in their given area of expertise.

Any martial artist suffering from the Dunning-Kruger Effect will get a reality check if they ever find themselves on the receiving end of a truly violent altercation. Ignorance may be bliss, however, in real-world personal protection it can get you killed.

Many martial artists profess to teach some form of real-world personal protection, yet too many of them continue to teach outdated and antiquated concepts. In a world where information is so easily attainable by anyone, how can instructors who continue to perpetuate falsehoods such as "Breaking someone's eardrums will cause them to not be able to walk" be taken seriously? Beliefs, concepts, and techniques that are passed down without ever verifying their veracity contributes to the lack of perceived professionalism in the martial arts. Scientists and scholars do research to test a hypothesis and prove a theory. Martial artists and martial scientists need to test techniques and concepts in a real "laboratory" environment. You cannot adequately test your defense against a rear naked choke if your training partner is not applying any direct pressure to your carotid arteries. For that to occur, they need to know where the carotid arteries actually lay, and what they do.

Sun Tzu explained in *The Art of War*, "If you know the enemy and know yourself, you need not fear the result of a hundred battles." How then do you "know your enemy?" By gaining intel, by study, by research, by reading. Taking this idea even one step further, rather than just understanding your assailant's or opponent's strategic and tactical abilities; you must also understand their actual physical vulnerabilities — their *anatomical* weaknesses. Learning to think as a martial *scientist* will provide the tools needed when evaluating the efficacy of techniques: Are the end results reproducible? Will that specific technique work in more than just a finite number of situations? Will this technique work against a non-compliant training partner, or an aggressive assailant, or someone of a larger size? If the answer to any of these questions is *No*, the martial scientist needs to reevaluate either the technique itself or the application in which it is being used.

▪ Be A Warrior-Scholar

Early in both my martial arts and medical careers, I understood the importance of knowing human anatomy, and *that* understanding enabled my martial arts techniques to be much more effective. It became clear that *that* specific knowledge could not only shorten my learning curve but also that of my students, and that specialized insight could assist them in achieving a higher degree of effectiveness and consistency when executing techniques. From that moment forward, I began my explorative journey into better understanding anatomical vulnerabilities to enhance not only my martial arts journey but that of others as well.

This quest for knowledge is the core of a warrior-scholar. My keen interest in using anatomical vulnerabilities is just one example of a warrior-scholar's quest.

The advantage a warrior-scholar has is gaining knowledge their enemy doesn't have or doesn't bother to learn. As a U.S. Army veteran, I know firsthand that soldiers (warriors) understand their lives depend on being better trained than their enemy. If they cannot be faster or stronger, they had better be smarter. Knowing their enemy's vulnerabilities is the first step to overcoming and surviving combat.

Warrior-scholars who know human anatomy are better able to apply biomechanics — the momentum and leverage needed to efficiently execute techniques on any plane in any given scenario. Understanding the anatomy and biomechanics of the pelvis and hip joint (i.e., how the femoral head articulates with the acetabulum) assists with proper *post-foot* positioning, thereby improving the height and power of kicking techniques.

Warrior-scholars research what works best based on hard evidence. When they gain new data or acquire a new skillset, they must be willing to change. *Evolve or become irrelevant.* Not evolving can have dire consequences when others have gained new insights.

• Good Intel

You can overcome a more powerful adversary with good intel. Over the duration of my martial arts career, I've seen it demonstrated numerous times in real-world self-defense scenarios, at martial arts tournaments, and in combat sports.

A student of mine had been competing in Sport Jujitsu tournaments for only three years before being selected for the USA National Jujitsu Team. At the World Jujitsu Championships, my student faced an opponent who was bigger, stronger, and had much more experience. By using their *knowledge* of anatomy and biomechanics, while fighting to apply a straight armbar, my student made a subtle adjustment to the forearm of the seasoned warrior and was able to apply the elbow lock efficiently and effectively. With that one small anatomical adjustment, my student had decisively locked the opponent's elbow and got the Win over a much more experienced and worthy opponent.

Good intel or specialized knowledge is how warriors improve their odds of winning battles. Martial artists win bouts, and everyday people survive violent self-defense situations, by using knowledge against their adversary.

Becoming a warrior-scholar or a martial scientist is simply the act of enhancing your education in a desired field. *Knowing* your enemy is more than simply understanding their strategic and tactical capabilities. It is also about understanding their actual physical vulnerabilities — their *anatomical weaknesses*.

• Scientific Method

The *scientific method* is the inquiry and testing of a hypothesis through achieving empirical and measurable data as evidence. This is achieved with a deliberate observation of what is being evaluated. Understanding the potential for cognitive bias, careful skepticism is applied to what was observed during the evaluation. Re-evaluation and reproducible results are paramount. As *martial scientists*, we have the moral obligation to evaluate the efficacy of what we teach. Therefore, we must evaluate the effectiveness and practicality of techniques. Understanding the anatomical and biomechanical principles governing individual techniques aids in the testing of their application in real-world scenarios.

From a science-based center, I assert that certain dogma (practices and beliefs) thought to be true needs to be reevaluated when new data is presented. That is often hard to do in a *traditional* environment, where honoring traditions is valued over evolving; and modifying techniques (and concepts) needed to meet today's self-defense realities are met with suspicion. Not evolving can be dangerous and even deadly when personal safety is at stake.

Initially it was difficult for me to admit that some of the techniques (and concepts) I had been taught were ineffective (or inaccurate) in real-world conflict. I do not place blame. I know that the vast majority of martial arts instructors are doing their best at passing down information previously taught to them. I understand why some martial arts instructors find it hard to accept they may have been mistaken and need to modify the way in which certain techniques are being taught. However, in scientific research, the goal is to find the truth; if "past truths" are proven wrong in that quest, you mustn't get offended and take it personal.

Applying a scientific approach to my life-long passion of martial arts, and based on my background in sports medicine and orthopedic surgery, I am convinced that having a strong understanding of scientific principles and human anatomy is vitally important for modern-day warriors. Being able to readily identify vulnerable targets is extremely important in mounting effective and efficient self-defense tactics and strategies. No matter how long a martial artist has been training, it is never too late to adopt and integrate new information. That is the joy of being a life-long learner and warrior-scholar. It is to that end that I present the material offered in *Comprehensive Anatomy for Martial Arts*.

SECTION ONE

BIOMECHANICS

Chapter 1

BIOMECHANICS

Biomechanics is the application of mechanical principles to human movement. Applying engineering concepts and the laws of physics to the study of the human body provides a better understanding of the relationship between external environments and the muscles, tendons, bones, and joints during locomotion.

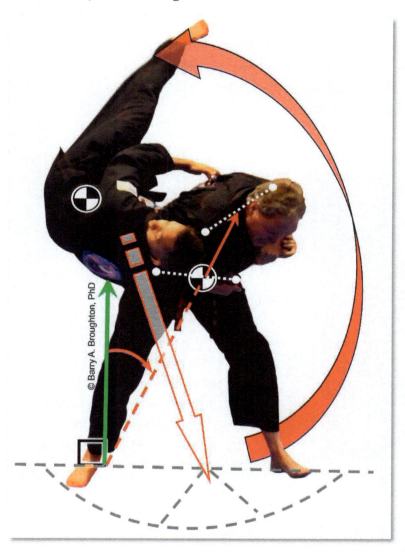

Human movement occurs when an external or internal force is applied to the body. The force required for movement depends on the mass on which the force is exerted, with the extremities, muscles, and joints interacting to create the desired movement. External factors such as gravity can vary the force required to produce any given movement.

PRINCIPLES OF BIOMECHANICS

It is important to know several biomechanical principles and terms to better understand the role of biomechanics in martial arts training. Understanding how these principles work is important to improve the effectiveness of techniques while executing throws, grappling, and strikes.

Fig. 1.1 - The application of biomechanics in executing a throw.

Kinetics and Kinematics

Two distinct areas known as kinetics (the forces by which movement is initiated) and kinematics (how the body moves) are crucial in studying biomechanics. For example, the kinematic data obtained from an analysis of roundhouse kicks detail the angles of motion that occur at each joint at different time points throughout the kicking cycle. Kinetic information from this type of analysis may be used to calculate the force generated from a muscle to control leg movements during the kick. Understanding both the kinematics and kinetics of human movement can allow for more efficient and effective movements during martial arts activities. It can also allow healthcare providers to gain a greater understanding of how best to prevent, reduce, and rehabilitate injuries.

Newton's Laws of Motion

Our current understanding of how forces act upon the human body is derived from Sir Isaac Newton's principles of physics. Newton published the three-volume classic text in 1687 which detailed the three laws of motion along with the universal law of gravitation. These laws explain how forces create motion in martial arts related activities.

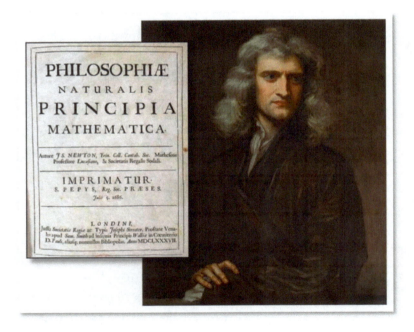

Newton's First Law- Law of Inertia

"Every object persists in a state of rest or uniform motion unless it is compelled to change that state by forces impressed upon it."

Newton's first law explains how objects tend to resist change and remain at rest unless a force is exerted upon it. The second consideration of this law is that once an object is moving it will remain moving at the same velocity unless another force acts upon it.

Fig. 1.2 - Sir Isaac Newton published his famous work Philosophiæ Naturalis Principia Mathematica, which lays out the laws of universal motion in 1687.

In human motion each movement must be initiated by force, but it will also take a force to stop or change that move.

In sports, the first law of motion can be demonstrated by a penalty kick in soccer. Before the kick, the ball is in a state of rest; however, once a ball is kicked, a force acts upon it and movement is initiated.

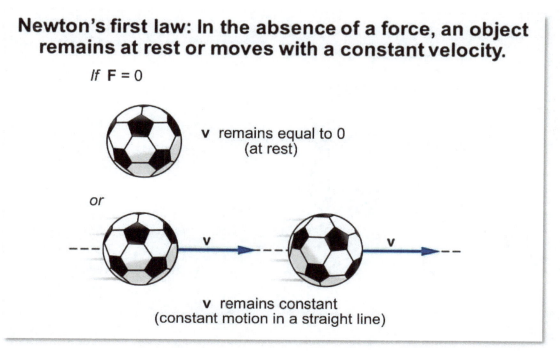

Fig. 1.3 - Diagram of Newton's First Law explained.

Newton's Second Law — Law of Acceleration

> "The relationship between an object's mass (m), its acceleration (a), and its applied force (F) is $F = ma$. The direction of the force vector is the same as the direction of its acceleration vector."

The second law of motion is important when analyzing the forces involved in movement. Newton's Second Law explains how much motion a force creates. The acceleration (tendency of an object to change speed or direction) an object experiences is proportional to the size of the force, and inversely proportional to the object's mass (F=ma).

In sports, the second law can be understood by envisioning a basketball player attempting to make a foul shot with either a basketball or a bowling ball. Because the bowling ball has greater mass than the basketball, a greater amount of force must be exerted to cause acceleration at the same rate toward the hoop.

As the mass of an object increases so does the force required to propel it at a given acceleration. Knowledge of an object's mass and acceleration makes it possible to measure the force applied to it.

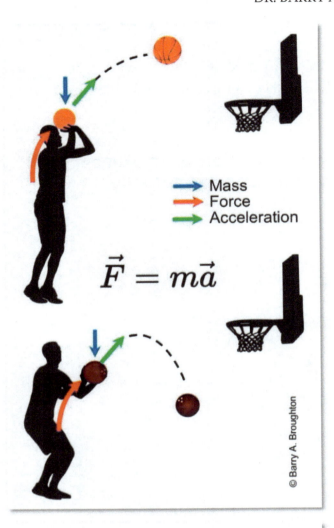

Fig. 1.4 - Newton's second law can be expressed mathematically through the equation F=ma where F is the resultant force, m is the mass of the object, and a is the acceleration of the body.

Newton's Third Law — Law of Action and Reaction

"For every action, there is an equal and opposite reaction."

The third law can be demonstrated by bouncing a tennis ball on the floor. The ball has mass and is accelerating toward the floor, making impact with a certain amount of force. At the point of contact, the ball is met with an equal and opposite reaction force, which causes the ball to rebound. The equal and opposite reaction from the floor is known as the ground reaction force.

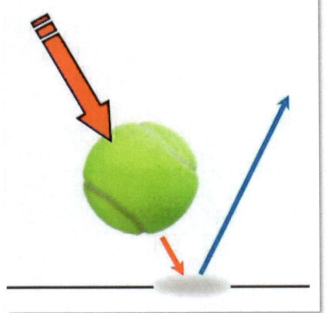

Fig. 1.5 - Every action has an equal and opposite reaction.

FORCE

What is force?

Force is simply the push or pull action required for an object to move, stop, or change shape. Force is measured in Newtons (N), with one newton defined as the force required to accelerate one kilogram of mass at the rate of one meter per second squared. Understanding forces at work and the actions they have on the body is essential when trying to understand human movement.

In physics there are four types of forces present in nature: *gravitational* force, *electromagnetic* force, *weak nuclear* force, and *strong nuclear* force. When evaluating the biomechanics of human movement, the effect of gravitational force is most often considered.

> *"Two bodies attract each other with a force that is proportional to the product of their masses and inversely proportional to the square of the distance between them."* ~Newton's Law of Gravitation.

Gravity is an attraction force that occurs between any two objects that have mass. The more mass an object has, the greater its attraction force. In the study of biomechanics, it is essential to consider the constant action that gravity has on the human body during movement. Near to the earth's surface, gravity is continually causing an accelerating effect on the body that is roughly equivalent to 9.81 meters/s^2 (approximately 32 feet/second squared). At ground level this is not always apparent, due to the opposite and equal force being applied by the ground. When free falling from an airplane, a skydiver accelerates towards Earth, achieving a maximum speed (terminal velocity) of roughly 120 mph (200 kph). Gravity could accelerate the skydiver to greater speeds; however, the effects of other forces, such as air resistance, limits overall velocity.

Air Resistance

The Earth's atmosphere is made of a dense array of gas particles. Although mostly invisible to the human eye, the atmosphere provides a resistance force, which a moving body must overcome. This concept can be illustrated in sports such as running and cycling, where athletes commonly adjust their body positions to become more aerodynamic. By manipulating their body position, athletes can become less susceptible to the force applied by air resistance. Much of this resistance comes from friction that occurs between the moving body and the gas particles that surround it.

Friction

Friction can be defined as the resistance to motion that one surface encounters when moving over another. Excessive friction is most often viewed as harmful and in some cases may be a cause of injury. However, friction can be a benefit to some athletic endeavors. Martial artists can use the friction generated between their feet and the mat or floor to generate enough force required to push off to execute a kick or in cutting the angle to avoid getting hit. However, if they attempt this same action on a surface that offers less friction, such as an ice-skating rink, they would not be able to propel themselves at the same rate of speed.

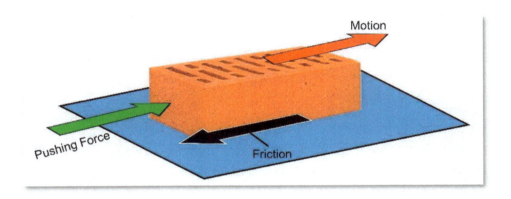

Fig. 1.6 - Motion of two surfaces causing friction.

Mass and Weight

The mass of an object is the amount of matter in an object, whereas weight is the force exerted on an object by gravity. The mass of an object is constant and does not change in different environments, whereas an object's weight is dependent on its mass and the acceleration effect that gravity has in a particular environment. On Earth's surface, gravity generally accelerates matter at 9.81 m/s2, causing 1 kg of matter to weigh 9.81 newtons. In other environments, such as the surface of the moon, where gravity causes a lower level of acceleration, the same kilogram of matter would weigh less. During the analysis of human movement both the mass of the body and its subsequent weight are important factors.

MOMENT, MOMENT ARM, AND TORQUE

Human movement occurs by the contraction of muscles. In turn, those contractions pull on tendons that cross joints and insert into bones, causing motion. The *moment of force* is the application of a force at a perpendicular angle to a joint or point of rotation. The *moment arm* is the distance between the application of the *moment of force* and the *axis of rotation*.

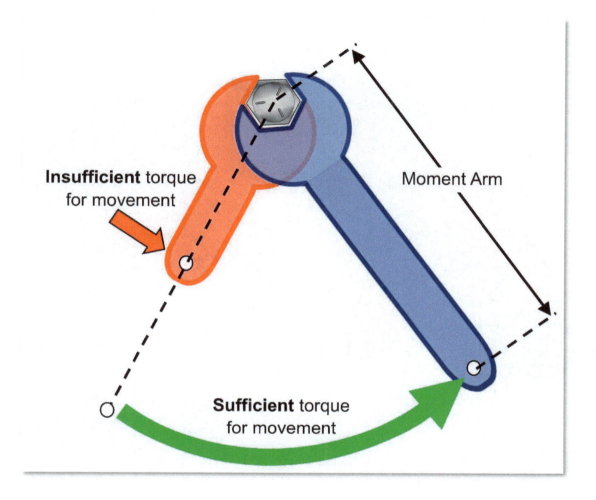

Fig. 1.7 - The greater the distance from the point of rotation to the moment of force (indicated by the moment arm), the greater the torque.

Torque is the twisting force causing rotation around its axis. For torque to occur, both a moment of force and a moment arm must be present. In the human body, the *axis of rotation* is a joint, and a *moment of force* is the pulling force applied by a contracting muscle and tendon on a bone. The moment arm is the distance between the muscle's insertion and the joints center of rotation.

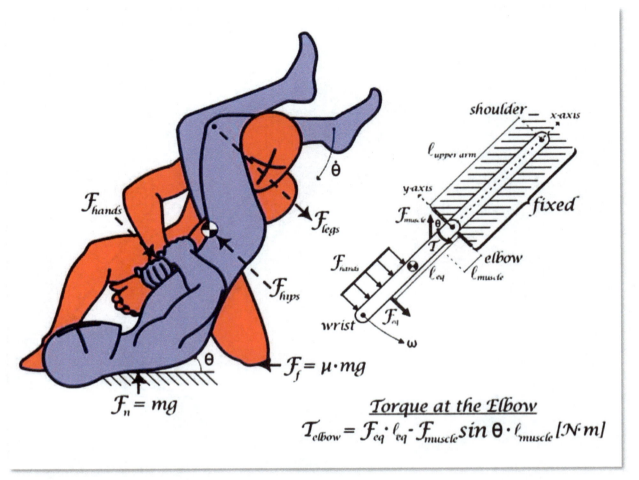

Fig. 1.8 - Biomechanics of an Armbar. By using the legs to stabilize the opponent's upper arm and shoulder, and using the opponent's forearm as the moment arm, torque is applied to the elbow joint.
Image Credit: Rakus, 2014. Used with the artist's written permission. Not for reuse.

Joint and Muscle Moment

The principles of moment of *force*, *moment arm*, and *torque* can be demonstrated by evaluating the mechanics required to push open a door. If a pushing force is applied at the hinged edge of the door, it will not open. However, if the same pushing force is applied on the opposite edge of the door, it will open by spinning around its fixed axis. In the second scenario, the door opens because of the presence of a moment arm. As previously explained, for torque to occur, a moment arm must be present. When pushing at the hinged edge of the door, there is no distance between the axis of rotation (hinges) in moment of force (push), meaning there is no moment arm.

When the force is applied at the opposite edge of the door, a moment arm is present, causing torque to be generated. When considering human movement, this offers some key considerations. A muscle and tendon's insertion must be at a sufficient distance (moment arm) from a joint's axis of rotation to generate movement and subsequent torque. Furthermore, muscles with an attachment located farther away from a joint require less force than muscles with a closer attachment.

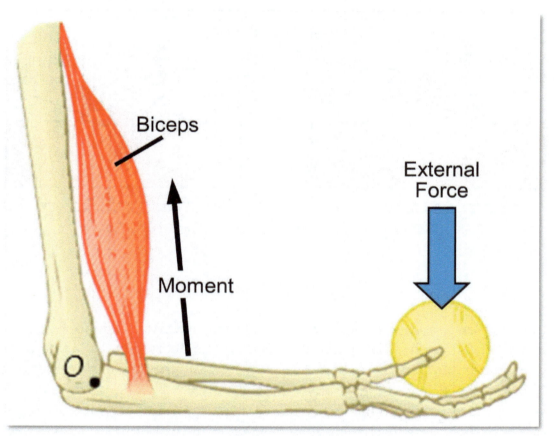

Fig. 1.9 - Muscle Moment: *The proximity of the muscle to the joint affects the force required to perform a particular function.*

Pressure

Pressure is the perpendicular force applied over the surface of an object. If a large force is applied over a large surface area, the relative pressure will be low. Alternatively, if the same force is applied over a much smaller area, the pressure will be high. *Center of Pressure* is the point at which the total sum of pressure acts on an object, causing a force to act through that point.

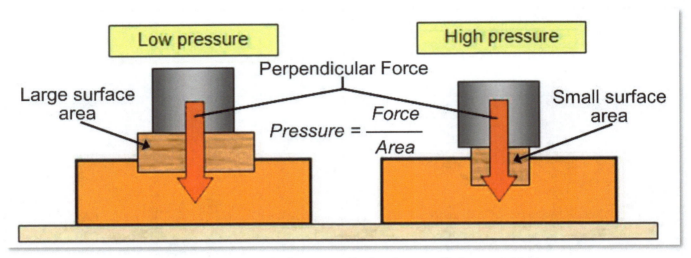

Fig. 1.10 - Pressure is the perpendicular force applied on an object.

Center of Mass

Although not completely accurate, the term "*center of mass*" (COM) is commonly interchanged with the term "*center of gravity*." The center of mass is an imaginary point on an object where its mass is evenly distributed. The center of mass is not always in the geometric center of an object; rather, it is the average location of that body's mass.

The center of gravity of the human body can change significantly because the segments of the body can move their mass by changing the position of the extremities. However, with the body in a stationary position, the COM is generally considered to approximately one inch below the umbilicus centered half-way between the spine and the anterior abdomen. The center of mass is usually lower on a female than it is on a male.

Base of Support

The *base of support* refers to the area enclosed by the points at which an object contacts a supporting surface. In human movement, this is commonly considered to be somewhere between both feet. When standing, the base of support is small in comparison to a four-point position (hands and knees), which is a larger base of support. The base of support is a key factor when evaluating stability and equilibrium.

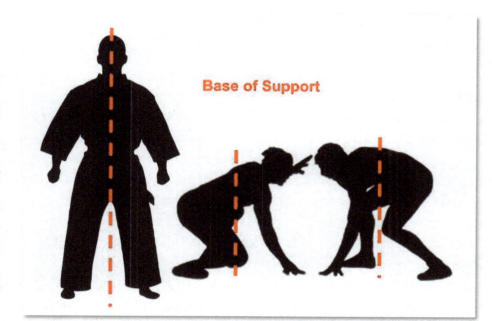

BASE AND BALANCE

The body's resistance to linear and angular forces is termed stability, or equilibrium. Balance is known as the ability to return the body to equilibrium after experiencing displacement from an external force. Balance and stability are vital when executing martial arts techniques.

Fig. 1.11 - *Base of Support for human standing upright is roughly midway between their two feet.*

Input from peripheral receptors such as vestibular organs within the inner ear, the eyes, muscles, and joints are sent to the brain, which interprets the information and sends motor response to the relevant muscles.

Factors that affect stability include location of the center of mass (COM), base of support, anticipation of the approaching force, weight, and friction between the two contact surfaces. If the COM falls within the base of support, then the body is stable. A stable body is less likely to fall or be injured when an external force is applied.

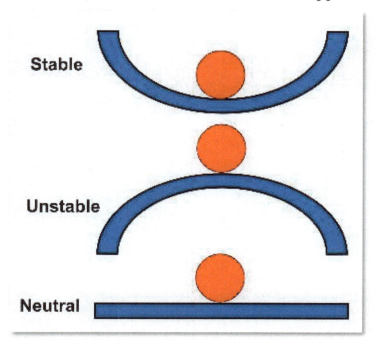

Balance and stability can be categorized into three states: stable, unstable, and neutral. A *stable state* of balance or equilibrium is when an object is moved and returns to its original position. When an object is moved, and it continues to move, it is classified as *unstable*. For example, a ball on top of a sloped ramp that is displaced (moved) to either side will increase its displacement. *Neutral stability* happens if an object is moved to a new position and remains balanced.

Fig. 1.12 - *Stable, unstable, and neutral states of equilibrium.*

Martial Arts Relevance:

- **Throws and Takedowns**

Successfully applying the principles of biomechanics and the laws of motion to martial arts throws and takedowns boils down to accomplishing several tasks. This is achieved by moving the opponent's *center of mass* away from their base (usually their feet) or moving their *base* away from their center of mass. Once the center of mass is disrupted the opponent must either adjust to rebalance or fall to the ground. The countless variations of takedowns and throws almost always include some method of either grasping, pushing, pulling, or moving the opponent that prevents them from adjusting and correcting their loss of balance. In doing so, it prevents the opponent from re-aligning their center of mass and reestablishing their base.

A simplified explanation using Newton's Third Law may be applied to the process of executing a shoulder throw. One martial artist resists the pushing force of a second martial artist; the first can suddenly redirect the second's pushing force — allowing gravity to aid in throwing the second martial artist over their shoulder.

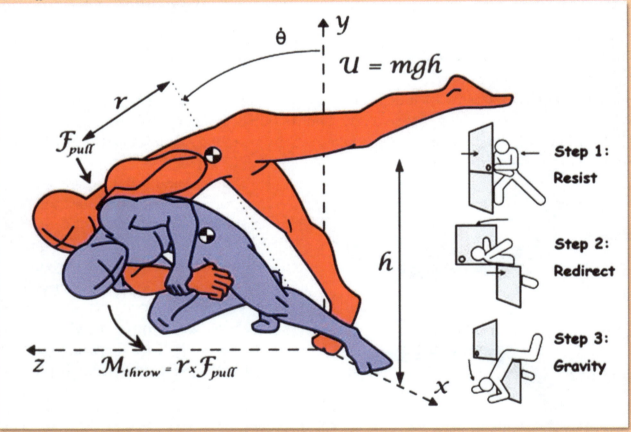

Fig. 1.13 - Biomechanics of a Shoulder Throw (Seoi-Nage). Image Credit: Rakus, 2014. Used with the artist's written permission. Not for reuse.

To more thoroughly analyze these principles in action, consider the requirements needed to execute a successful hip throw (Harai-goshi). The opponent would most likely be standing and facing you, which places their center of mass at approximately waist level centered between their spine and navel. (Note: an adult female COM is slightly lower than that of an adult male.) You must initially close the gap and acquire a grip on the opponent to be able to shift their center of mass. You must push or pull the opponent in one direction or another to force them off balance. While off balance, the opponent will try to move their feet or body in some fashion in an attempt to realign the center of mass and base. As the opponent attempts to readjust, you simultaneously drop your COM lower and swing one of your posterior hips (buttock) into their anterior hip, under their center of mass. Once you have displaced their center of mass with your pelvis and take away their ability to reset their legs, continue pulling and turning as the opponent becomes airborne.

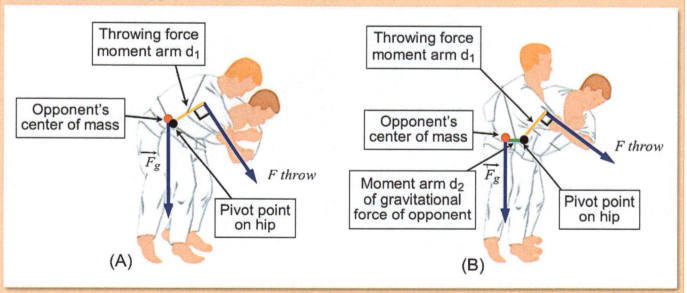

Fig. 1.14 - Hip Throw (A) <u>Correctly</u> executed, (B) <u>Incorrectly</u> executed.

The torque of the throw must overcome the resistant given by the opponent. The more off balance the opponent is, the longer the lever arm will be. This means that the more you can move their center of mass away from the supports (legs/feet) the more energy the throw will have. The more off balance you make them, the easier they will fall.

Variations of different throws and takedowns are all essentially different methods of manipulating and affecting biomechanical forces. Most throws have the same basic principles. By looking at the science behind why an opponent can be easily thrown to the mat, one can begin to implement the concepts in different scenarios. Applying the principles of biomechanics provides limitless possibilities for the informed martial artist.

The Science of Punching (and Striking) Power

When discussing the science behind delivering powerful punches, there are numerous factors to consider. Understanding the physics of executing a more powerful strike will aid martial artists in proper training and instruction. When executing a punch, it should not be considered just a hand technique, just as a kick is not just a leg technique; they are both total body techniques. The entire body is involved with moving the required mass to the target.

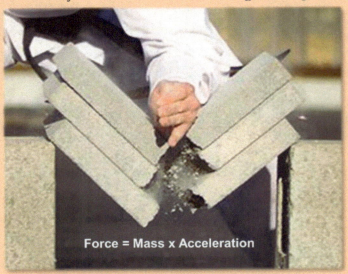

Fig. 1.15 - Newton's Second Law of Motion is one of several principles that aids in breaking cement blocks.

The Impulse-Momentum Theorem

The *Impulse-Momentum Theorem* states that the impulse applied to an object is equal to the change in momentum of that object; or the change in momentum experienced by an object under the actions of a force is equal to the impulse of the resistant force. If you have more mass, *and* you can move it quickly, you can create more impact on the target. Think of it as the combination of the speed of the punch and the strength behind it.

This concept is derived from Newton's second law when evaluating the mass and velocity of a punch. As discussed previously, the Second Law of Motion is expressed as Force = Mass x Acceleration.

In considering striking power, the factors in that equation can be more accurately expressed as Kinetic Energy (KE) = 1/2 mass x velocity^2. This equation is referred to as the *Impulse-Momentum Theorem*. It allows us to be more specific with exactly what is happening to generate the force of a punch. The impulse-momentum theorem shows that because the velocity is squared, the overall speed (velocity) has a more significant impact on the energy of a punch than the weight (mass in the punch). The science shows that it is more important to throw a fast punch than a heavy-handed punch when you are trying to generate power. Obviously *both* mass and velocity are important, however, velocity carries the mass; that is why a punch must be a total body technique. Placing proper footwork and body weight behind the punch is important.

Therefore, punches (and other strikes) will be more powerful when a punch's mass is maximized by engaging the whole body- shoulders, hips, and legs. But more importantly, maximize the speed (velocity) of the punch.

The Impulse-Momentum Theorem in Action: Boxing Gloves

The use of boxing gloves in combat sports is an example of the impulse-momentum theorem. The padding in boxing gloves increases the time it takes the fist, within the glove, to stop. If a boxer throws consistent punches with the same speed, the gloved hand takes longer to stop, resulting in a lower force. If the same punch was thrown without a glove, the shorter stopping time would result in an increased force. This would result in more damage to the face being punched, as well as to the fist throwing the punch. *Note*: the downside of using boxing gloves is that more strikes are delivered to the head potentially causing cumulative injuries. See Clinical Significance and Martial Arts Relevance: Concussions in the *Introduction to the Nervous System chapter*.

The Kinetic Chain

While the impulse-momentum theorem provides a mathematical basis for explaining the forces that make up a punch, it does not fully explain what creates those factors. In an attempt to maximize the mass behind a punch, the kinetic chain must be engaged. Anatomically, a kinetic chain describes the interrelated group of body segments, connecting joints, and muscles together to perform movements. When one segment of the body is in motion, it creates a chain of events that affects the movement of the neighboring joints and segments.

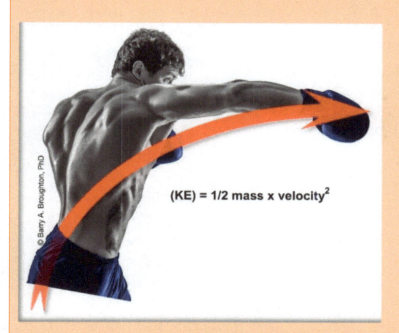

The trick to delivering a powerful punch is to activate multiple muscle groups and link them together in one fluid motion. Training every muscle from the foot to the fist to engage seamlessly in the single action of moving the punch to the target. The more efficiently the muscle movements are linked together the faster the strike will be, resulting in maximum velocity and force.

Fig. 1.16 - To deliver the most kinetic energy, the kinetic chain of the punch begins at the feet.

$(KE) = 1/2\ mass \times velocity^2$

Torque and Power

Intuitively, most people understand that to produce a stronger kick, they either need to apply more force to the kick, or kick faster. Therefore, the question remains — *How* is that accomplished? By taking advantage of the anatomical pulleys and levers throughout our body, torque can be introduced to increase the velocity of the mass of the punch or kick, thereby delivering more kinetic energy at the target.

The roundhouse kick is probably the most common kick across all martial arts disciplines. No matter the system or style, the fundamental principles of all roundhouse kicks employ the concepts of *torque* (rotational force) and *angular velocity* (speed).

The force required to overcome the mass of the leg and allow it to rotate is *torque*. Torque is expressed as: T = length of the lever arm (r) x magnitude of the force applied (F) <u>or</u> T = r x F.

A roundhouse kick is executed by essentially swinging the lower extremity around in an arcing-type motion while standing on the post foot. However, torque is inconsequential in terms of impact unless one applies a speed measurement to it. The *push-off* of the kicking foot produces the forward momentum of the kicking leg and the movement of the center of mass (COM). That is where the equation for power comes in, which is expressed as: Power (P) = torque (T) x angular velocity (ω) <u>or</u> P = T x ω.

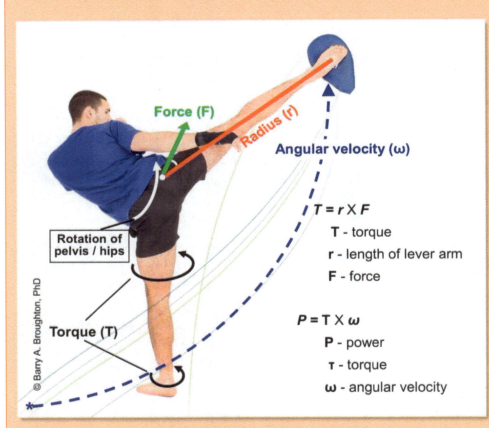

When executing a kick, in addition to the push-off, the power comes from the hips. The amount of torque produced is determined by how quickly and how much the hips and post foot are rotated.

A study published in 2017 by Gavagan and Sayers measured the various roundhouse kicking techniques of 24 expert level Karate, Tae Kwon Do, and Muay Thai practitioners (8 participants from each

Fig. 1.17 - The biomechanics involved in executing a roundhouse kick.

style). The purpose of this study was to determine if there were differences in the roundhouse kicking leg kinematics, and if so to identify the kinematic determinants of effective roundhouse kicking performance.

Although there were indeed some differences in the execution of the roundhouse kick among the three styles, they found that there was no statistical difference in the impact force once the foot hit the target. The average impact force of a roundhouse kick in the study was nearly 1400 N. Their data confirmed that linear foot velocities, as well as the anterior pelvic tilt and axial rotation velocities, combined with rapid movements of the COM towards the target play a major role in the production of impact force.

LEVERS

Over time the human body has evolved into an extremely efficient organism. Our built-in biomechanical levers illustrate this efficiency. A lever is a simple machine that uses leverage to multiply force. As force multipliers, the use of levers in martial arts are extremely valuable in helping to exert more force upon a given target than would otherwise be possible. The mechanical advantage assists in moving someone, or something, more easily.

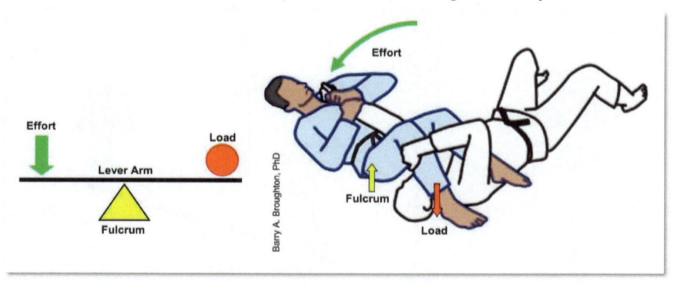

Fig. 1.18 - Example of a lever while executing an armbar.

The four main components of a lever include: a *fulcrum* (pivot point), a *lever arm*, an *effort force*, and a *resistance force*. In the human body, these components are represented as joints, bones, muscles, and body weight.

There are three types of levers that can be found in the human body: first-class levers, second-class levers, and third-class levers.

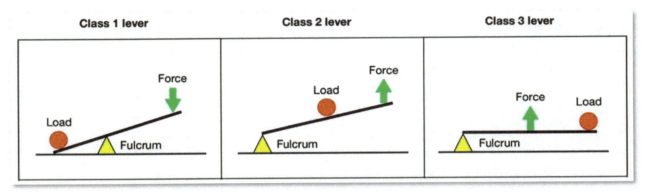

Fig. 1.19 - The Three Types of Levers.

A **first-class lever** has the fulcrum placed between the resistance force and the effort force on the lever (i.e., a seesaw). An example of a first-class lever in human anatomy is the skull as it sits atop the first cervical vertebra (the atlas). The weight of the head is the resistance force, the posterior cervical muscles are the effort force, and the craniovertebral joint acts as the fulcrum.

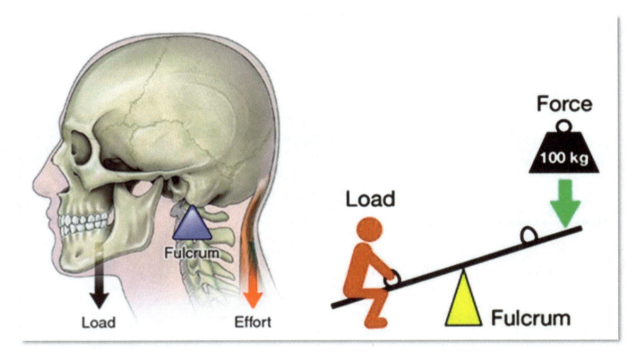

Fig. 1.20 - First-Class Levers. Left Image Credit: Mark Dutton: Dutton's Orthopaedic Examination, Evaluation, and Intervention 4th Ed.

A **second-class lever** has both the resistance force and the effort force on the same side of the fulcrum. In this class of lever, the resistance force is always between the effort force and the fulcrum (i.e., a wheelbarrow). In human biomechanics a second-class lever can be demonstrated while executing a heel raise. The metatarsophalangeal joints (ball of the foot) act as the fulcrum, with the effort force applied via the muscles of the posterior lower leg to help to overcome body weight (resistance).

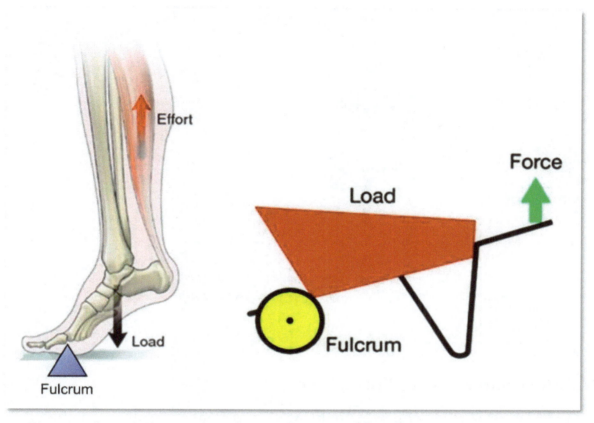

Fig. 1.21 - Second-Class Levers. Left Image Credit: Modified by Barry A. Broughton, PhD, Original by Mark Dutton: Dutton's Orthopaedic Examination, Evaluation, and Intervention 4th Ed.

A **third-class lever** also has both forces on the same side of the fulcrum; however, the effort force is acting in between the fulcrum and the resistance force (i.e., a baseball bat). This is the most common type of lever found in the human body. The most obvious example in human anatomy is the elbow joint: the resistance (weight held in hand) is farthest away, with the effort force (biceps) closest to the fulcrum (elbow joint).

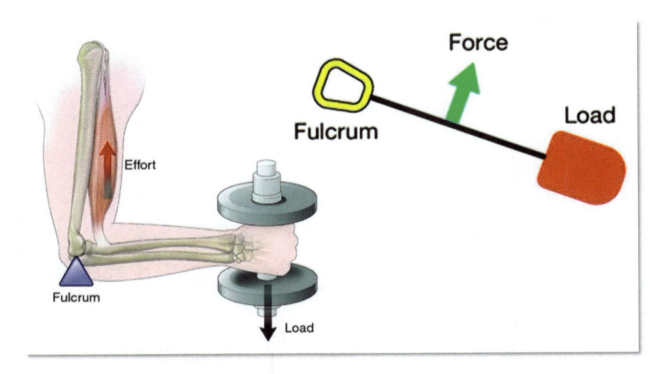

Fig. 1.22 - Third-Class Levers. Left Image Credit: Mark Dutton: Dutton's Orthopaedic Examination, Evaluation, and Intervention 4th Ed.

MOTION

Classifications and Practical Applications

Motion is the process or action of moving or being moved from one plane to another. *Linear motion* relates to movement along a straight or curved pathway where all points of the body move the same distance in the same amount of time. The individual's *center of mass* (COM) is usually the point in the body that is used for monitoring this movement. The COM is the point on the body at where the distribution of mass is equal in all directions and is independent of the gravitational field. However, in sports, other parts of the body may be used as the point to be monitored.

Angular motion refers to a motion of an object around a fixed point in which different regions of the same body do not move the same distance in a set time. This usually refers to motions around an axis, an example in sports would be gymnast swinging around a high bar. The gymnast's arms do not move as far as their legs during the entire rotation.

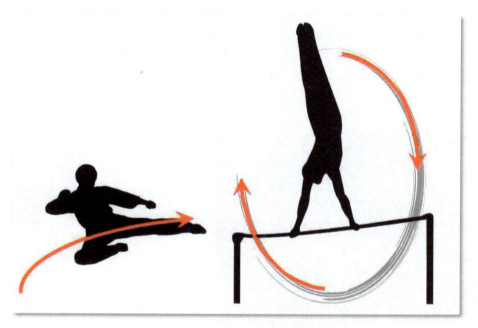

Fig. 1.23 - Linear (left) and Angular (right) Motion

Acceleration and Momentum

Acceleration refers to the change in velocity of an object relative to time. Acceleration is most often recorded as meters per second and is calculated as:

Acceleration = Change in velocity / Change in time

In human motion, the velocity of a body or segment is rarely constant. Velocity often changes, even if it appears that it remains the same.

Momentum is the quantity of motion an object possesses, the product of its mass. Momentum can be transferred from one object to another. Linear momentum is the quantity of motion of a moving object in a straight line. If a body is moving, it has momentum and will move in the direction in which a force is applied to it. The heavier the object (or person), the greater the momentum. Angular momentum is the quantity of rotation of a body or object. If gravity is the only external force acting on an object, the angular momentum remains constant throughout the duration of the movement. During the act of walking with a normal gait, there is forward, lateral, in vertical momentum, as there are forces acting on the body from different directions, i.e., gravity, ground reaction forces, and muscle forces.

FRAMES

Frames are rigid structures that provide support to a heavy object. Creating a skeletal frame while grappling, either standing or on the ground, helps to create space between individuals. Forming skeletal frames with the extremities helps support a significant amount of weight without the need for brute force and muscle strength.

Frames are formed by connecting two extremities; either both arms, both legs, or an arm and a leg to build a rigid barrier.

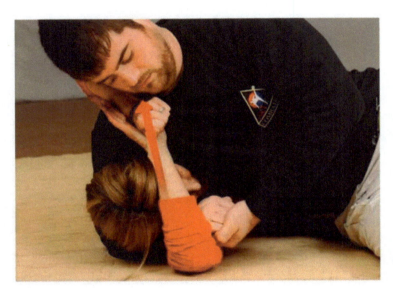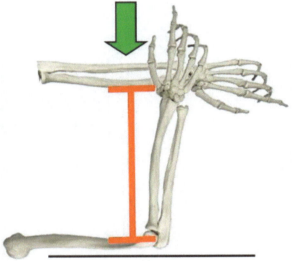

Fig. 1.24 - Forming a skeletal frame to create space.

Forming a frame with the upper extremities, while using the floor as a base for the arm and elbow is very effective. A rigid frame can prevent someone from getting too close and controlling you with their weight.

SECTION TWO

TERMINOLOGY

Chapter 2

TERMINOLOGY

Martial Arts Relevance: Talking The Language

Because martial arts techniques frequently have different names among different arts, I am often asked after teaching seminars to distinguish the names of specific techniques that I have presented. If we as martial artists could agree on the certain vernacular that we use in describing techniques, we would all have a better understanding of what is being presented without preconceived ideas regarding efficacy. Such is the case of me being asked to clarify the difference between what some people refer to as an Americana and a Kimura. Because one specific technique may be called numerous things by differing factions, I tend to refrain from using names such as Americana or Kimura, instead favoring more descriptive terms such as Bent Arm Bar from the Mount (or from Side Control Position, Scarf Hold, Half-Guard, etc.) and Reverse Bent Arm from the Guard (or Side Shoulder Mount, Side Control Position, etc.).

Both named techniques are joint locks that generally attack the shoulder (glenohumeral) joint. However, the elbow may be secondarily injured depending on the position of the attacker and the defender during execution of the technique, the defender's shoulder joint laxity, the physical size and strength of both, and how aggressively the lock is being executed. Additionally, one can attack the wrist simultaneously while attacking the shoulder or elbow joint.

My version of a Bent Arm Bar (from whatever position - frequently referred to as an Americana) has the opponent's elbow flexed (bent — usually while on their back) so that their affected hand is pointed up towards their head; after adducting the arm towards the torso, lifting the elbow causes external rotation of the humeral (upper arm bone) head within the glenohumeral joint. Of course, due to the limited space here, this is not a full description of all the nuances required in executing a Bent Arm Bar.

On the other hand, my version of a Reverse Bent Arm Bar (from whatever position) (often referred to as a Kimura — someone's name — when executed from the Closed Guard) has the opponent's elbow flexed (bent down in a Reversed position) so that their affected hand is pointed down towards their hip/feet direction. Using the Radius and Ulna (forearm bones) as a lever, the Humerus (upper arm bone) is abducted away from the torso and internally rotated within the glenohumeral joint. Of course, due to the limited space here, this is not a full description of all the nuances required in executing a Reverse Bent Arm Bar. The better understanding of true musculoskeletal, neurovascular, and gross anatomy that martial artists have, the better practitioners they will be. I understand that my background in orthopedic surgery and sport medicine has given me a distinct advantage in the execution of certain techniques; my goal is to share my knowledge and experience to help others be more proficient and hopefully prevent injuries.

THE ANATOMICAL POSITION

Before defining any specific terms, the human body must be given an accepted reference point from which all anatomical terms are referred. This universal way to position the human body is known as the *anatomical position*.

The modern anatomical position is similar to Leonardo da Vinci's famous Vitruvian Man.

- A person standing upright, facing forward.
- Arms are straight down with hands held by the hips, with palms facing forward.
- Feet are parallel and toes pointing forward.

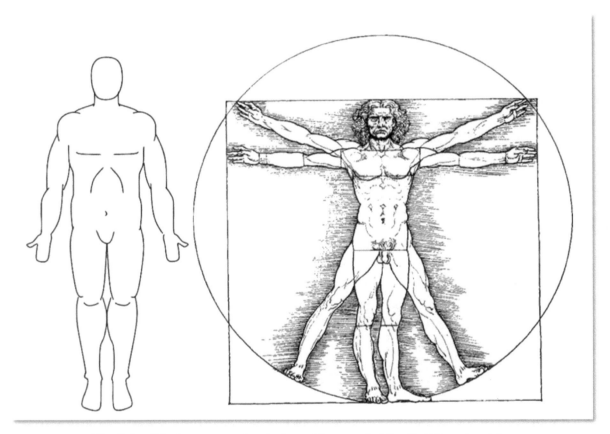

Fig. 2.1 – The human anatomical position vs. da Vinci's Vitruvian Man.

THE ANATOMICAL PLANES

An anatomical plane is essentially a flat slice through the human body, which can be thought of as a sheet of glass. The anatomical planes divide the human body in sections. The use of anatomical planes provides for accurate descriptions of a specific location, allowing for more precise communication and understanding.

The three most commonly used planes are: sagittal, coronal and transverse.

- **Sagittal plane** – a vertical line dividing the body into a left section and a right section.

- **Coronal plane** – a vertical line which divides the body into a front (anterior) section and back (posterior) section.

- **Transverse plane** – a horizontal line, parallel to the ground, which divides the body into an upper (superior) section, a lower (inferior) section.

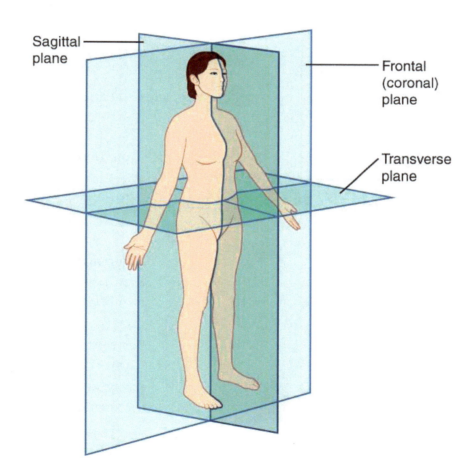

Fig. 2.2 – The anatomical planes of the human body.
Image Credit: Connexions [CC- by-3.0], via Wikimedia Commons

Supine and Prone

In general, the terms **supine and prone** describes opposing positions of the body; with a person lying on their back with chest up is in a supine position, and a person lying chest downward is in a prone position.

ANATOMICAL TERMS OF MOVEMENT

Anatomical terms of movement are used to describe the way in which the body moves due to muscles acting upon the skeleton. Muscle contraction produces the movement of joints; and the subsequent movements can be accurately described by using this precise terminology. Incorporating these terms into the vernacular of martial artists would aid in a better understanding of how techniques are taught, learned and executed.

The terms presented here assumes that the body begins in the anatomical position. Most movements have an opposing antagonistic movement. For ease of understanding, terms here are described in antagonistic pairs.

Flexion and Extension

The movements of flexion and extension occur in the sagittal plane and refer to increasing and decreasing the angle between two body parts.

Flexion refers to a movement that decreases the angle between two body segments. Flexion at the elbow decreases the angle between the forearm and the (upper) arm. Flexion of the knee moves the foot and ankle closer to the buttock, reducing the angle between the thigh and (lower) leg.

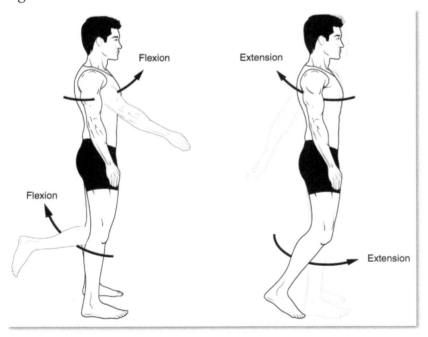

Extension refers to a movement that increases the angle between two body segments. Extension at the elbow is increasing the angle between the forearm and the (upper) arm. Extension of the knee straightens the lower extremity, increasing the angle at the knee.

Fig. 2.3 – Flexion and extension. Image Credit: Connexions [CC-by-3.0], via Wikimedia Commons

Abduction and Adduction

Abduction and adduction are opposing terms that describe movements towards or away from the midline of the body.

Abduction moves something laterally away from the midline. For example, abduction of the shoulder raises the arms out away from the sides of the body.

Adduction is a movement that brings something towards the midline. Adduction of the hip squeezes the lower extremities together.

In fingers and toes, the midline used is *not* the midline of the body, but of the hand and foot, respectively. Therefore, abducting the fingers spreads them out, while adduction brings them together.

Medial and Lateral Rotation

Medial and lateral rotation describe movement of the entire extremity around their long axis.

Medial rotation is a rotational movement towards the midline, sometimes referred to as internal rotation. Medial rotation of the hip is achieved by internally rotating the lower extremity with the toes pointed inward towards the midline of the body.

Lateral rotation is a rotational movement away from the midline, sometimes referred to an external rotation. This is in the opposite direction to the movements described above.

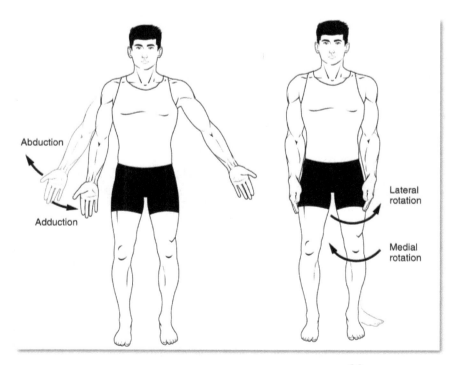

Fig. 2.4 – Adduction, abduction and rotation. Image Credit: Connexions [CC-BY-3.0], via Wikimedia Commons

Depression and Elevation

Depression and elevation movements occur in the coronal plane.

Depression refers to a lowering movement in an inferior direction, while **elevation** refers to movement in a superior direction (e.g., shoulder shrug).

Supination and Pronation

Supination and pronation define movements and relative orientation of the hand and forearm, and the foot in space. These movements are often confused with medial (internal) and lateral (external) rotation. However, there is a subtle difference. Internal and external rotation usually refers to the movement of the entire upper or lower extremity, whereas supination and pronation refers to either just the hand and forearm, or the foot.

With the elbow flexed, the act of rotating the hand and forearm into a position of palm facing up is referred to as **supination**. Again, keeping the elbow flexed, **pronation** is the act of turning the hand into a palm down position.

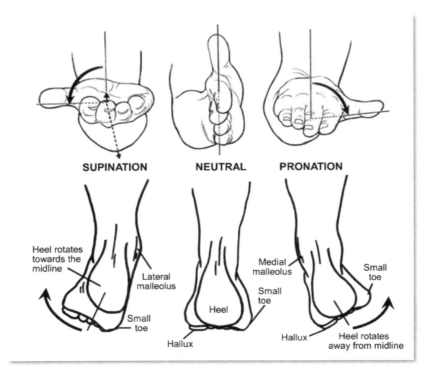

Fig. 2.5 - Supination, neutral, and pronation positions of the right hand and foot.

Keeping in mind that *supine* is lying flat on the back, the similarity in terms may assist you in remembering the supination is the back of the hand facing down.

Dorsiflexion and Plantar Flexion

In reference to the two surfaces of the foot; dorsiflexion and plantar flexion are terms used to describe movements at the ankle.

Dorsiflexion refers to flexion at the ankle towards the dorsum (superior surface), so that the foot points more superiorly.

Plantar flexion refers extension at the ankle towards the plantar surface (the sole), so that the foot points inferiorly.

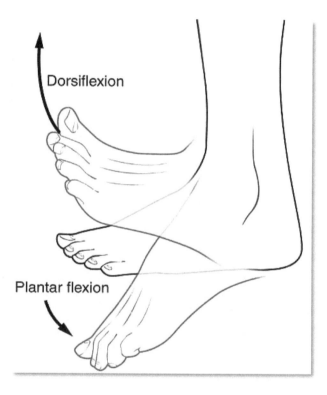

Fig. 2.6 - Dorsiflexion and plantar flexion. Image Credit: Connexions [CC-BY-3.0], via Wikimedia Commons

Inversion and Eversion

Inversion and eversion are movements which occur at the foot and ankle.

Inversion involves the movement of the plantar surface of the foot towards the median plane – so that the sole faces in a medial direction.

Eversion involves the movement of the plantar surface of the foot away from the median plane – so that the sole faces in a lateral direction.

Opposition and Reposition

Opposition and reposition refer to movements of the fingers and thumb that are limited to humans, some primates, and only a few other species.

Opposition brings the thumb and little finger together.

Reposition is a movement that moves the thumb and the little finger away from each other, effectively reversing opposition.

Circumduction

Circumduction can be defined as a conical (cone-like) movement of a limb extending from the joint at which the movement is controlled.

The movement is often thought to be a circular motion; however, it is more accurately conical in nature due to the *cone* formed by the moving limb.

Protraction and Retraction

Protraction describes the anterolateral movement of the scapula on the posterior thoracic wall that allows the shoulder to move anteriorly. This movement is accomplished by reaching for something.

Retraction is the posteromedial movement of the scapula on the posterior thoracic wall, which causes the shoulder region to move posteriorly, i.e., picking something up.

ANATOMICAL TERMS OF LOCATION

The use of anatomical terms of location are vital in discussing and understanding human anatomy. They help to avoid confusion and ambiguity that can arise when describing the location of anatomical structures and lesions. These terms are often relative, i.e., the location being described must be referenced to another point on the body.

Medial and Lateral

The midline is an imaginary line in the sagittal plane evenly splitting the body into right and left halves. **Medial** means towards the midline, **lateral** means away from the midline.

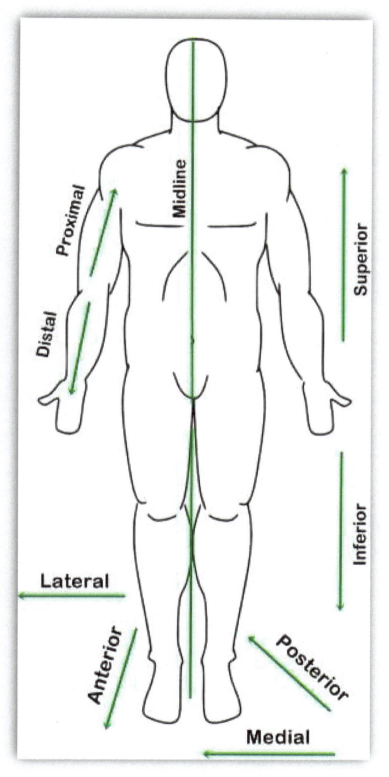

Examples:

- *The small toe is lateral to the big toe.*
- *The nose is medial to the ears.*

Bilateral, Contralateral, and Ipsilateral

Bilateral refers to something occurring on both sides of the body. **Contralateral** refers to something on the other side of the body. **Ipsilateral** is considered the opposite of contralateral and occurs on the same side of the body.

Bilateral: On both sides.
   Example: He sustained bilateral clavicle fractures (He broke both his right and left collar bones).

Ipsilateral: On the same side.
   Example: The left leg is ipsilateral to the left arm.

Contralateral: On the opposite side.
   Example: The right leg is contralateral to the left arm.

Fig. 2.7 – Anatomical terms of location labelled on the anatomical position.

Anterior and Posterior

Anterior refers to the *front*, while **posterior** refers to the *back*. For context, the sternum is anterior to the heart because it lies in front of it. Equally, the heart is posterior to the sternum because it lies in behind it.

Examples:

- *The trachea is anterior to the cervical spine.*
- *The patella is located anteriorly in the knee joint.*

Volar refers to the palmar aspect of the hand and forearm, and less frequently to the plantar aspect of the foot.

Dorsal or **dorsum** refers to the back of the hand or the top of the foot.

Superior and Inferior

These terms are used in reference to a vertical axis. **Superior** refers to *higher than*, while **inferior** means *lower than*.

Examples

- *The skull is superior to the cervical spine.*
- *The lumbar spine is inferior to the thoracic spine.*

Because the upper and lower extremities are very mobile, and what is superior in one position is inferior in another, we need another descriptive pair of terms:

Proximal and Distal

Proximal and **distal** are terms used in in describing locations of anatomical structures that are considered to have a beginning and an end (such as the upper and lower extremities). They describe the position of a structure in reference to the anatomical position and its origin. Proximal means closer to its origin, while distal means further away.

Examples:

- *The ankle joint is distal to the knee joint.*
- *The elbow joint is proximal to the wrist.*

BODY CAVITIES

A body cavity is a space or compartment that contains internal organs or other structures. The two primary cavities are called the dorsal and ventral cavities. The larger ventral cavity is divided by the diaphragm into two smaller cavities known as the thoracic and abdominopelvic cavities.

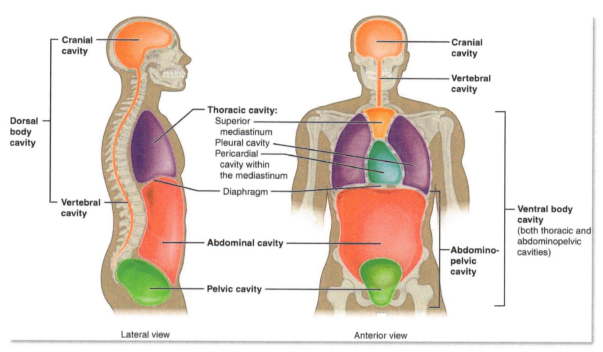

Fig. 2.8 - Cavities of the human body.

Thoracic Cavity

The thoracic cavity contains the heart, lungs, trachea, esophagus, large blood vessels, and nerves. The thoracic cavity is surrounded laterally by the ribs, anteriorly by the sternum, posteriorly by the spine, with the diaphragm forming the inferior boarder.

Abdominopelvic Cavity

The lower ventral, abdominopelvic cavity can be subdivided into two cavities: the abdominal cavity and pelvic cavity. The abdominal cavity contains most of the gastrointestinal tract (including the stomach, liver, gallbladder, pancreas, small intestine, large intestine), as well as the spleen, kidneys and adrenal glands. The abdominal cavity is bound superiorly by the diaphragm, laterally by the body wall, and inferiorly by the pelvic cavity.

The pelvic cavity contains most of the urogenital system (such as urinary bladder, distal ureters, urethra, reproductive organs), as well as the sigmoid colon and rectum. The pelvic cavity is bounded superiorly by the abdominal cavity, inferiorly by the sacrum, and laterally by the pelvis.

Dorsal Cavity

The smaller of the two main cavities is called the dorsal cavity. As its name implies, it lies in the posterior aspect of the body and contains the primary organs of the nervous system, including the brain and spinal cord.

The dorsal cavity can be divided into two portions. The upper portion consists of the cranial cavity which houses the brain. The lower portion includes the vertebral canal which houses the spinal cord.

SECTION THREE

Introduction to the Human Body

Introduction to the Human Body

Consider the vastness of billions of microscopic parts, each with its own function, working in a synchronized fashion to benefit the total being. The human body is a single structure, made up of billions of smaller structures, making Homo sapiens one of the most complex organisms on this planet. There are several levels of organization to human beings, with each level being more complex than the previous.

Cells, the basic building blocks of the human body, make up *tissue*, which form specialized structures called *organs*. Organs and tissues that function together for a single purpose forms a *system*. Many organ systems working together to perform multiple functions of an independent being is an *organism*.

Cells

The human body contains more than 30 trillion cells. In human biology, cells are considered the smallest units of living matter that can maintain life and reproduce themselves. They are comprised of the cell membrane, the nucleus, and the cytoplasm. The cell membrane surrounds the cell, controlling the substances that go into and out of the cell. The cytoplasm is the fluid inside the cell which contains other tiny cell parts that have specific functions. The cytoplasm is where most chemical reactions take place, and most proteins are made. The nucleus is a structure inside the cell that contains the nucleolus and most of the cell's DNA.

Tissues

Tissues are a group of many similar cells or layer of cells that work together to perform a specific function.

Organs

An organ is a group of several different kinds of tissues which together perform a specific function. For example, the stomach is a group of epithelial, connective, muscle, and nerve tissues all working together. Muscle and connective tissues form the stomach wall, epithelial and connective tissues form the lining, and nervous tissue extends throughout both the stomach wall and its lining.

Systems

A system is an organization of various organs working together to perform complex functions for the body as a whole. The ten major systems of the human body presented in this text include:

- Integumentary
- Skeletal
- Muscular
- Nervous
- Respiratory
- Cardiovascular
- Lymphatic
- Digestive
- Genitourinary
- Endocrine

The Human Organism

Just as the organs in a particular system function together to accomplish a specific task; all organ systems must work together for the survival of the larger organism. For an organism, such as humans, to maintain homeostasis and overall health, no individual organ system can work independently of other systems.

For example, the circulatory system and the respiratory system work together to deliver oxygen to cells, while simultaneously removing carbon dioxide that the cells produce. The circulatory system picks up oxygen from the lungs and delivers it to tissues such as the brain, while transporting carbon dioxide back to the lungs. The lungs expel the carbon dioxide and bring in new oxygen-containing air.

Oxygenated brain tissue receives impulses from the neurological system that innervates the muscular system. The stimulated nerve cells within the skeletal muscles contract to move a particular joint, allowing for body movement. Additionally, the blood in the circulatory system receives nutrients from the digestive system which undergoes filtration in the kidneys, an organ of the urinary system.

Only when all systems are working together can the human organism accomplish the complex feats of martial arts training.

Chapter 3

Introduction to the Integumentary System

As the largest organ system of the human body, the integumentary system is comprised of the skin and its accessory structures. Not typically thought of as an organ, the skin is a group of tissues that work together as a single structure to perform critical functions. Forming the body's outermost layer, it provides a physical barrier between the external environment and the body's internal environment, while also helping to maintain homeostasis. The skin acts as the first line of defense from the elements that surround us. It keeps bacteria and other pathogens out, while keeping water and heat in. It contains the sites of numerous sensory receptors, as well as autonomic and sympathetic nerve fibers allowing communication to and from the brain.

Made of multiple layers of cells and tissues, the skin is secured to underlying structures by connective tissue. The deeper layer of skin is well vascularized and highly innervated, both important factors for the knowledgeable martial artist.

LAYERS OF SKIN

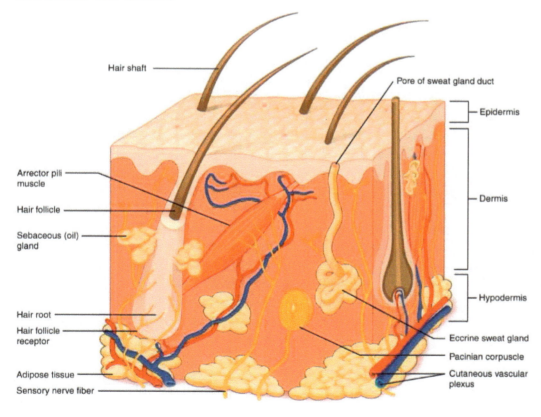

Fig. 3.1 - The three layers of skin include the epidermis, dermis, and hypodermis. The outer layer called the epidermis is made of closely packed epithelial cells; while the dermis is comprised of dense, irregular connective tissue that supports blood vessels, sweat glands, hair follicles, and other structures. The hypodermis, which lies beneath the dermis, is composed primarily of fatty and loose connective tissues.

The Epidermis

Composed of keratinized, stratified squamous epithelial cells, the epidermis is the thin outer layer of the skin that is visible. Because it is avascular (without blood vessels), it receives nutrients via diffusion of the tissue fluid from the dermis.

Depending on its location on the body, the epidermis is composed of four or five layers of epithelial cells. Most of the body's skin is considered "thin skin"; having only four layers. These layers are, from deep to superficial: the stratum basale, stratum spinosum, stratum granulosum, and stratum corneum. The fifth layer that makes up "thick skin", called the stratum lucidum, is located between the stratum corneum and the stratum granulosum. "Thick skin" is found of the soles of the feel and the palms of the hands.

Layers of the Epidermis

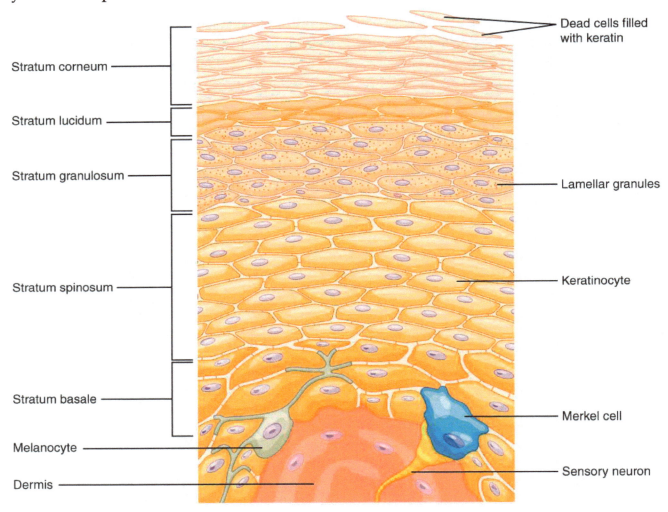

Fig. 3.2 - Five layers of the epidermis: stratum basale, stratum spinosum, stratum granulosum, stratum lucidum, and stratum corneum.

Stratum Basale

The deepest layer called the stratum basale, meaning basal layer, is attached to the dermis. It is made of a single row of rapidly dividing cells, called keratinocytes, pushing new cells up into the layers above to help regenerate dead skin. This is vital because millions of dead keratinocytes are rubbed off the skin every day. So that the skin always remains intact, these constantly dividing cells in the stratum basale ensure that a new epidermis forms every few weeks.

The stratum basale also contains melanocytes (that produce melanin), and tactile cells which act as the sensory receptor for touch. The pigment molecule melanin is one of the components of the skin that determines its color and protects the skin from ultraviolet radiation. Other pigments responsible for skin color are carotene, which is yellow-orange, and hemoglobin, which is red when oxygenated.

Skin Pigmentation

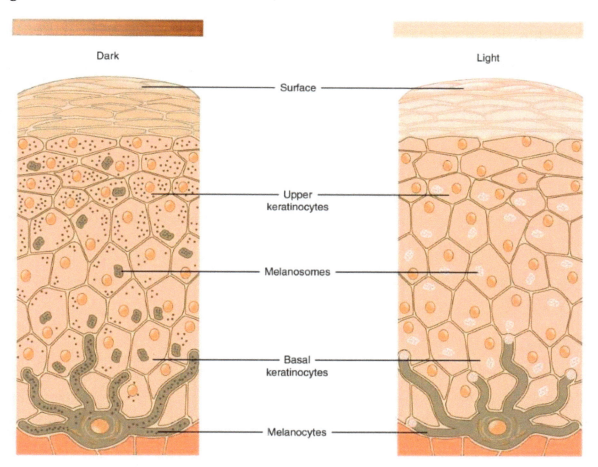

Fig. 3.3 - The relative coloration of the skin depends on the amount of melanin produced by melanocytes in the stratum basale and taken up by keratinocytes.

Stratum Spinosum

Above the stratum basale is the stratum spinosum, meaning spinous or prickly layer. This section is several layers of cells thick and is full of cells with a weblike system of intermediate filaments attached to desmosomes. Desmosomes are specialized adhesive protein complexes that are responsible for maintaining the mechanical integrity of tissues. Also contained within the stratum spinosum are dendritic cells, which ingest foreign substances and activate the immune system against foreign pathogens.

Stratum Granulosum

The stratum granulosum, or granular layer, is four to six cell layers thick. It is in this section that keratinization begins as cells move their way upwards from the basal layer. When the cells move far enough away from the dermal capillaries below to receive sufficient nutrients, the cells fill with keratin as they die. During this process, the cells flatten as the organelles within the cells disintegrate. The keratinization process makes the cell tougher and scalier, allowing for the outer layers to better protect the body.

Stratum Lucidum

The "thick skin" of the palms of the hands and soles of the feet contains the stratum lucidum, or clear layer, sandwiched between the stratum granulosum and the stratum corneum. This layer is two or three cell layers thick, made of dead keratinocytes that have become flat and clear. The stratum lucidum is where they begin to aggregate into arrays called tonofilaments that binds the pieces of the cytoskeleton to each other and to the cell membrane.

Stratum Corneum

The stratum corneum, or horny layer, is the outermost section of the epidermis, marking the final stage of keratinocyte development and maturation. At twenty to thirty cell layers thick, all of the cells of the stratum corneum are anucleated, meaning the nucleus has disintegrated.

This complex network of dead cells protects all the living cells inside the body from all the potential dangers outside of it.

The Dermis

The dermis is the inner layer of skin containing a rich supply of blood vessels and nerves. This layer of fibrous connective tissue also houses oil and sweat glands, hair follicles, and other structures. The dermis is divided into two sections, the papillary layer and the reticular layer.

Layers of the Dermis

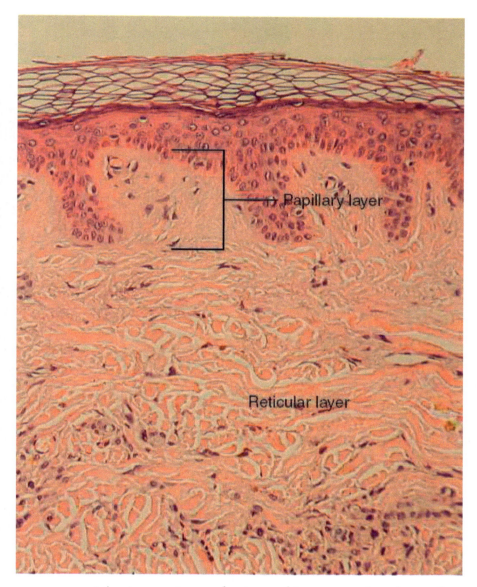

Fig. 3.4 - This stained slide shows the two components of the dermis — the papillary layer and the reticular layer. Both are made of connective tissue with fibers of collagen extending from one to the other, making the border between the two somewhat indistinct. The dermal papillae extending into the epidermis belong to the papillary layer, whereas the dense collagen fiber bundles below belong to the reticular layer. LM × 10. Image Credit: modification of work by "kilbad"/Wikimedia Commons

Papillary Layer

Descending from the epidermis is the thin papillary layer, made of highly vascular loose connective tissue and a network of collagen and elastic fibers. This loose meshwork greatly increases the surface area over which oxygen, nutrients, waste products, and immune signals can be exchanged between the epidermis and dermis.

The word papillary refers to the dermal papillae which project into the epidermis above. In areas of significant friction, such as the hands, these papillae form dermal ridges, causing ridges in the epidermis. Enhancing the gripping ability of the fingers, the ridges form the visible lines on the fingertips which provide unique fingerprints.

Reticular Layer

Forming the bulk of the dermis, the reticular layer sits just below papillary layer. The dense irregular fibrous connective tissue serves to strengthen the skin while providing its elasticity. Within the reticular layer are the roots of the hair, sebaceous glands, sweat glands, nerve receptors, nails, and blood vessels.

The Hypodermis

The hypodermis, or subcutaneous layer, is the innermost (deepest) and thickest layer of skin. Made predominately of adipose tissue (fat cells), the hypodermis contains fibroblasts (cells which make up connective tissue), larger nerves and blood vessels, and macrophages (cells that are part of the immune system involved in the detection and destruction of bacteria and other harmful organisms).

Anchoring the skin to the structures below it, the thickness of the hypodermis varies in different regions of the body and varies considerably between different people.

Clinical Significance and Martial Arts Relevance

Scalp Lacerations and Facial Lacerations

Deep lacerations to the scalp tend to bleed profusely for several reasons:

- The occipitofrontalis muscle of the scalp pulls on the wound, preventing the closure of the bleeding vessel and surrounding skin.
- The blood vessels of the scalp form an anastomosis, which contributes to the profuse bleeding.
- The blood vessels to the scalp adhere to dense connective tissue, preventing the vasoconstriction that normally occurs in response to trauma.
- Because of the significant vascularity of the head and face, scalp and facial lacerations tend to bleed more profusely than comparable wounds elsewhere, frequently giving the initial appearance that the wound is much worse than it really is.

Understanding these details gives the informed martial artist an advantage during real-world self-defense scenarios. It also aids the martial arts instructor who may need to care for a student who receives an unintentional injury while training.

Appendages of the Integumentary System

The epidermal and dermal derived components of the integumentary system are called skin appendages. The skin appendages include hair, nails, sweat glands, and sebaceous glands. Each component has a unique structure and function.

Hair

Hair is the component of the integumentary system that extends out from the dermal layer where it sits within the hair follicle. Humans have hair on their head in addition to hair all over their body, including eyelashes and nasal hair. Hair serves as a sensory function, as well as specific protective functions from cold and UV radiation. Hair follicles are found in most regions of skin, excluding the lips, palms of the hands, soles of the feet, glans penis, clitoris, and labia minora.

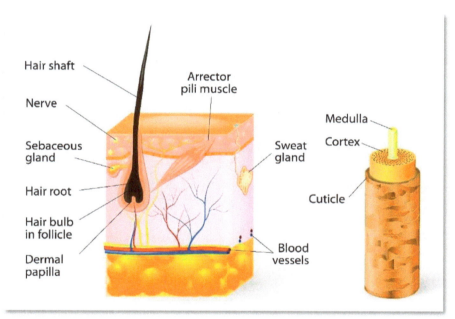

Fig. 3.5 - Hair Anatomy

Hair is a flexible thread-like strand of largely dead, keratinized cells formed by the hair bulb within the follicle. The hair bulb has a rich supply of nerves and capillaries. The bundle of nerve endings that attach to the bulb act as a receptor, responding to any bending of the hair and alerting the brain. Each hair follicle has an arrector pili muscle attached to it. When cold or afraid, this small bundle of muscle cells contracts and pulls on the follicle, which in turn causes the surface of the skin to dimple out, producing what is commonly referred to as goose bumps.

Each individual hair consists of three layers of cells; the medulla, cortex, and cuticle. The medulla is the innermost layer, containing large cells and soft keratin. The middle layer is the cortex, consisting of several layers of flattened cells. The outermost layer is the cuticle, a single layer of overlapping keratinized cells. Body hair can either be vellus hair, which is pale and fine; or terminal hair, which is darker and coarser, like hair of the eyebrows and scalp. Hair color is produced by melanin granules deposited by nearby melanocytes.

Nails

The nails found on fingers and toes are also part of the integumentary system. Much like hair, nails contain hard keratin (as opposed to the soft keratin of the skin), making them great tools for picking up objects. Each nail has a free edge at the distal tip. The visible nail plate is called the body of the nail.

The nail root is embedded proximally under the skin of the eponychium, or cuticle. The nail plate sits on is the nail bed. As the cells divide, growing out of the nail matrix, it pushes the existing nail outwards across the nail bed.

The skin folds overlapping the borders of the nail are called nail folds. At the edge of the finger, under the distal nail is the hyponychium.

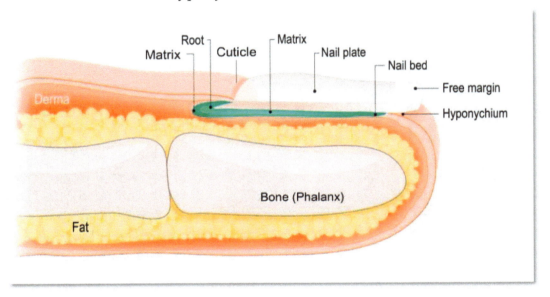

Fig. 3.6 - Structure of the Nail.

Glands

There is a vast collection of four types of exocrine glands in the integumentary system: *sudoriferous* glands, *sebaceous* glands, *ceruminous* glands, and *mammary* glands.

There are two types of sudoriferous glands, also known as sweat glands, totaling around three million glands found almost everywhere on the surface of the skin. Most of the sweat glands are eccrine glands, which consists of a coiled tube. Secretions occur within the dermis; the resulting fluid (or sweat) travels through the tube, towards a funnel-shaped opening at the surface of the skin called a pore. Sweat is ninety-nine percent water, but also contains some salts and metabolic wastes.

Sweat is also secreted by *apocrine* sweat glands, which are much fewer in number, and are found only in certain areas of the body. In addition to the sweat mixture, apocrine glands secrete fat and protein components which is the cause of body odor.

Sebaceous glands, also known as oil glands, secrete a substance called sebum. Sebum is made of oily lipids that soften and lubricate hair and skin, slows water loss, and kills certain bacteria.

Mammary glands and ceruminous glands are also types of apocrine glands, which produce breast milk and earwax, respectively.

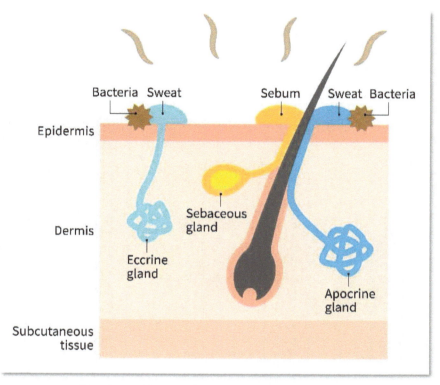

Fig. 3.7 - Glands of the integumentary system.

Clinical Significance and Martial Arts Relevance:

Skin Infections

Gyms are notorious for being places that harbor the perfect storm for spreading skin infections.

Because of the significant potential for extended periods of skin-to-skin contact in jujitsu and grappling related arts, skin infections can be a common and unfortunate occurrence in martial arts training. The most common cause for the spread of skin infections in a martial arts academy or gym is the lack of education about skin infections, especially in preventing them if cleaning standards are subpar. Most skin infections associated with athletic endeavors are minor and usually only become major health issues if they are not treated properly. However, an outbreak of skin infection in a martial arts academy can cause considerable concern not only for fellow students and training partners, but health officials as well.

Most of the pathogens (infectious organisms) that are of concern to martial artists require only minimal direct contact for transmission. Therefore, avoid training while infected, or suspected of being infected, until fully treated. These highly infectious organisms require warm moist areas to live, breed, and grow; therefore, it is important to ensure that training equipment, personal gear, uniforms (including belts), rash guards, and mats are cleaned and dried on a daily basis when used.

The most common types of skin infections associated with combat sports include Ring worm, Impetigo, Staph/MRSA, and Herpes simplex.

Ringworm

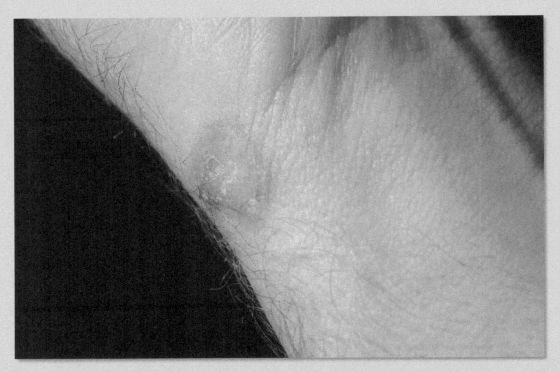

Fig. 3.8 - Ringworm infection on the wrist.

Ringworm (tinea corporis) is a rash caused by a fungal infection. It usually itches and appears as a slightly raised, red circular scaly rash with clearer skin in the middle. Ringworm gets its name because of its appearance, not because a worm is involved.

The fungus tinea, which causes ringworm, also causes athlete's foot (tinea pedis), jock itch (tinea cruris) and ringworm of the scalp (tinea capitis). Ringworm often spreads by direct skin-to-skin contact with an infected person.

Mild ringworm often responds to antifungal medications applied to the skin. More severe infections may require antifungal pills for several weeks.

Impetigo

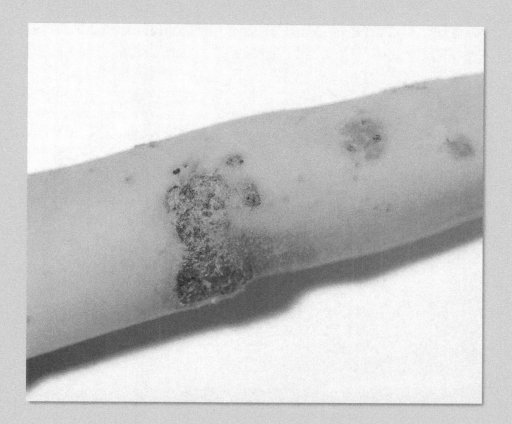

Fig. 3.9 - Impetigo infection on upper extremity.

Impetigo is a common and highly contagious bacterial skin infection. The bacteria *Staphylococcus aureus* (staph) or *Streptococcus pyogenes* (strep) infect the epidermis, causing sores most often on the face, arms, and legs.

Although impetigo is more common in young children, adults who participate in contact sports requiring skin-to-skin contact can be infected as well. However, because of its highly contagious nature, impetigo can spread through any close contact.

The symptoms of impetigo in adults are usually clustered reddish sores around the nose and mouth, or any other exposed areas of skin on the body. The blisters break open, ooze, and then form a golden/yellow crust around the affect area.

Impetigo is generally considered a mild skin infection; however, adults have a higher risk of complications than children: including lymphangitis, cellulitis, sepsis, and acute post-streptococcal kidney disease.

Staph and MRSA

Commonly referred to "gym staph" by athletes, staphylococcus aureus (staph) is a group of bacteria that can cause several different skin infections. Staph usually enters the body through hair follicles and small open wounds. However, it can cause an infection without a break in the skin. The bacteria usually target the layers of the skin, but in severe cases it can penetrate deeper into the fascia, muscles, and even bones. Staph is almost always transmitted by skin-to-skin contact. However, unclean facilities and training equipment are also known causes for infection.

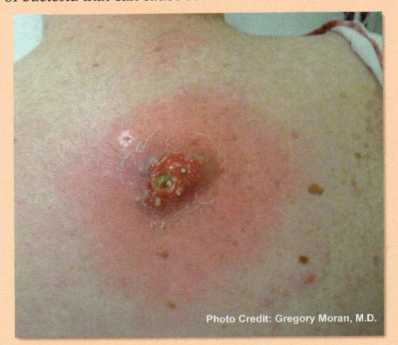

Fig. 3.10 - A cutaneous abscess located on the back, which had been caused by methicillin-resistant Staphylococcus aureus bacteria, referred to by the acronym MRSA. Image credit: Gregory Moran, M.D.

Staphylococcus aureus and its subsequent infections are considered to be opportunist. With up to 25% of people carrying the organism with no symptoms or ill-effects, it only develops into an infection when the circumstances are right. Worse, however, than your daily garden-variety staph infection is methicillin-resistant staphylococcus aureus (MRSA). This troublesome mutated version of staph does not respond to the usual prescribed antibiotics and can be extremely difficult to cure. There are numerous factors that have contributed to the emergence of MRSA, such as inappropriate use of antibiotics, but being irresponsible and not seeking early treatment are contributing factors as well.

Early symptoms of a staph infection may vary significantly, but some are quite predictable if not addressed. Staph infections often develop as a reddish rash that progresses into a pimple-like blister that is commonly confused with acne. It may become a larger boil and an open sore if it bursts on its own. There is usually accompanying tenderness, inflammation, increased warmth, and redness around wound. Common areas for staph and MRSA infections include the back of the neck, underarms, groin, legs, and the beard area in men. In addition to skin related symptoms, a fever is almost always present as the rash worsens in more severe cases.

Herpes Simplex

Herpes gladiatorum ("wrestler's herpes" or "mat herpes") is a skin infection caused by herpes simplex virus type 1 (HSV-1). HSV-1 is the same virus that causes cold sores on the lips. With around 66.6% of the world's population being exposed to herpes by adulthood; HSV-1 infections are very common. However, many people never develop symptoms.

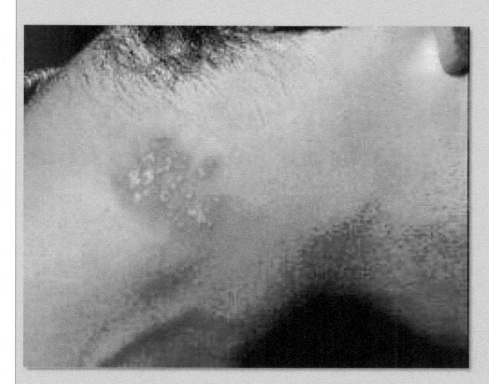

While the symptoms of herpes gladiatorum (HSV-1) can be treated, once someone is infected with the virus, they are infected for life. People with herpes gladiatorum can have periods where the virus is inactive and cannot be spread to others. However, the virus can be reactivated at any time and be transmitted to others, even if there are no symptoms such as blisters or sores.

Fig. 3.11 - Herpes Gladiatorum of the neck. Image Credit: OrthoBullets.com

Martial artists with herpes gladiatorum may develop lesions anywhere on the face or body and are highly contagious while the lesions remain open. HSV-1 infection of the eye is very serious and requires immediate medical attention. The herpes virus is most commonly spread to others through direct skin-to-skin contact with the lesions, or by the sharing of inanimate objects such as: beverage containers, cell phones, and eating utensils.

Initial symptoms of herpes gladiatorum usually begin about 8 days after exposure to HSV-1. The outbreak often begins as a tingling sensation at the affected area accompanied by swollen lymph nodes. The presence of fever is common, especially during the first episode. A cluster of clear, fluid-filled blisters develop that may be surrounded by an area of redness. The blisters may be painful, and the lesions usually dry up and heal within 7 to 10 days.

Prevention

Unfortunately, there is a subculture of ill-informed martial arts practitioners who consider "gym infections" to be a badge of honor. Not only is this irresponsible, but it is also avoidable. The primary focus for martial arts instructors and practitioners, regarding skin infections, is prevention. Because they are easily transmissible, and do have the potential for long term complications, preventing skin infections are much easier than treating them. Proper hygiene, to include washing personal training gear and uniforms after each workout; and daily cleaning and disinfecting of mats and public use training equipment goes a long way in avoiding an outbreak in your facility.

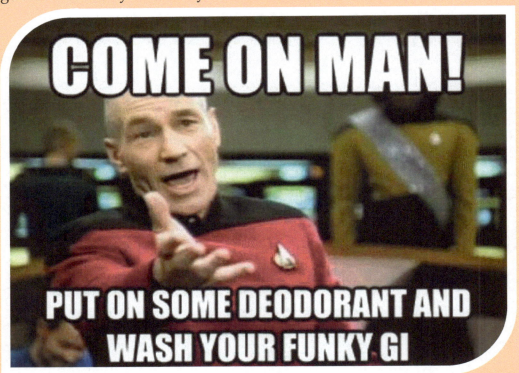

Fig. 3.12 – Prevention is key in avoiding gym infections.

Chapter 4

Introduction to the Skeletal System

Humans are vertebrates, animals that have a vertebral column (spine/backbone) and a sturdy internal skeletal frame. The human skeletal system consists of bones, cartilage, and ligaments that provides support for the body. Accounting for about 20 percent of the body weight, living bones contain active tissues that require a blood supply, use oxygen, consume nutrients, and remodel to change shape in response to injury or mechanical stress.

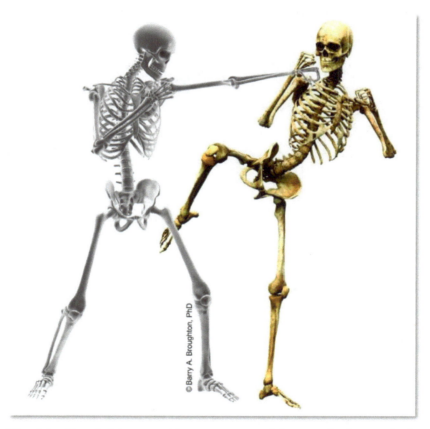

Fig. 4.1 - The skeleton provides structure and form to the human body.

The skeleton provides a rigid framework that supports and protects the soft structures within the body cavities. The fused bones of the cranium form a bony vault that surrounds the brain, making it less vulnerable to injury. Bones of the rib cage help protect the heart and lungs within the thorax, while vertebrae surround and protect the spinal cord.

The large bones of the lower extremities support the trunk, keeping it upright while standing. Bones function together with muscles to form mechanical lever systems that produce body movement.

The intercellular matrix of bone contains large amounts of calcium which is released when blood calcium levels decrease below normal, thus, providing an appropriate supply of calcium needed for metabolic processes. If serum calcium levels increase above normal levels, excess calcium is stored within the bone matrix. The formation of blood cells and platelets (called hematopoiesis) takes place primarily within the red marrow of the bones. In adults, red marrow is found within the spongy cancellous bone of the long bones, skull, sternum, vertebrae and pelvis. In infants, red marrow is found in all the bone cavities; with age, it is largely replaced by yellow marrow for fat storage.

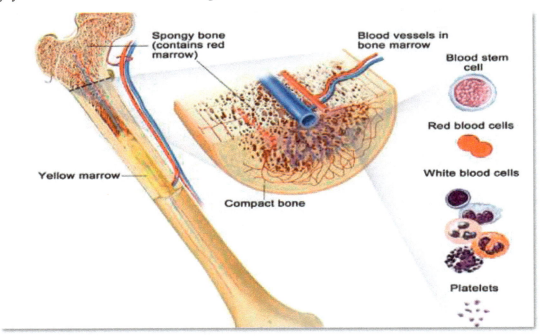

Fig. 4.2 - Hematopoiesis occurs in the red marrow of bones.

Structure of Bone Tissue

There are two types of bone tissue: cortical (compact) and cancellous (spongy). As the names imply, the two bone types differ in their density and in how tightly the tissue is packed together.

Cortical (Compact) Bone

Cortical bone is the dense outer surface of the bone that forms a protective layer around the internal cavity. Cortical (compact) bone makes up nearly 80% of the skeletal mass. Because of its high resistance to torsion and bending, it is crucial for maintaining body structure and weight-bearing.

Cortical bone consists of tightly packed canal systems to form what appears to be a solid mass. However, bony canals within the bone contain blood vessels that run parallel to the long axis of the bone. These blood vessels interconnect with vessels on the surface of the bone by way of perforating canals.

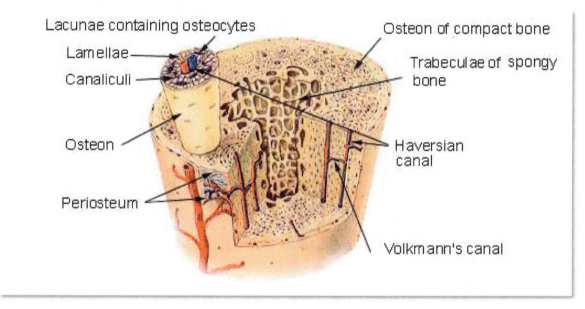

Fig. 4.3 - Cortical and Cancellous Bone.

Cancellous (Spongy) Bone

Cancellous bone is lighter and less dense than the exterior cortical bone. The cancellous (spongy) bone is formed by trabeculae (plates and bars of bone) adjacent to small, irregular cavities that contain red bone marrow. The trabeculae appear to be arranged in a haphazard manner; however, they are organized to provide maximum strength to the bone. The trabeculae of cancellous bone follow the lines of stress and can realign over time if the direction of mechanical stress changes.

Bone Development & Growth

As mentioned previously, bones have a blood supply and are a living tissue. A healthy human skeleton is consistently producing new bone, replacing itself every 7-10 years.

Early in human fetal development, the skeleton is made entirely of cartilage. Through the process of ossification, the relatively soft cartilage gradually turns into hard bone as mineral deposits replace cartilage. During this time, ossification of long bones, which are found in the arms and legs, begins at the center of the bones and continues toward the ends. Several areas of cartilage remain in the skeleton at birth, including the epiphyseal plate (growth plates) at the ends of the long bones. So that the bones can keep increasing in length during childhood, this cartilage continues to grow as the long bones grow.

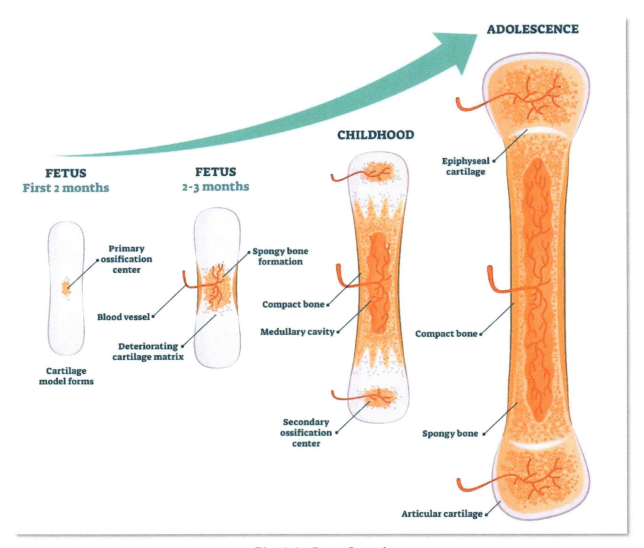

Fig. 4.4 - Bone Growth.

Long bones ossify and get longer as they develop and grow. In the presence of the epiphyseal plate, these bones grow from their ends, known as the epiphysis. The epiphyseal line on x-ray signifies that the bone is still growing. In the late teens or early twenties, humans reach skeletal maturity. After puberty, all of the cartilage in the growth plates are replaced by bone, so no further growth in bone length is possible. However, bones can still increase in thickness. This may occur in response to injury, increased muscle activity, or skeletal stress such as weight training.

Classification of Bones

The bones of the human body are divided by sizes and shapes. The four primary types of bones are long, short, irregular, and flat.

Long Bones

Long bones are hard, dense bones that are longer than they are wide; and provide strength, structure, and mobility. Long bones include bones of the thigh, leg, arm, and forearm.

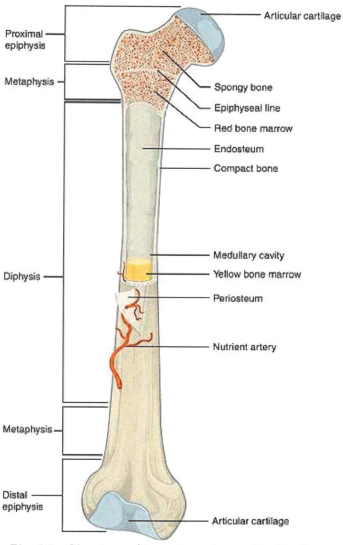

Fig. 4.5 - Structure of Long Bone. Image Credit: chegg.com

Long bones have a diaphysis (shaft) in the middle between two prominent epiphyses (ends). The metaphyseal junction is the widened area between the diaphysis and the epiphysis. They are primarily composed of cortical bone but may have a large amount of cancellous bone at the epiphysis. The outside of the bone is covered with a tough membrane called the periosteum.

Short Bones

Short bones are cube-like shaped bones with approximately equal horizontal and vertical dimensions. Short bones are comprised primarily of cancellous bone, which is covered by a thin layer of cortical bone. Short bones include the bones of the ankle and wrist.

Irregular Bones

Like short bones, irregular bones are primarily cancellous bone covered with a thin layer of cortical bone; however, they have an irregular shape and contour. Some of the bones in the skull and the vertebrae and are classified as irregular bones.

Flat Bones

Flat bones are flattened, thin, and usually curved. Most of the bones of the cranium are considered flat bones.

All bones have certain characteristics and surface markings that make a specific bone unique. There are projections, depressions, holes, smooth facets, lines, and other anatomical features. These features usually represent points of attachment for tendons and ligaments, points of articulation with other bones, or canals for the passage of nerves and vessels.

Joints

A joint is an articulation formed between two or more bones of the skeletal system. Joints can be broadly classified by the tissue which connects the bones (fibrous, cartilaginous or synovial), or by the degree of movement permitted (synarthrosis, amphiarthrosis or diarthrosis).

Classification of Joints

Fibrous Joints

Fibrous joints are bound by a tough fibrous tissue. These joints typically require strength and stability rather than range of movement.

Fibrous joints are further sub-classified into sutures, gomphoses, and syndesmoses.

- **Sutures**

Sutures are immovable joints (synarthrosis) that are only found between the flat bones of the skull. The bones of the skull are not fused at birth, allowing for deformation of the skull as it passes through the birth canal. The suture lines begin to close throughout infancy and adolescence, however they do not begin to fully fuse together until early adulthood and into the 3rd decade.

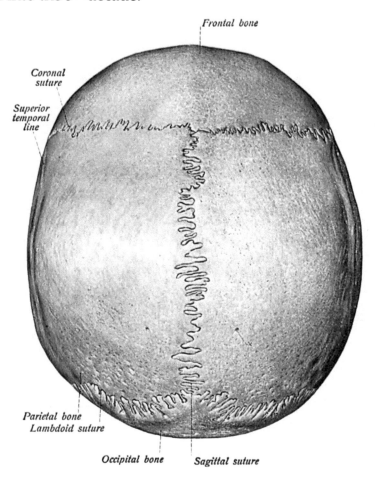

Fig. 4.6 – Sutures of the cranium.

- **Gomphoses**

Gomphoses are immovable joints where the teeth articulate within their sockets in the maxilla (upper teeth) and the mandible (lower teeth). The tooth is secured in its socket by the strong periodontal ligament.

- **Syndesmoses**

Syndesmoses are slightly movable joints that are formed by an interosseous membrane that holds bones together. The middle tibiofibular joint in the leg is an example of a syndesmosis joint.

Cartilaginous Joints

Joints in which bones are united together by fibrocartilage or hyaline cartilage are called cartilaginous joints.

The two types of cartilaginous joints include: synchondrosis (primary cartilaginous) and symphysis (secondary cartilaginous).

- **Synchondrosis**

A synchondrosis joint is immovable and the bones are connected by hyaline cartilage. The joint between the diaphysis and epiphysis of growing long bones are considered a synchondrosis joint.

- **Symphysis**

Symphysial joints are slightly movable (amphiarthroses). The joint between the bones of a symphysis is united by a layer of fibrocartilage.

The pubic symphysis, and the joints between vertebral bodies are symphysis joints.

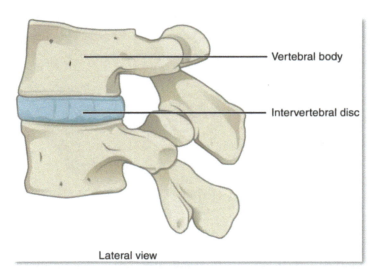

Fig. 4.7 – Example of a symphysis type joint. Adjacent vertebral bodies are connected by fibrocartilage. Image Credit: OpenStax College [CC by 3.0], via Wikimedia Commons

Synovial Joints

A synovial joint is a freely movable (diarthrosis) fluid-filled joint cavity enclosed within a fibrous capsule. They are the most common type of joint found in the body and permit the greatest range of movement.

Synovial joints are sub-classified into several different types of joints; depending on the shape of their articular surfaces and the movements permitted:

- **Gliding joints**, also known as plane joints, are formed by relatively flat articular surfaces, allowing the bones to glide over one another.

    i.e., subtalar joint, sternoclavicular joint.

- **Hinge joints** permit movement in one plane, usually flexion and extension.

    i.e., ankle joint, knee joint, elbow joint.

- **Pivot joints** allow only rotation. They are formed by a central bony pivot, which is surrounded by a bony-ligamentous ring.

    i.e., cervical atlantoaxial joint, proximal radioulnar joint.

- **Ellipsoid joints**, also known as condyloid joints, contains a convex surface which articulates with a concave elliptical cavity.

    i.e., wrist joint, metacarpophalangeal joint, metatarsophalangeal joint.

- **Saddle joints** are characterized by opposing concave-convex articular surfaces that allows for articulation by reciprocal reception. Both bones have concave-convex articular surfaces which interlock like two saddles opposed to each other. Saddle joints allow movement with two degrees of motion like condyloid joints. They allow for flexion and extension, and abduction and adduction, which therefore allows circumduction. Unlike ball and socket joints, saddle joints do not allow axial rotation.

    i.e., carpometacarpal joints.

- **Ball and Socket** joints are formed by the ball-shaped surface of one rounded bone which fits into the socket-like depression of another bone. Ball and socket joints allow for free movement in numerous axes.

    i.e., shoulder joint, hip joint.

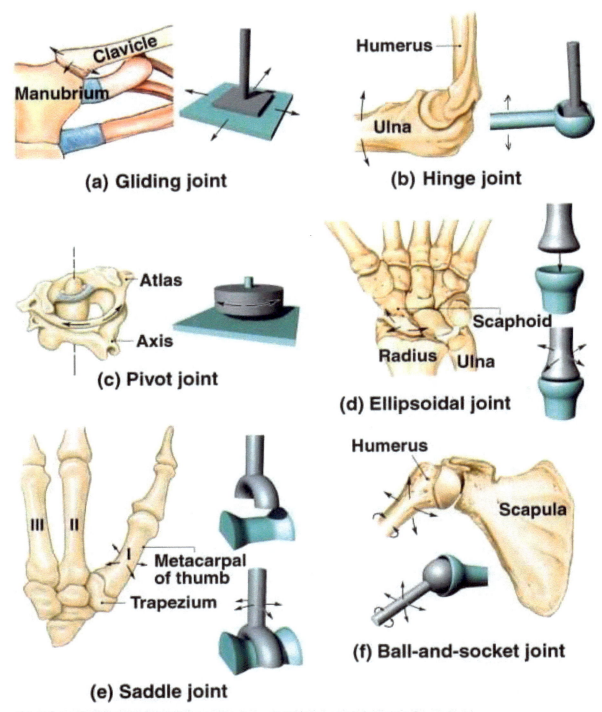

Fig. 4.8 – Different types of synovial joint.
Image Credit: Pearson Education, Inc. publishing as Benjamin Cummings, 2007

Structures of a Synovial Joint

There are three main features of a synovial joint which are not seen in fibrous or cartilaginous joints. They include an articular capsule, articular cartilage, and synovial fluid.

- **Articular capsule** - As a continuation of the periosteum of the articulating bones, the articular capsule surrounds the joint into a closed space.

The capsule consists of two layers:

> **Fibrous layer (outer)** – known the capsular ligament, consists of white fibrous tissue that holds the articulating bones together and supports the underlying synovium.
>
> **Synovial layer (inner)** – known as the synovium, is a highly vascularized layer of serous connective tissue that secretes synovial fluid.

- **Articular Cartilage**

The articulating surfaces of a synovial joint are covered by a thin layer of hyaline cartilage. The articular cartilage minimizes friction that occurs during joint movement and provides for shock absorption during activity.

- **Synovial Fluid**

The synovial fluid within the joint acts has three primary functions. It acts as lubrication for the joint surfaces, provides shock absorption during activity, and provides nutrients to the joint tissue. Articular cartilage is relatively avascular and is therefore dependent upon the passive diffusion of nutrients from the synovial fluid during motion of the joint.

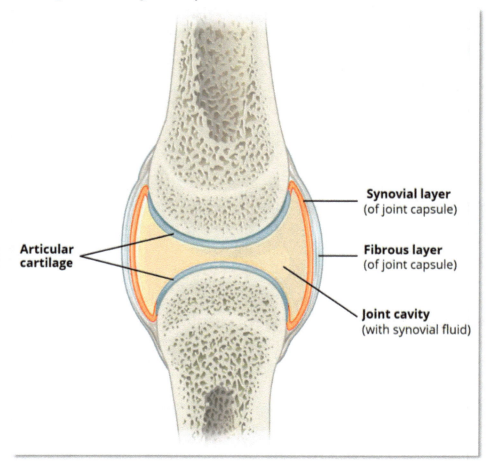

Fig. 4.9 – The basic structures of a synovial joint. Image Credit: Adapted from OpenStax College [CC by 3.0], via Wikimedia Commons

Accessory Structures of a Synovial Joint

▪ Accessory Ligaments

Accessory ligaments strengthen and reinforce the stability of synovial joints by connecting the articulating bones together. Intrinsic ligaments are formed within the joint capsule. Extrinsic ligaments are separate ligaments outside of the joint capsule or are localized thickenings of the joint capsule itself.

Ligaments consist of bundles of dense regular connective tissue, which are highly adapted for resisting strain. They resist any extreme ranges of movement that may damage the joint.

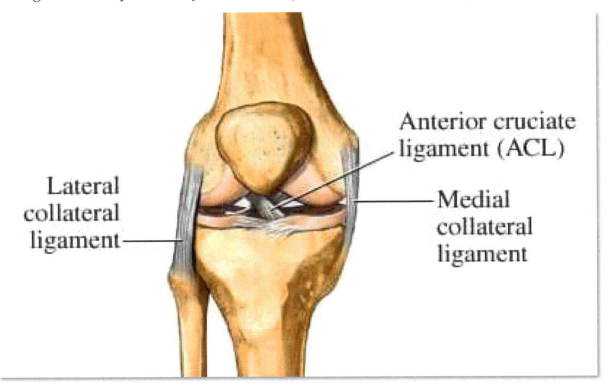

Fig. 4.10 – The lateral and medial collateral ligaments and the anterior cruciate ligament are examples of ligaments of a synovial joint.

▪ Bursa

A synovial bursa (plural- bursae) is a small fluid-filled sac lined by a synovial membrane. Most of the bursa are potential spaces and are not normally palpable or visualized on imaging.

The bursa provides a cushion between a bony prominence and the tendons or muscles around a joint. The bursa helps to reduce friction between the bones and allows free movement of the soft tissue.

In conditions such as over-use, excessive local friction, infection, or direct trauma, fluid collects within the bursa or fluid extends into the bursa from the adjacent joint.

Clinical Significance and Martial Arts Relevance:

• Bursitis

Inflammation of any of the bursae throughout the body can occur in martial arts training as a result of over-use, direct trauma from a blow or fall, or repeated pressure. The most common effected areas include the shoulder, hip, knee, and elbow.

The affected bursal area usually becomes red, swollen, warm, and tender to touch. Frequently, flexion of the neighboring joint is painful because more pressure is applied over the bursa.

Septic (infected) bursitis is most likely to occur in superficial bursae that lie just below the skin, such as the prepatellar bursa (at the kneecap), and the olecranon bursa (at the tip of the elbow). These bursae can be exposed to bacteria from the training mat or gym after an abrasion, "mat burn", or cut.

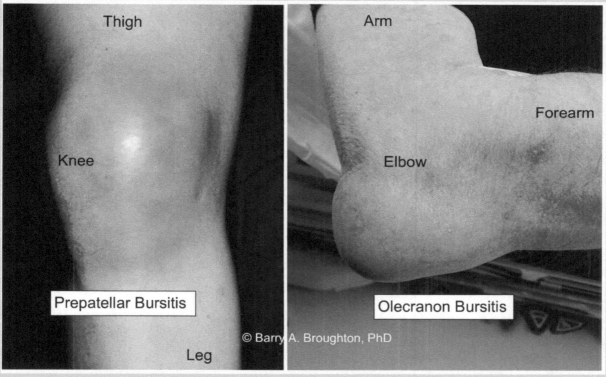

Fig. 4.11 - Left: Prepatellar bursitis of the knee. Right: Olecranon bursitis of the elbow.

• Post-traumatic Osteoarthritis

Osteoarthritis (OA) is the most common form of arthritis causing joint inflammation. It is often a result of heavy use of the effected joints over the course of many years, causing the wearing away of the articular cartilage, and the subsequent erosion of the underlying articulating surfaces of bones as well.

The arthritic changes that occur are degenerative and irreversible, resulting in decreased effectiveness of articular cartilage as a shock absorber. As a result of the degenerative process, repeated use can cause symptoms of joint pain and stiffness. Osteoarthritis usually affects weight-bearing joints, such as the hips and the knees, however it can also effect joints that undergo repeated trauma as well, i.e., hand and shoulders.

Participation in sports and martial arts training increases the potential risk of joint injuries that can lead to post-traumatic osteoarthritis. Post-traumatic arthritis is a clinical syndrome that is a result of trauma-initiated joint degeneration that causes permanent and often progressive joint pain and dysfunction.

Lifelong participation in sports that cause minimal joint impact and torsional loading by an athlete or martial artist with normal joints and neuromuscular function does not necessarily increase the risk of post-traumatic osteoarthritis. However, participation in training that exposes joints to high levels of impact and torsional loading does increase the risk of joint injury and subsequent joint degeneration.

Education of human anatomy, and awareness of proper training techniques are fundamental keys to injury prevention and increasing the longevity of martial arts careers.

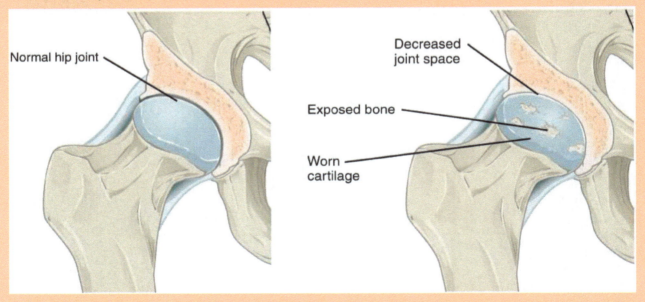

Fig. 4.12 - Example of osteoarthritis of the hip joint. Image Credit: OpenStax College [CC by 3.0], via Wikimedia Commons

THE HUMAN SKELETON

To better describe, communicate, and have an understanding of proper body movement and the kinetics involved with the proper execution of each technique, it is advantageous to have an understanding of basic skeletal anatomy and the terminology.

COMPREHENSIVE ANATOMY FOR MARTIAL ARTS

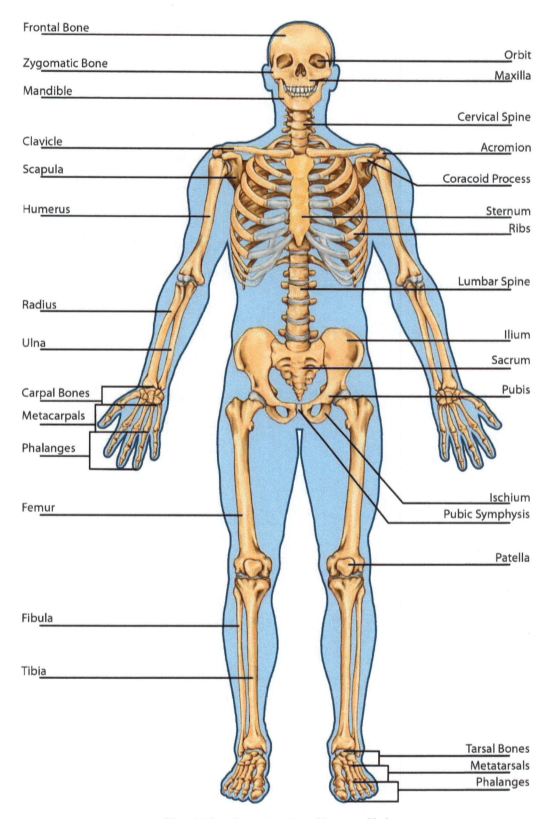

Fig. 4.13 - Anterior view Human Skeleton.

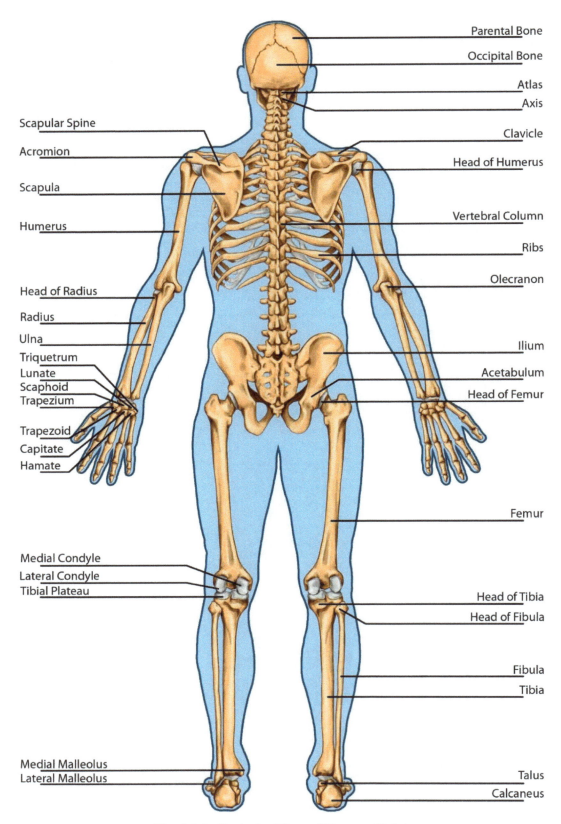

Fig. 4.14 - Posterior View of Human Skeleton.

SKELETAL TERMS

1. Skull- Also known as cranium, comprises the bony structures that form the head and houses the brain.

2. Orbit of the Eye- Refers to the bony socket in the skull that contains the eye and its associated structures.

3. Mandible- The lower jawbone.

4. Cervical- Refers to the neck region that consists of seven vertebrae.

5. Clavicle- Also known as the collar bone, which acts as a strut from the sternum to the acromion of the scapula/shoulder blade. The only long bones of the body that lie horizontal.

6. Humerus- The arm bone. The long bone of the upper extremity that runs from the shoulder to the elbow.

7. Ulna- One of the two bones of the forearm that runs from the elbow to the small finger side of the wrist.

8. Carpals- The eight small bones of the wrist.

9. Metacarpals- The five long bones of the hand.

10. Phalanges- the small bones that form the fingers and toes.

11. Radius- One of the two bones of the forearm that runs from the lateral side of the elbow to the thumb side of the wrist.

12. Sternum- The long flat bone in the center of the chest to which the ribs connect via cartilage. Also known as the breastbone.

13. Ribs- Twelve pairs of long curved bones that form the rib cage.

14. Floating Ribs- The two most inferior ribs of the rib cage that only attaches to the thoracic spine, and do not have a ventral attachment to the sternum, either directly or via cartilage.

15. Thoracic- Refers to the mid back region that consists of twelve vertebrae.

16. Lumbar- Refers to the lower back that consists of five vertebrae.

17. Sacrum- The wedge-shaped bone at the inferior end of the spine that intersects with the pelvis.

18. Coccyx- Also known as the tailbone. The distal tip of the spine inferior to the sacrum.

19. Pelvic Ilium- The largest and uppermost bone of the pelvis.

20. Pubic Ramus- Inferior most part of the pelvis.

21. Pubic Symphysis- The midline cartilaginous joint formed by the right and left superior rami of pubic bones.

22. Femur- Long bone of the thigh that runs from the hip to the knee.

23. Greater Trochanter- The irregular lateral prominence at the proximal end of the femur.

24. Femoral Head- The rounded proximal end of the femur that articulates with the pelvis forming the hip joint.

25. Femoral Neck- Connects the femoral head to the proximal end of the shaft of the femur.

26. Patella- Knee cap. The small circular-triangular shaped bone imbedded in the quadriceps tendon and articulates with the distal femur.

27. Fibula- The smaller of the two bones of the lower leg and is located lateral to the tibia.

28. Tibia- Also known as the shin bone it is the larger and stronger of the two bones of the lower leg.

29. Tarsals- Seven irregular shaped bones of the foot and ankle.

30. Metatarsals- The five long bones of the foot.

31. Calcaneus- Also known as the heel bone, it is the largest and strongest bone of the foot.

32. Upper Extremity- Referring to the anatomical structures between the shoulder and the fingers.

33. Arm- Referring to the anatomical structures between the shoulder and the elbow.

34. Forearm- Referring to the anatomical structures between the elbow and the wrist.

35. Lower Extremity- Referring to the anatomical structures between the hip and the toes.

36. Thigh- Referring to the anatomical structures between the hip and the knee.

37. Leg- Referring to the anatomical structures between the knee and the ankle.

38. Philtrum- The vertical groove from the base of the nose to the border of the upper lip overlying the teeth and gums.

39. Scapula- Also known as the shoulder blade.

40. Radial- Referring to the radius bone.

41. Ulnar- Referring to the ulna bone.

42. Vertebrae- The bony segments of the spine.

43. Pelvis- Refers to the bony structures that form the cavity of the lower torso.

44. Sciatic Nerve- The longest and widest single nerve in the human body, runs from the lumbar spine through the buttock down the posterior thigh and leg to the foot. The sciatic nerve provides innervations to the majority of the skin and musculature of the thigh and lower leg. (See *Introduction to the Nervous System*)

45. Lateral Femoral Cutaneous Nerve- The nerve that innervates the skin on the lateral aspect of the thigh. (See *Introduction to the Nervous System*)

46. Common Peroneal Nerve- A branch of the Sciatic Nerve that travels around the lateral knee to the foot, innervating the skin of the lateral knee and leg and the musculature of the anterior leg and foot. (See *Introduction to the Nervous System*)

47. Meniscus- Crescent shaped cartilaginous structure in the knee - both medial and lateral. Attached to the proximal tibia, it provides structural integrity to the knee throughout its range of motion as it articulates with the distal femur.

48. Medial Collateral Ligament (MCL)- The structure on the inner aspect of the knee that provides side-to-side stability. Because of its origin on the medial aspect of the distal femur, and its insertion on the medial aspect of the proximal tibia, it is the most commonly injured structure of the knee.

49. Anterior Cruciate Ligament (ACL) – One of a pair of structures (the other being the Posterior Cruciate Ligament) in the middle of the knee joint that provides forward and rotational stability by preventing the tibia from sliding forward on the distal femur.

50. Forefoot- The anterior aspect of the foot comprised of the phalanges and the metatarsals.

51. Midfoot- Refers to the bones and joints that make up the arch of the foot and connect the forefoot to the hindfoot.

52. Hindfoot- The posterior aspect of the foot that is formed by four of the tarsal bones including the calcaneus, talus, navicular, and cuboid.

53. Phalanx- Singular of the term phalanges.

Divisions of the Skeleton

The adult human skeleton usually consists of 206 named bones. The human skeleton is divided into two major divisions, the axial skeleton and the appendicular skeleton.

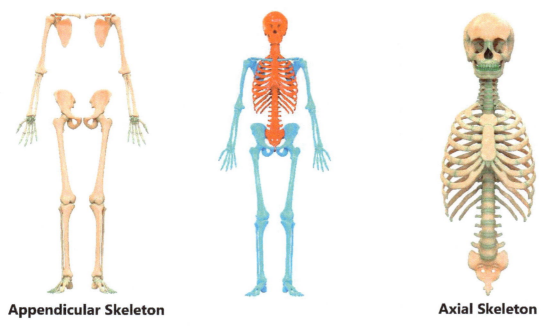

Fig. 4.15 - Anterior view of Appendicular and Axial Skeletons.

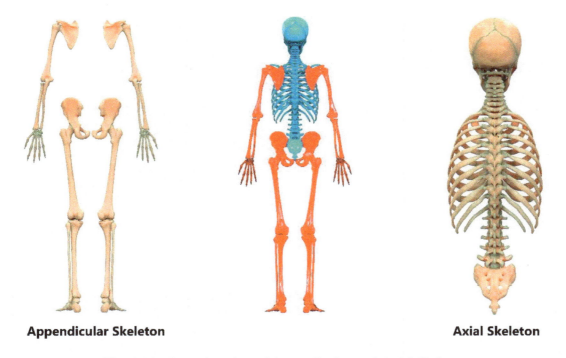

Fig. 4.16 - Posterior view of Appendicular and Axial Skeletons.

Axial Skeleton (80 bones)

The axial skeleton forms the main trunk and the vertical axis of the body. The 80 bones of the axial skeleton include the bones of the head, vertebral column, ribs, and sternum.

Skull

The cranial vault or skullcap consists mainly of flat bones: the paired parietal bones and temporal bones; frontal and occipital bone. Together with the base of the skull, they encase and protect the brain. The cranial vault and the base of skull together form the neurocranium.

Cranial Bones

The cranial bones include the parietal, temporal, frontal, occipital, ethmoid, and sphenoid bones.

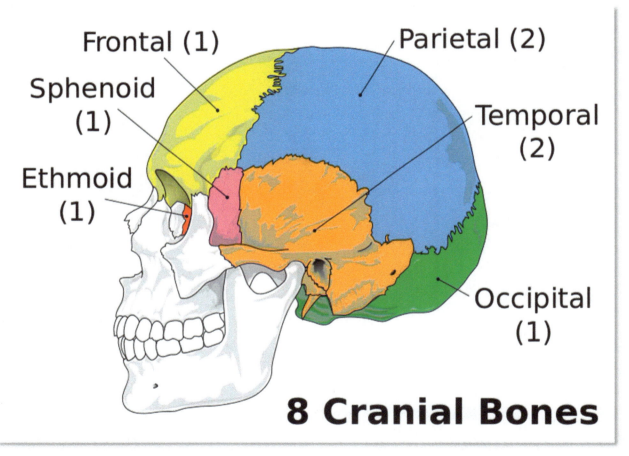

Fig. 4.17 - Eight bones of the cranium. Image Credit: Was a bee, [CC0 1.0], via Wikimedia Commons

Clinical Significance and Martial Arts Relevance:

- **Fractures of the Pterion**

The pterion is an H-shaped junction located on the side of the skull, just behind the temple, where the skull is at its weakest. It is the point where the frontal, parietal, sphenoid, and temporal bones meet. Blunt force or penetrating trauma in this area can injure the middle meningeal artery (MMA), causing an extradural hematoma (blood to accumulate between the skull and the dura mater). An extradural hematoma can cause a dangerous increase in intra-cranial pressure, which may lead to herniation of brain tissue and ischemia (loss of blood supply).

The increase in intra-cranial pressure can cause a host of symptoms to include nausea, vomiting, seizures, bradycardia (slowed heart rate), and extremity weakness. Extradural hematomas are treated by diuretics in minor cases, and drilling burr holes into the skull in the more extreme hemorrhages.

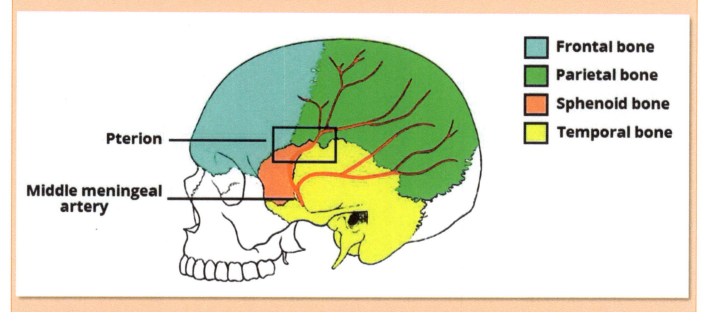

Fig. 4.18 - Lateral view of the skull, showing the path of the meningeal arteries. Note the pterion, a weak point of the skull, where the anterior middle meningeal artery is at risk of damage.

- **Fracture of the Cribriform Plate**

The cribriform plate of the ethmoid bone forms the roof of the nasal cavity. Because it is the thinnest part of the anterior cranial fossa, it may fracture with a significant blunt force trauma to the face.

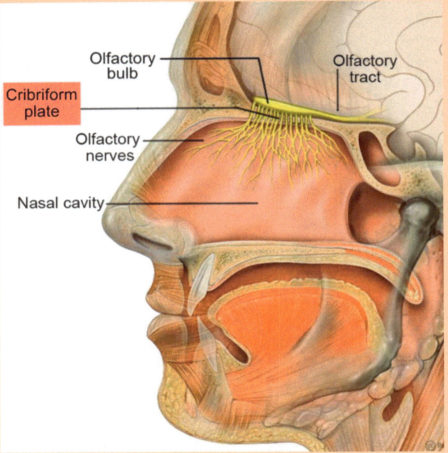

Fig. 4.19 - Cribriform Plate- Image Credit: Patrick J. Lynch [CC BY 2.5] via Wikimedia Commons

Rarely do cribriform plate fractures occur in isolation. Two major complications of cribriform plate fracture include:
- Anosmia – the loss of sense of smell, due to shearing of the olfactory nerve fibers that run through the cribriform plate.
- CSF Rhinorrhea – the leakage of cerebrospinal fluid into the nasal cavity, due to fragments of bone tearing the meningeal coverings of the brain. This is visible as a clear fluid from the nasal passage.

Facial Bones

The fourteen facial bones include the maxilla, zygomatic, mandible, nasal, palatine, inferior nasal concha, lacrimal, and vomer bones.

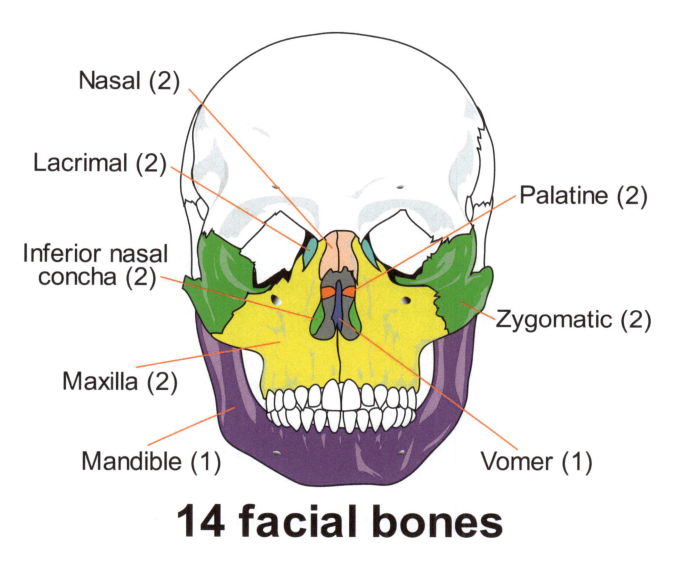

Fig. 4.20 - Facial Bones. Image Credit: Public domain, via Wikimedia Commons

Clinical Significance and Martial Arts Relevance:

- **Facial Fractures**

Fractures of the facial skeleton are relatively common and most frequently result from fights, falls, and motor vehicle accidents.

The four most common facial fracture types are:
- **Nasal fracture** – Due to the prominent position of the nasal bones at the bridge of the nose, nasal bone fractures are the most common facial fracture. There is often significant soft tissue swelling and epistaxis (nosebleed). Also See: *Clinical Significance and Martial Arts Relevance* in the Nose & Nasal Cavity section of the *Introduction to the Respiratory System* chapter.
- **Maxillary fracture** – A maxilla fracture often occurs from injuries to the face such as getting punched, a motor vehicle accident, sports, or from a fall. Because of the high-energy trauma, these injuries can be significant and require medical attention.
- **Mandibular fracture** – approximately 60% of mandibular fractures occur in two places. Clinical features include pain at the fracture site and may result in a decreased ability to fully open the mouth. There may be malocclusion (misalignment of the teeth) and bleeding of the gums.
- **Zygomatic arch fracture** – associated with trauma to the side of the face. Displaced fractures can damage the nearby infraorbital nerve, leading to ipsilateral paresthesia of the cheek, nose, and lip.

- **Fractures of the Eye Socket**

There are two major types of orbital (eye socket) fractures:

- **Orbital rim fracture** – A fracture of the bones forming the outer rim of the bony orbit of the eye. Fractures usually occur at the suture lines joining the three bones of the orbital rim – the maxilla, zygomatic, and frontal.
- **Blowout fracture** – refers to partial herniation of the contents within the orbit of the eye through one of its walls. With the medial and inferior walls being the weakest, the orbital contents may herniate into the ethmoid and maxillary sinuses. This usually occurs from blunt force trauma to the eye.

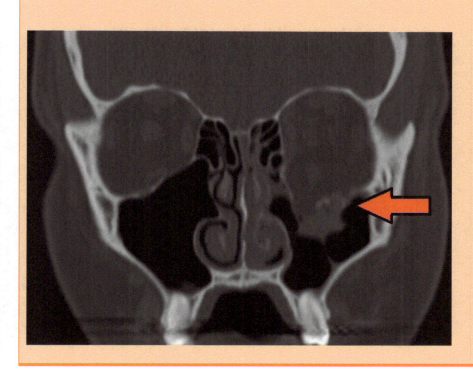

Fig. 4.21 - CT scan of a blowout fracture of the eye, through the inferior wall. The contents of the orbit have herniated into the maxillary sinus. Image Credit: James Heilman, MD [CC-BY-SA-3.0] via Wikimedia Commons

Any fracture of the orbit may result in increased intraorbital pressure within the orbit, causing exophthalmos (protrusion of the eye).

Auditory Ossicles

The auditory ossicles are a chain of three small bones in the middle ear. The bony chain transmits mechanical vibration (sound waves) from the outer ear to the inner ear converting it to sound.

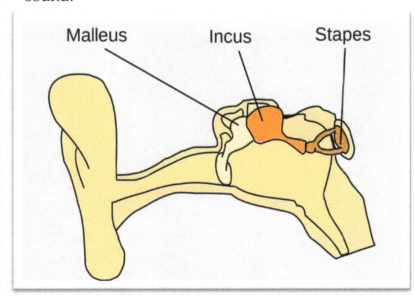

The three bones include the malleus (hammer), incus (anvil), and stapes (stirrup). The malleus is shaped like a hammer and sits between the eardrum and the incus. The incus is anvil-shaped and transmits vibrations between the malleus and stapes. The stapes, a small stirrup-shaped bone, transmit vibrations from the incus to the oval window of the inner ear.

Fig. 4.22 - Auditory ossicles

Hyoid

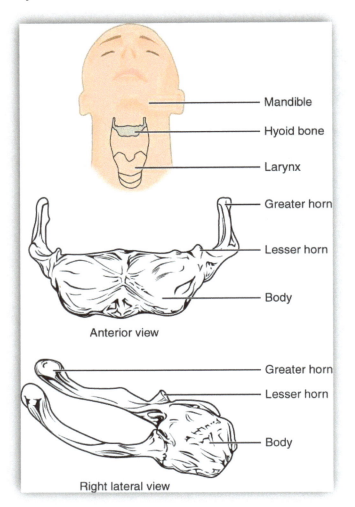

The hyoid bone is a "U" shaped structure located at the base of the mandible (at approximately C3 level), in the anterior neck. It is unique because it does not articulate with any other bones. The hyoid is suspended in place by the anterior neck muscles and ligaments that attach to it.

Fig. 4.23 - Hyoid bone. Image Credit: OpenStax College, [CC BY 3.0] via Wikimedia Commons

Clinical Significance and Martial Arts Relevance:

Fracture of the Hyoid Bone

The hyoid bone is well protected by the mandible and cervical spine; therefore, fractures are relatively rare.

Hyoid bones fractures are characteristically associated with strangulation (present in approximately 1/3 of all strangulation homicides), making it a significant post-mortem finding.

Hyoid fractures can also occur as a result of direct trauma to the anterior neck, such as from strikes or airway chokes. Clinical features include pain on speaking, painful swallowing (odynophagia), and difficult breathing (dyspnea).

Vertebral Column

The vertebral (spinal) column consists of 26 vertebrae with an intervertebral disc between each. The spinal column functions to protect the spinal cord, while the intervertebral discs act as a shock absorber between each vertebra.

Intervertebral Discs

The *intervertebral discs* make up approximately one fourth of the spinal column's overall length. There are no discs between the first and second vertebra, and sacrum and coccyx. Discs do not have their own blood supply, therefore depend on the end plates to diffuse their required nutrients. The cartilaginous layers of the end plates anchor the discs in place on the vertebrae.

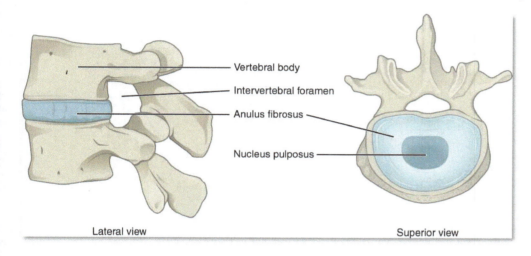

Fig. 4.24 - Intervertebral discs. Lateral and superior views. Image Credit: OpenStax College, [CC BY 3.0], via Wikimedia Commons

The intervertebral discs are fibrocartilaginous cushions that act as shock absorbers, protecting the vertebrae, spinal nerves, and other soft tissue structures. The disc at the individual level allows for minimal extension and flexion, however considerable motion is possible when several discs move in concert.

Intervertebral discs are composed of an annulus fibrosus and a nucleus pulposus.

- *Annulus Fibrosus:* The *annulus fibrosus* is a tough radial tire–like structure made up of concentric sheets of collagen fibers that connect to the vertebral end plates. The collagen fiber sheets are orientated at various angles which provide its strength. The annulus fibrosus encloses the nucleus pulposus.

Although both the annulus fibrosus and nucleus pulposus are composed of water, collagen, and proteoglycans, there is more fluid in the nucleus pulposus. The proteoglycan molecules attract and retain water within the structures.

- *Nucleus Pulposus:* The *nucleus pulposus* also contains a hydrated gelatinous–like substance that resists compression. The amount of water within the nucleus varies throughout the day depending on activity.

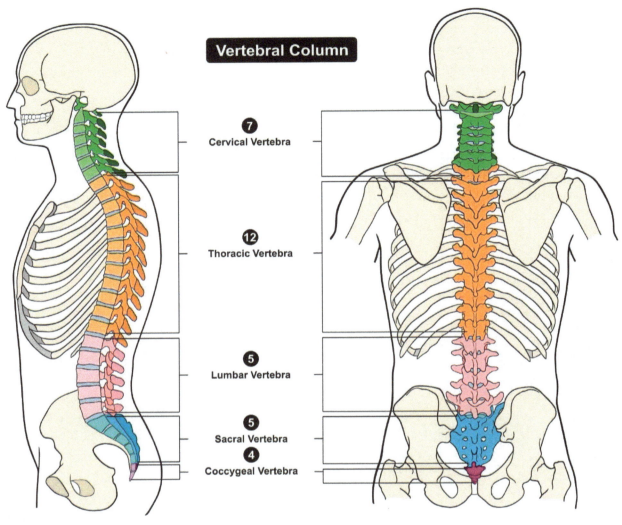

Fig. 4.25 - Five sections of the Vertebral Column.

▪ Cervical Spine

There are a total of 7 vertebrae that comprise the cervical portion of the vertebral column. Along with the hyoid bone, they form the skeleton of the neck extending superiorly from the base of the skull inferiorly to the 1st thoracic vertebra.

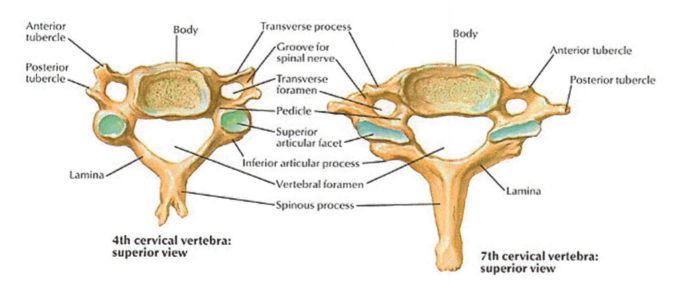

Fig. 4.26 - Structure of cervical vertebrae – Image Credit: TheArtofMedicine.com

The first two cervical vertebrae, C1 and C2, are uniquely different from the remaining five. The first cervical vertebra is called the Atlas — derived from Atlas of Greek mythology who held up the sphere of the earth on his shoulders. The atlas (C1) has a rounded shape that the skull rests upon. It consists of an anterior and a posterior arch with elongated transverse processes and does not have a body or spinous process. The second cervical vertebra has an upward projecting bony dens (odontoid) that articulates with the anterior arch of the atlas. The atlas and axis support the head on top of the vertebral column while providing significant mobility in flexion, extension, rotation and lateral bending.

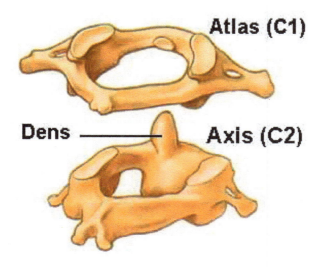

Fig. 4.27 - Cervical vertebrae C1 (Atlas) sits on C2 (Axis). Image Credit: SpineUniverse.com

Clinical Significance and Martial Arts Relevance:

Injuries to the Cervical Spine

▪ **Fracture of the Atlas**

A fracture to the first cervical vertebra can occur when a high-energy axial load is applied to the head while the cervical spine is hyperextended. Mechanisms of injury can include: an inverted vertical fall on the head during a martial arts throw; diving head-first into excessively shallow water; or hitting the head on the roof of a vehicle during a motor vehicle accident. The axial load force can compress the two wedge-shaped lateral masses of the atlas (C1 vertebra), between the occipital condyles (of the skull) and the axis (C2 vertebra), causing them to be driven apart, fracturing one or both anterior/posterior arches.

If the fall occurs with enough force, the transverse ligament of the atlas may also be ruptured. Since the vertebral foramen is large, it is unlikely that there will be damage to the spinal cord at the C1 level. However, there may be damage further down the vertebral column.

Refer to Fig. 4.28 - Fractures of first cervical (C1) vertebra on next page.

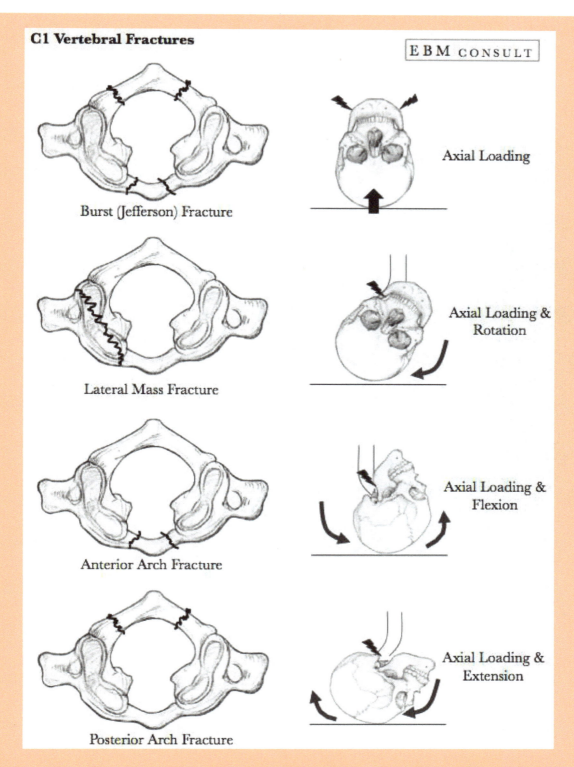

Fig. 4.28 - Fractures of first cervical (C1) vertebra. Image Credit: Evidence Based Medicine Consult

▪ Fracture of the Dens

Fractures of the dens (odontoid process) represent approximately 40% of all C2 fractures, which oftentimes may be unstable. Because of the isolation of the distal fragment from any blood supply, the dens is at high risk of avascular necrosis (death of bone tissue due to a lack of blood supply). As with any fracture of the vertebral column, there is a risk of spinal cord involvement.

▪ Hyperextension (Whiplash) Injury

Whiplash injuries are due to forceful, rapid back-and-forth movement of the head and neck. The whipping motion during injury is similar to the cracking of a whip, hence the name. Hyperextension injuries to the cervical spine can occur during throws, incorrect breakfalls, uppercuts, and certain chokes.

The subsequent injuries may involve strains or sprains (to muscles or ligaments), intervertebral joint injuries, injured nerve roots, or herniated discs. In minor cases, the anterior longitudinal ligament of the cervical spine is sprained, causing acute neck pain. In more severe cases, a fracture may occur to any cervical vertebrae as they are suddenly compressed by rapid deceleration. Because the vertebral foramen is large there is less chance of spinal cord involvement.

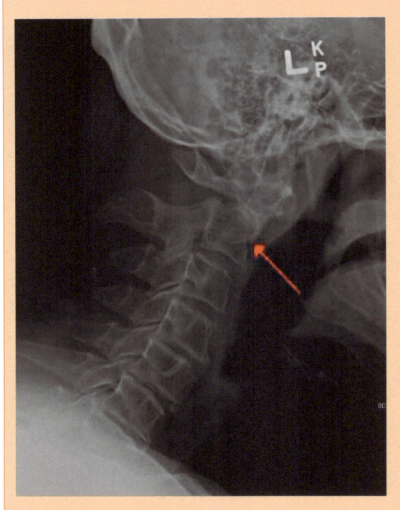

Fig. 4.29 – *A fracture of the base of the dens. Image Credit: James Heilman, MD [CC-BY-SA-3.0], via Wikimedia Commons*

In worst-case whiplash scenarios, a subluxation or dislocation of the cervical vertebrae may occur. Most often this occurs when the body of C2 vertebra moves anteriorly on the C3 vertebra. This type of injury can lead to spinal cord involvement, resulting in quadriplegia or even death. More commonly however, 50% of traumatic cervical subluxation occurs at the C6-C7 level.

▪ Neck Cranks

The neck, and its associated structures are one of the most vulnerable parts of the human body. Typically, in martial arts and during self-defense scenarios, it is susceptible to strikes, strangles, and chokes. It is also vulnerable to neck cranks (or cervical cranks) that can be applied from multiple positions. With numerous variations (such as Full Nelson, Half Nelson, Can Opener, Twister), most cranks that affect the spine are performed on the cervical spine, however thoracic and lumbar cranks are also options.

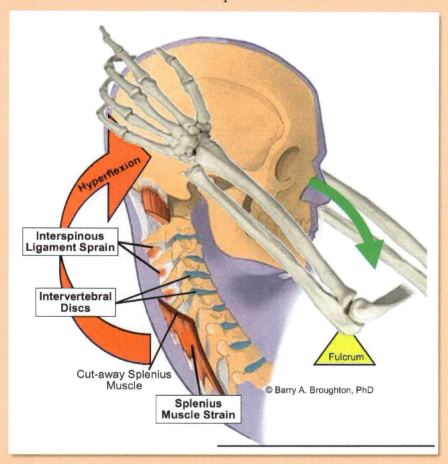

Fig. 4.30 - Neck cranks can cause injury to numerous soft tissue structures.

There are several ligaments throughout the cervical spine that provide stability and protection from extremes of movement that could injure the spinal cord. The *interspinous ligament* connects the spinous processes of adjacent vertebrae preventing hyperflexion. The *ligamentum flavum* connects the ventral aspect of the laminae of adjacent vertebrae. The *supraspinous ligament* attaches to the tips of the spinous processes of C1 though C7. It extends superiorly as the nuchal ligament to the external occipital protuberance, and inferiorly to the fourth lumbar vertebra. The *anterior* and *posterior longitudinal ligaments* run the length of the vertebral column, covering vertebral bodies and intervertebral discs.

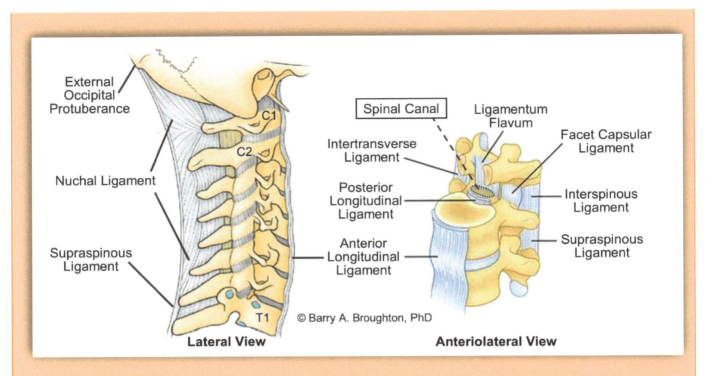

Fig. 4.31 - Ligament of the spinal column.

Most neck cranks involve flexing the cervical spine by pushing the head down towards the chest. During hyperflexion of the cervical spine, the ligaments, especially the interspinous ligament and posterior longitudinal ligament, are being stretched and possibly torn. The nuchal and interspinous ligaments are very proficient at resisting extreme flexion. However, lateral bending limits their ability to effectively protect the cervical spine.

The primary movement of the atlanto-axial (C1 on C2) joint is rotation, allowing for 60% of cervical rotation (50 degrees). There is limited flexion, extension, and lateral flexion (side bending) at C1-C2. Lateral flexion only occurs when combined with rotation. As the joint is rotated, a slackening of the ligaments allows for a subtle lateral shift of the atlas on the axis. This subtle movement allows for greater stretch of the cervical ligaments making it more difficult to resist the neck crank.

Additionally, forced anterior flexion of the spine compresses the intervertebral discs posteriorly, possibly causing it to herniate and impinge upon the spinal nerve or spinal cord (see *Introduction to the Nervous System* chapter).

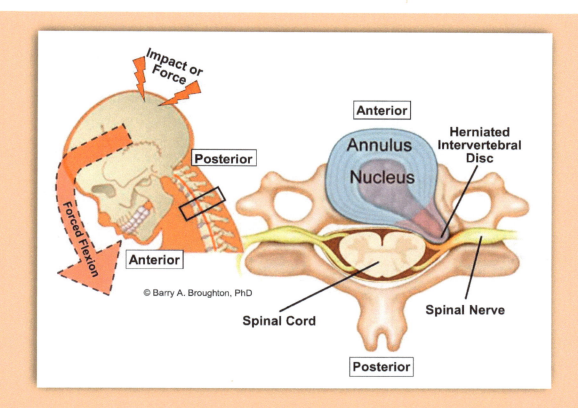

Fig. 4.32 - Cervical spine herniated intervertebral disc via force hyperflexion.

▪ Thoracic Spine

Consisting of 12 vertebrae, the thoracic spine is the longest region of the vertebral column. Stacked between the cervical spine superiorly and the lumbar spine inferiorly, the thoracic spine is the most complex segment of the spinal column. With its inherent stability, the thoracic spine helps keep the body upright, and is the only spinal region attached to the rib cage.

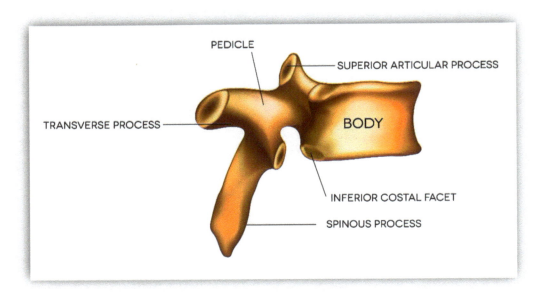

Fig. 4.33 - Lateral view of thoracic vertebra.

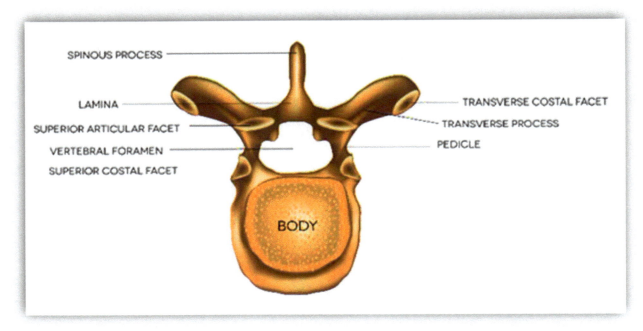

Fig. 4.34 - Superior view of thoracic vertebra.

▪ Lumbar Spine

The lumbar spine (lower back) consists of five vertebrae in the lower part of the spine, inferior to the thoracic spine and superior to the sacrum. The largest of the vertebral column the lumbar vertebrae supports the upper spine and torso. The lumbar spine bears most of the body's weight as well as the stress of lifting and carrying items.

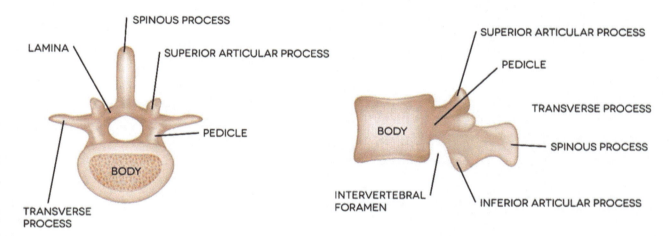

Fig. 4.35 - Left: Superior view of lumbar vertebra. Right: Lateral view of Lumbar vertebra.

Sacrum

The sacrum is the triangular bone just below the lumbar vertebrae. Five bony segments fused together into one large bone, the sacrum fits between the two halves of the pelvis, connecting the axial skeleton to the lower extremities of the appendicular skeleton.

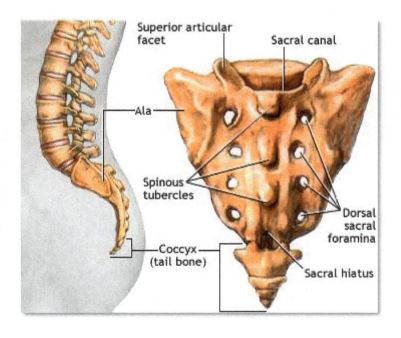

Coccyx

The coccyx consists of three to five different bones (depending on an individual's development) connected by fused, or semi-fused, joints. The coccyx represents a vestigial tail, hence the common term tailbone.

Fig. 4.36 - Lateral and posterior view of sacrum and coccyx. Image Credit: Medlineplus.gov

Clinical Significance and Martial Arts Relevance:

Fractured Coccyx

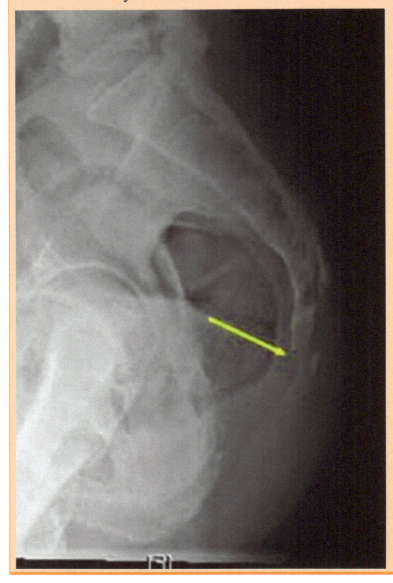

An abrupt fall onto the buttocks, from a throw, takedown, or via stumbling backwards can fracture the coccygeal vertebrae (tailbone). Although this injury may be very painful, it is usually managed with conservative care (i.e., rest), although severe displaced fractures may require in-patient treatment.

Fig. 4.37 - X-ray Lateral view of coccyx fracture

The Thoracic Cage

The thoracic cage is formed anteriorly by the sternum; posteriorly by the thoracic spine, and laterally by twelve pairs of ribs, and the associated costal cartilages. The thoracic cage protects vital organs such as the lungs and heart, the major blood vessels, and provides support for the upper extremities. It also assists in respiration; during inhalation the ribs become elevated, and during exhalation the ribs return to a relaxed position. The bones of the thoracic cage are also responsible for the production of blood (hematopoiesis).

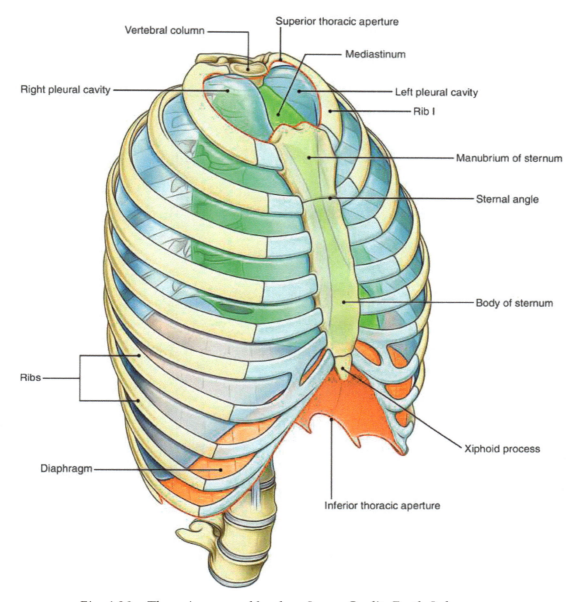

Fig. 4.38 – Thoracic cage and borders. Image Credit: EarthsLab.com

The Sternum

The sternum, or breastbone, is a narrow flat bone located in the middle of the anterior chest. The sternum protects the organs of your thorax from injury, and also serves as an articulation point for the ribs, clavicles, and musculature. The three regions of the sternum include the manubrium, the body, and the xiphoid process.

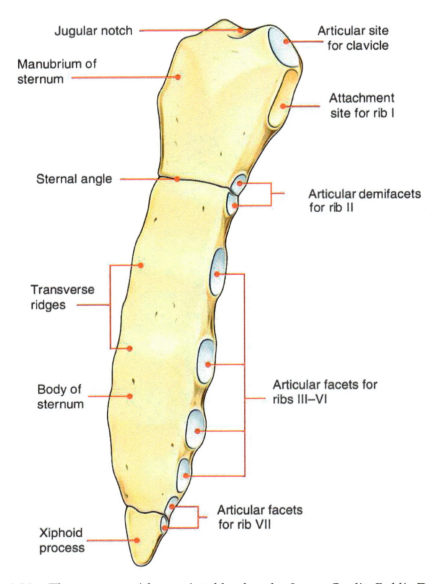

Fig. 4.39 – The sternum with associated landmarks. Image Credit: Public Domain

The Ribs

The ribs are a set of twelve paired bones which form the curved aspect of the thoracic cage. All 24 ribs articulate posteriorly to the thoracic spine. The first seven pairs of ribs are true ribs, meaning that they articulate directly to the sternum via their costal cartilages. The next three sets of ribs are considered false ribs as they are attached to the sternum by costal cartilage links.

The last two pairs of ribs are considered floating because they are not attached anteriorly to the sternum. The floating ribs are more mobile because they only attachment posteriorly to the thoracic spine.

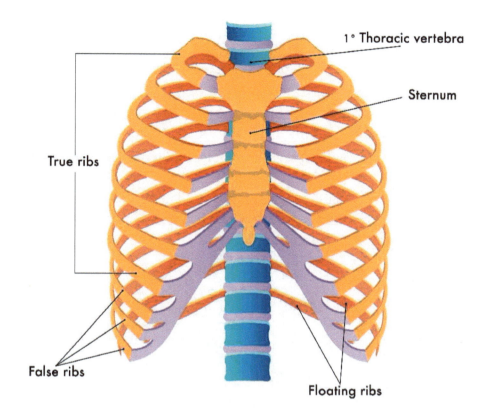

Fig. 4.40 – Overview of the ribs and costal cartilage.

Rib Structure

Ribs are classified as either typical or atypical. The typical ribs have similar characteristics, while the atypical ribs have variations in their structure. Each rib contains a costal groove on the inferior surface of its body that contains the intercostal artery, vein, and nerve.

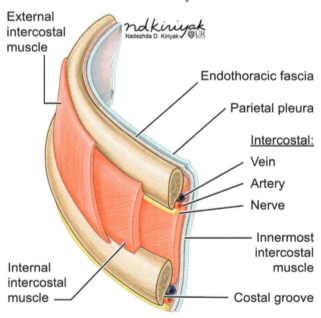

Fig. 4.41 – Rib structure with neurovascular bundle. Image Credit: Nadezhda D. Kiriyak

Typical Ribs

Rib sets 3-9 are considered typical ribs. Each of the typical ribs have a characteristic head, neck, tubercle and body. The wedge-shaped head articulates with the body of the thoracic vertebrae by two articular facets. One of facet articulates with the numerically corresponding thoracic vertebrae, while the other facet articulates with the vertebrae above.

The neck of the rib connects the rib head with the body of the rib. At the junction of the rib neck and body is a raised tubercle with a facet which articulates with the transverse process of the corresponding vertebrae.

The body, or shaft, of the rib is curved and flattened. The internal surface of the body contains a groove along the inferior edge of the shaft. This costal groove protects the neurovascular supply of the thorax from injury.

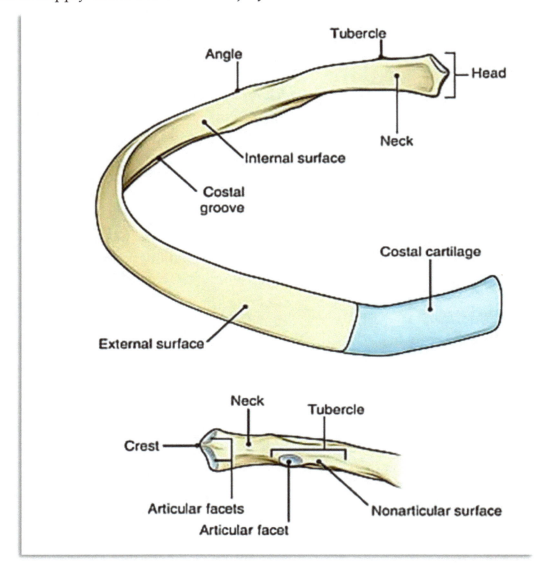

Fig. 4.42 – The bony landmarks of a typical rib. Image Credit: Public Domain

Atypical Ribs

Ribs 1, 2, 10, 11, and 12 are considered atypical ribs because they have features that are not common to all the ribs.

Rib 1 is shorter and wider than the other subsequent ribs. Because it articulates with only the first thoracic vertebrae, it only has one facet on the head of the rib. The superior surface of the body has two grooves across it, allowing for the subclavian vessels.

Rib 2 is longer and thinner than rib 1 and has a roughened area on its upper surface where the serratus anterior muscle originates.

Rib 10 only has one facet that articulates with only the tenth thoracic vertebrae.

Ribs 11 and 12 have no neck, and contain only one facet, which articulates with their corresponding vertebrae.

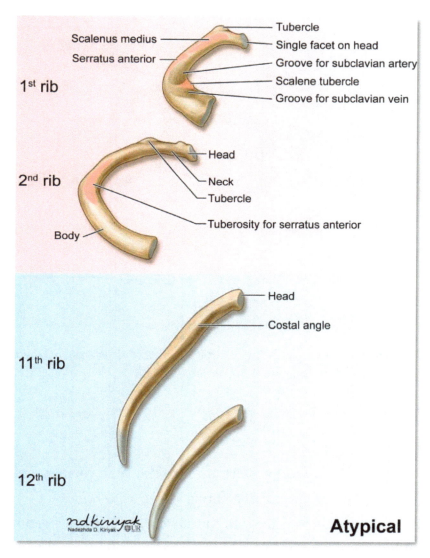

Fig. 4.43 - Atypical Ribs. The first and second ribs are considered atypical because of their specialized shapes and attachments. The 11th and 12th ribs are considered atypical because they lack the anatomic distinctions of the typical ribs. Image Credit: Nadezhda D. Kiriyak

Rib Articulations

The majority of the ribs have an anterior and posterior articulation.

▪ Posterior Rib Articulations

All twelve rib pairs articulate posteriorly with the thoracic spine. Each rib forms two joints, the costotransverse joint and the costovertebral joint.

The costotransverse joint is the articulation between the tubercle of the rib and the costal facet of the transverse process of a thoracic vertebra.

The costovertebral joint is the articulation between the head of the rib, the superior costal facet of the corresponding vertebrae, and the inferior costal facet of the vertebrae above.

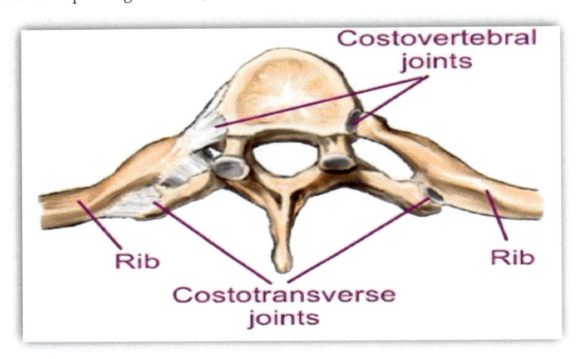

Fig. 4.44 – Posterior articulations between a typical rib and its corresponding vertebrae.
Image Credit: Public Domain

▪ Anterior Rib Articulations

The anterior attachment of the ribs varies:

- Ribs 1-7 attach independently to the sternum via their own costal cartilage.
- Ribs 8 – 10 attaches to the costal cartilage links superior to them.
- Ribs 11 and 12 do not attach anteriorly to the sternum. They are supported within the musculature of the thorax and are therefore considered floating ribs.

Clinical Significance and Martial Arts Relevance:

Rib Fractures

Rib fractures most commonly occur in ribs 7-10 as a result of direct blunt force trauma and are usually fairly benign when they are nondisplaced. Common rib fracture complications include pain and additional soft tissue injury from the broken fragments. More severe complications may include acute vascular injury, pneumothorax, hemothorax, pulmonary contusion, pulmonary laceration, and abdominal solid-organ injury to the liver, spleen, or diaphragm.

Flail chest is a condition in which two or more fractures occur in two or more adjacent ribs, resulting in an unstable area of the thoracic wall. It displays as a paradoxical movement (moving in opposite direction) during inhalations and exhalation. It impairs full chest wall excursion (expansion of the ribcage), thus decreases the oxygen content of the blood.

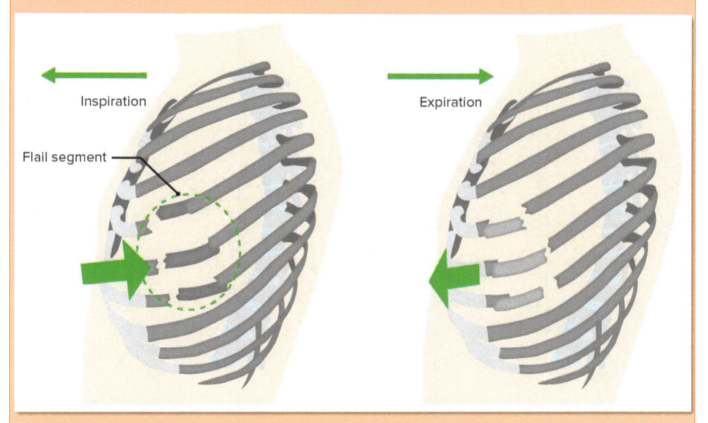

Fig. 4.45 -Flail chest. Multiple rib fractures causing disruption of the structural components of the chest wall (i.e., bone, cartilage, muscle) leading to a free-floating segment of the chest. The separated segment moves opposite to the rest of the chest wall during breathing (paradoxical movement), creating ineffective ventilation. Image Credit: Lecturio.

Ribs 1-3 are well protected by the scapula and clavicles. While ribs 7-10, by virtue of their location and anatomy, are the most prone to fracture as a result of blunt trauma. Ribs 11 and 12 (Floating ribs) are more mobile and therefore *more* difficult to fracture. This has significant **Martial Arts Relevance** because it is often taught by many martial arts instructors that a punch or kick to the floating ribs will cause it to fracture and puncture an internal organ. The misnomer "floating rib" often gives the uninformed practitioner the perception that by only having a posterior bony attachment, that 11th and 12th ribs are actually *"floating"*. However, each of the ribs are also attached to the intercostal muscles between each of the ribs, and the surrounding musculature of the thorax. Numerous studies have shown that because of their mobility the 11th and 12th ribs are the *least* frequent ribs to fracture during blunt force trauma. A study published in 2020 by Bauman, et. al., in the *European Journal of Trauma and Emergency Surgery* confirmed that floating rib fractures occur much less frequently and have the least likelihood of becoming displaced. Should a fracture of the floating ribs occur during a high-energy blunt force trauma event; and injury to adjacent viscous structures, i.e., the kidneys, liver, or spleen be present, the resultant organ injury is most likely due to the high-energy of the trauma and not the subsequent rib fracture.

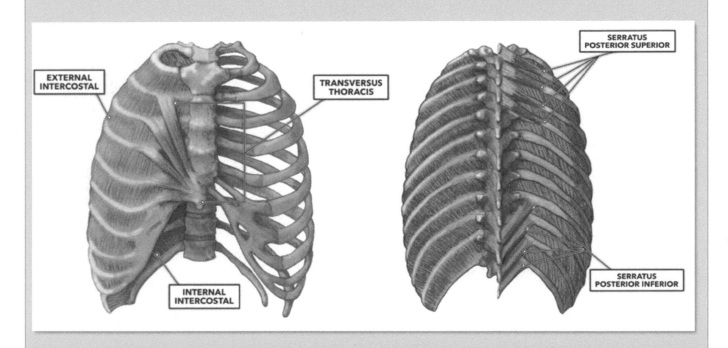

Fig. 4.46 – Muscular of the thoracic cage. Left- Anterior View, Right- Posterior View. Image Credit: Public Domain

Appendicular Skeleton (126 bones)

The second major section of the skeletal system is called the appendicular skeleton. The appendicular skeleton consists of 126 bones and includes the upper and lower extremities, and their attachments to the axial skeleton. The shoulder girdle attaches the upper extremity to the axial skeleton, while the pelvic girdle attaches the lower extremity.

Shoulder Girdle

The shoulder girdle, or pectoral girdle, is the set of bones in the appendicular skeleton which connects to the upper extremities to each side of the thoracic cage. The shoulder girdle consists of the clavicle and scapula bilaterally.

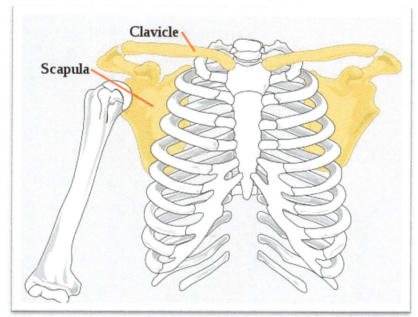

- **Clavicle**

The clavicle, or collarbone, is an S-shaped bone which lays horizontally in the anterior shoulder. The clavicle is the only direct connection between the shoulder girdle and axial skeleton. It acts as a strut between the sternum and the shoulder while allowing full range of motion of the glenohumeral joint. Because it does provide lateral stability to the shoulder, the clavicle is one of the most commonly fractured bones in the body.

Fig. 4.47 - The shoulder girdle includes the clavicle and scapula bilaterally.
Image Credit: LadyofHats, Public domain, via Wikimedia Commons

The clavicle has a secondary function of protecting the nerves and blood vessels that pass between the thorax and upper extremity.

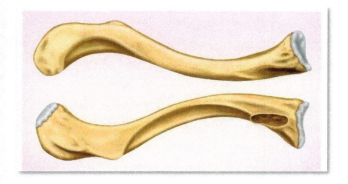

The clavicle is divided into three parts: the medial end, the shaft, and the lateral end.

The medial end of the clavicle attaches to the sternum forming the sternoclavicular joint.

Fig. 4.48 – The clavicle is an S-shaped bone with a distinct medial end, shaft, and lateral end.

The shaft, or body, of the clavicle is divided into medial and lateral regions. The medial region has a convex curvature (with an anterior apex), while the lateral region is concaved with a posterior apex).

The Lateral end of the clavicle attaches to the scapula forming the acromioclavicular (AC) joint.

- **Scapula**

The scapula, or shoulder blade, is a large triangular-shaped bone that lies in the posterior shoulder and articulates the clavicle and humerus. The scapula provides an attachment point for 17 different muscles in the shoulder, upper extremity, and back.

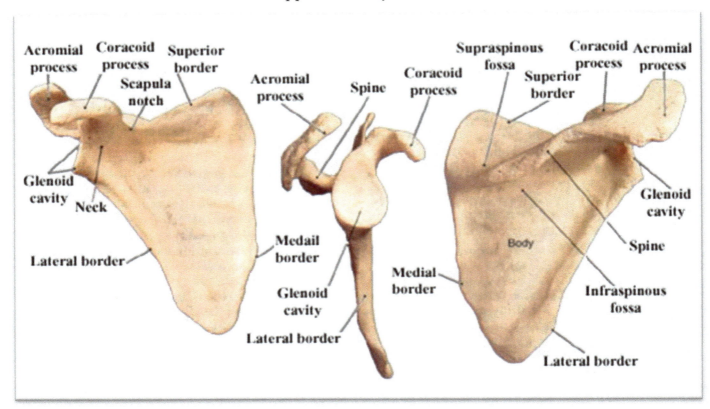

Fig. 4.49 - The scapula: anterior, lateral, and posterior views. Image Credit: Бекемгул, [CC BY-SA 4.0] via Wikimedia Commons

    The scapula is divided into three borders: the medial, lateral, and superior borders.
    The medial border runs parallel to the thoracic vertebrae while the lateral border is on the side of the axilla. The superior border is the uppermost edge and is the thinnest and shortest of the three borders.
    The spine of the scapula is an oblique prominent ridge that crosses the posterior surface. The two concave fossae formed by the spine provides attachments for muscles to rotate the upper extremity. The distal end of the spine forms the acromion, a process that articulates anteriorly with the clavicle.

The apex of the lateral border broadens to produce a shallow cavity, the glenoid fossa (cavity), which articulates with the head of the humerus, to form the glenohumeral joint (shoulder joint). The coracoid process is a beak-like projection that overhangs the glenoid cavity, providing attachment sites for ligaments and muscles.

Because of the significant muscular support, fractures to the scapula are uncommon, however they can occur with direct blows during high-energy trauma such as motor vehicle accidents and sports related injuries.

Joints of the Shoulder Girdle

There are four main joints in the shoulder girdle: the sternoclavicular, acromioclavicular, glenohumeral, and the scapulothoracic joints.

The **sternoclavicular joint** is formed by the clavicle and the sternum, providing the direct attachment between the upper extremity and axial skeleton.

The **acromioclavicular joint** (AC joint) is the point where the clavicle meets the acromion of the scapula.

The **glenohumeral joint**, also known as the shoulder joint, is the ball-and-socket connection between the glenoid fossa of the scapula and humerus.

The **scapulothoracic joint**, or scapulocostal joint, is where the anterior surface of the scapula meets the ribs of the posterior thoracic cage. This joint is formed by the surrounding musculature attachments on the scapula and the posterior thoracic wall.

Clinical Significance and Martial Arts Relevance:

- **Acromioclavicular Dislocation**

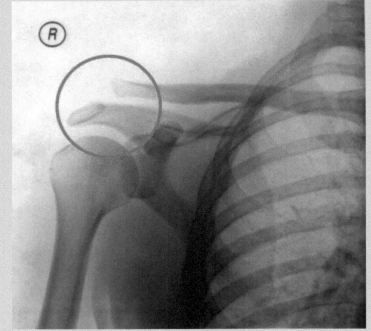

Fig. 4.50 – Radiograph of shoulder AC joint separation. Image Credit: Jay F. Cox [CC-BY-2.5], via Wikimedia Commons

Acromioclavicular (AC) joint separation, or sprain, occurs when the two articulating surfaces of the joint are injured and separated. It commonly occurs from a sweep, being thrown, or a fall causing a direct blow to the point of the shoulder, or a fall on an outstretched hand. In the absence of an associated fracture, an AC joint separation is considered a soft tissue injury.

The injury is more serious if ligament (acromioclavicular and/or coracoclavicular) rupture occurs. If the coracoclavicular ligament is torn there is an increased prominence of the clavicle. AC joint separations are graded by the severity of injury, with Grade (type) 1 - 3 being the most common.

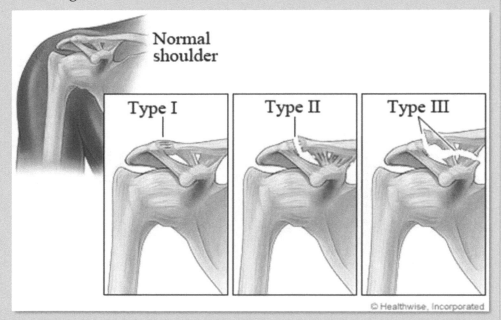

Fig. 4.51 - AC joint separations: Grade I – mild sprain of the acromioclavicular ligament; Grad II – complete rupture of acromioclavicular ligament and some tearing of the coracoclavicular ligament; Grade III - Complete rupture of the acromioclavicular and coracoclavicular ligaments. Image Credit: Healthwise, Inc.

Management of AC joint separation is dependent upon the severity of the injury and impact on quality of life. The treatment options range from ice and rest, to ligament reconstruction surgery.

▪ Clavicle Fracture

As the clavicle acts a strut for the shoulder, it transmits forces from the upper extremity to the axial skeleton. Given its relative size, it is particularly susceptible to fracture. Like AC joint injuries, the most common mechanism of injury for a clavicle fracture is a fall onto the shoulder or onto an outstretched hand.

With the clavicle divided into thirds: 80% of fractures occur in the middle third, 15% occur in the lateral third, and 5% of clavicle fractures occur in the medial third.

After a complete fracture, the medial end of the clavicle is pulled superiorly by the sternocleidomastoid muscle. The lateral end of the clavicle is held down by the coracoclavicular ligament (if the fracture does not involve the lateral third), and the shoulder displaces inferiorly by the weight of the arm.

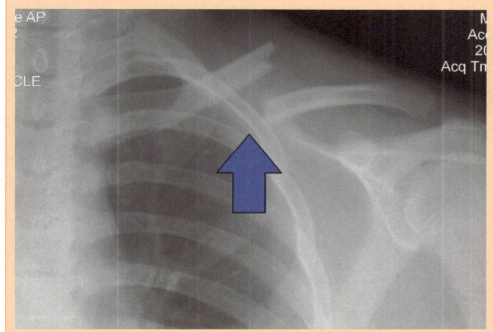

Management of a clavicular fracture can be conservative (i.e., Figure 8 splint or sling immobilization) or operative (i.e., open reduction and internal fixation).

Fig. 4.52 – X-Ray of a clavicular fracture. Note how the medial end is raised and the lateral end lowered. Image Credit: Majorkev [CC BY 3.0], via Wikimedia Commons

▪ Dislocation of the Sternoclavicular Joint

A dislocation of the sternoclavicular (SC) joint is quite rare, comprising less than 1% of all joint dislocations and only 3% of shoulder girdle injuries, and requires significant force. The costoclavicular ligament and the articular disc are highly effective at absorbing forces and transmitting them away from the joint into the sternum.

Two major types of SC joint dislocation:

- **Anterior dislocations** are the most common and can happen following a blow to the anterior shoulder which rotates the shoulder backwards. These injuries most often result in a minor cosmetic defect of an anterior bump at the sternoclavicular joint, with minimal functional impairment. Anterior SC joint dislocations are most often treated conservatively.
- **Posterior dislocations** are much less common than anterior SC joint dislocations. Resulting from a posterior force driving the shoulder forwards, or from direct anterior impact to the SC joint, 30% of posterior dislocations are associated with life-threatening complications due to associated injuries to the mediastinum. Posterior SC joint dislocations reductions are best performed by orthopedic specialists in the operating room, with vascular surgery available.

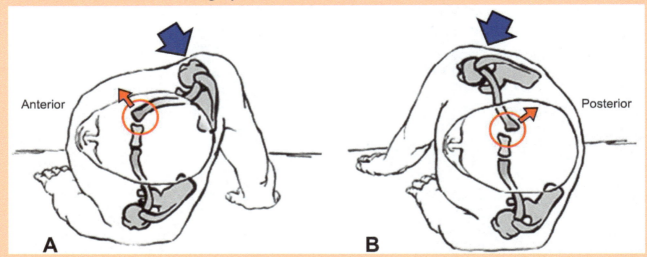

Fig. 4.53 - Mechanisms that produce (A) anterior or (B) posterior dislocations of the sternoclavicular joint. Image Credit: modified by Barry A. Broughton, PhD. Original by Bucholz RW, Heckman JD, Court-Brown C, et al., eds. Rockwood and Green's Fractures in Adults, 6th ed. Philadelphia: Lippincott Williams & Wilkins, 2006.

(A) Force applied to the anterolateral aspect of the shoulder: When the lateral compression force is directed from the anterior position, either while on the ground or resulting from a throw, the medial end of the clavicle is dislocated anteriorly.

(B) Force applied to the posterolateral aspect of the shoulder: If the martial artist is lying on the ground and posterolateral compression force is applied; or they are thrown and land on the posterolateral aspect of the shoulder, the medial end of the clavicle will be displaced posteriorly.

Because the epiphyseal growth plate on the sternal end of the clavicle has not fully closed in younger people, a SC joint dislocation is usually accompanied by a fracture through the growth plate.

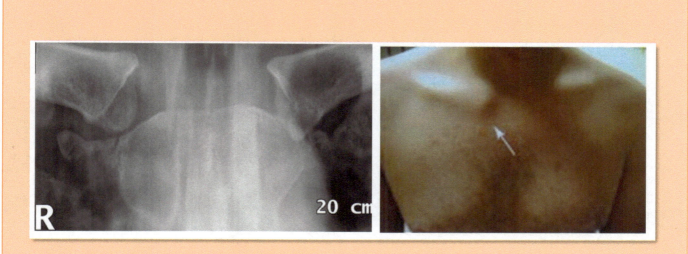

Fig. 4.54 – Radiograph and image of a right sternoclavicular joint dislocation. Image Credit: Life in the Fast Lane [CC BY-SA 4.0] via Wikimedia Commons

Martial Arts Relevance:

As described above, clavicle fractures, and acromioclavicular joint and sternoclavicular joint dislocations may all occur by falling directly onto the point of the shoulder. They may also occur by falling on an outstretched hand while executing an incorrect breakfall during a throw or takedown. Learning how to breakfall properly can go a long way in preventing long term sequela (adverse effects) from what could have been a benign fall.

Upper Extremity

The skeleton of the upper extremity includes 60 bones that are divided into three separate regions. The arm is located between the shoulder and elbow joints; the forearm is located between the elbow and wrist joints, while the hand is located distal to the wrist. The uppermost long bone of the arm is the humerus. The two bones of the forearm are the radius (laterally) and the ulna (medially). There are eight carpal bones in each wrist. Both hands include 5 metacarpal bones; while there are 14 bones in the fingers and thumb called phalanges.

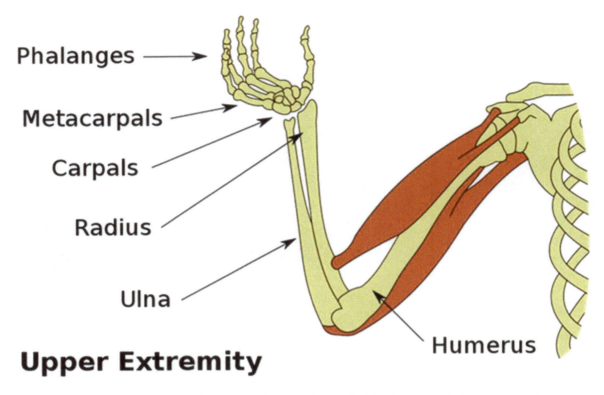

Fig. 4.55 - Bones of the Upper Extremity. Image Credit: Public domain, via Wikimedia Commons

Arm

The arm extends proximally from the glenohumeral (shoulder) joint to the elbow joint distally.

- **Humerus**

The humerus is a long bone of the upper extremity, which extends from the shoulder to the elbow. The proximal humerus articulates with the glenoid fossa of the scapula, forming the glenohumeral joint. Distally, the humerus articulates with the head of the radius and trochlear notch of the ulna forming the elbow joint.

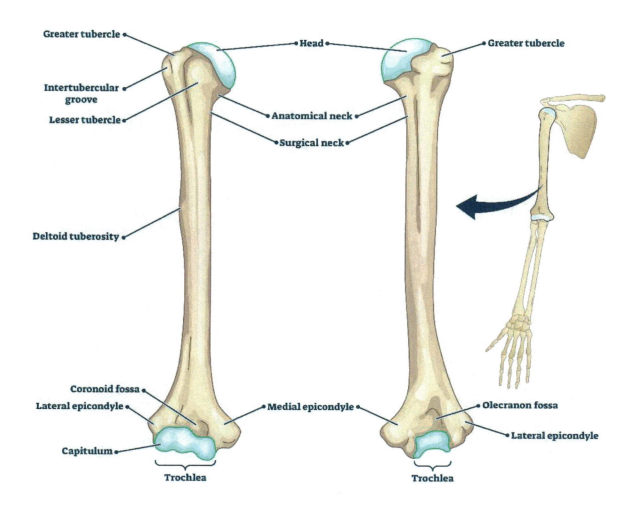

Fig. 4.56 - Humerus: Right Anterior (on Left) and Posterior (on Right) Views.

Glenohumeral Joint

The glenohumeral, or shoulder, joint is a synovial joint which attaches the upper extremity to the axial skeleton. A ball-and-socket joint is formed by the glenoid fossa of the scapula (gleno) and the head of humerus (humeral).

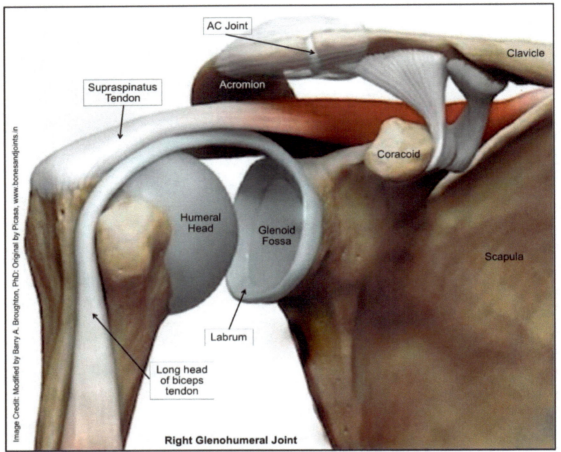

Fig. 4.57 - Shoulder (Glenohumeral) joint: Right Anterior View. Image Credit: Modified by Barry A. Broughton, PhD: Original by Picasa, www.bonesandjoints.in

As the most mobile joint of the human body, the shoulder is highly vulnerable to joint locks and subsequent injury. Acting in conjunction with the shoulder girdle, it allows for a wide range of motion of the upper extremity, i.e., extension, flexion, adduction, abduction, internal/medial rotation, external/lateral rotation, and circumduction. This joint mobility, however, comes at the cost of less stability as the shallow bony surface of the glenoid offers little support. Overcoming this deficiency, the glenoid labrum is a fibrocartilaginous ring that encircles the glenoid fossa. By deepening the glenoid socket, it provides static stability and shock absorption within the glenohumeral joint.

Dynamic stability of the shoulder is also provided by the muscles of the rotator cuff. The four rotator cuff muscles pull the humeral head into the glenoid cavity, providing integrity to the shoulder joint through its entire movement range. See the next chapter, *Introduction to the Muscular System,* for more in-depth details regarding the individual muscles of the rotator cuff.

Clinical Significance and Martial Arts Relevance:

Dislocation of the Shoulder Joint

Because of the mobility-stability compromise referenced above, the glenohumeral joint is one of the most frequently injured joints of the body. The most common causes of shoulder dislocations are sports related injuries and accidents that result in falling on an outstretched arm or shoulder. Martial artists must protect their own shoulder from falling prey to its vulnerability, while also exploiting it to their advantage. This is achieved by knowing at what point the shoulder joint is at its most stable and where is has the highest potential for dislocation.

Shoulder dislocations are described by where the humeral head lies in relation to the glenoid fossa. Anterior dislocations are the most prevalent, at 95% of all glenohumeral joint dislocations. Posterior shoulder dislocations occur in 4% of cases, while inferior dislocation account for only 1%. Superior displacement of the humeral head is prevented by the bony architecture of the coracoacromial arch.

An anterior dislocation is usually caused by excessive extension and lateral rotation of the humerus. This may occur from an improperly executed breakfall onto an outreached hand, or from a *bent armbar* forcing the humeral head anteriorly and inferiorly – into the weakest part of the joint capsule.

The force applied during a *bent armbar* exerts excessive external rotation of the shoulder beyond its normal 90° range of motion.

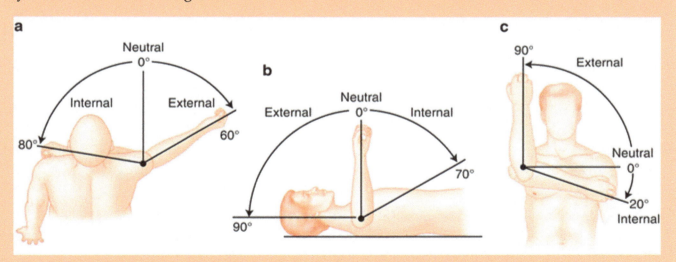

Fig. 4.58 - Normal shoulder range of motion. Image Credit: Warth, R., Millet, P., (2015). Range of Motion. In: Physical Examination of the Shoulder. Springer, New York, NY.

In addition to the excessive rotational motion that is applied during a *bent armbar*, a shearing force is also applied that forces anterior translation of the humeral head on the glenoid fossa. This combined motion is ideal in causing a shoulder dislocation.

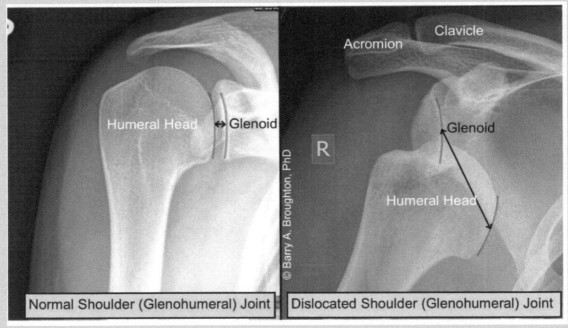

Fig. 4.59 – Left Image- Normal x-ray with humeral head seated on the glenoid of the scapula. Right Image- Anterior dislocation of the shoulder (glenohumeral) joint.

A *reverse bent armbar* primarily forces the shoulder joint in excessive internal rotation beyond the normal 70° of normal range of motion. To increase the efficacy of any armbar variation, isolate the motion to the glenohumeral joint by using the arm and forearm as the lever, while minimizing movement of the opponent's torso.

Tearing of the joint capsule during a shoulder dislocation may be associated with an increased risk of future dislocations. An impaction fracture on the humeral head (Hill-Sachs lesion) caused by the posterolateral humeral head hitting against anteroinferior glenoid may occur during an anterior shoulder dislocation. Additionally, a tear and detachment of the anteroinferior labrum (Bankart lesion), with or without an avulsion fracture, may also occur following shoulder dislocation.

The axillary nerve runs near the shoulder joint and around the surgical neck of the humerus and can be damaged during the dislocation or during an attempted reduction. Injury to the axillary nerve causes paralysis of the deltoid muscle, and loss of sensation over lateral deltoid area of the shoulder.

Because of the potential for exacerbating injuries to the glenohumeral joint and the upper extremity, do not attempt to reduce a presumed shoulder dislocation unless there is neurovascular compromise caused by the dislocation; <u>and</u> immediate transport to healthcare providers is not available.

Elbow Joint

The elbow is a complex joint formed by the distal aspect of the humerus, and the proximal radius and ulna bones of the forearm. The elbow joint is actually comprised of three separate joints:

- **Ulnohumeral joint** is where movement between the humerus and ulna occurs.
- **Radiohumeral joint** is where the radius connects to the capitellum of the distal humerus.
- **Proximal radioulnar (RU) joint** is formed by the articulation between the radius and ulna, allowing for pronation and supination of the hand and forearm.

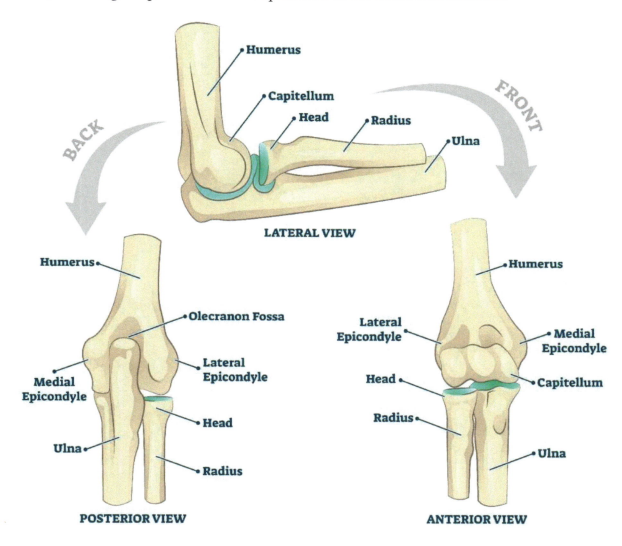

Fig. 4.60 - Right elbow joint: Lateral, Posterior, and Anterior Views.

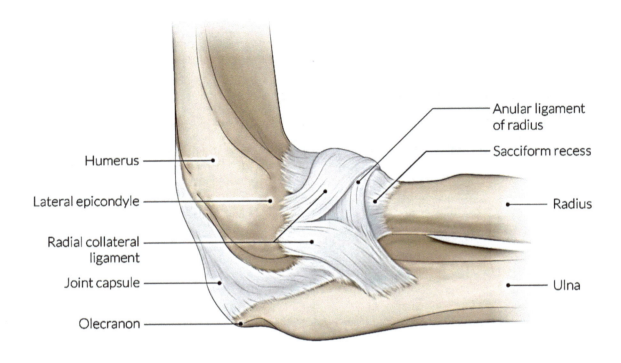

Fig. 4.61 - Lateral View of Elbow soft tissue structures. Image Credit: amboss.com

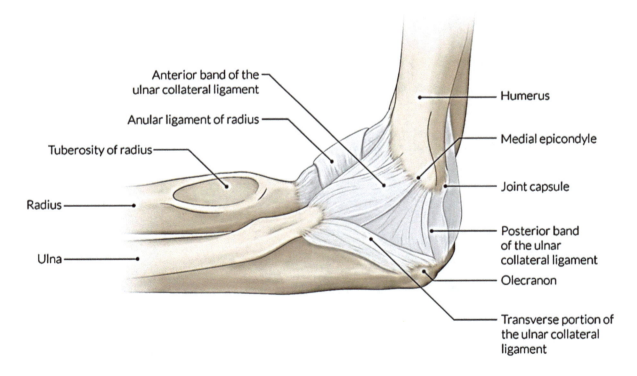

Fig. 4.62 - Medial View of Elbow soft tissue structures. Image Credit: amboss.com

Clinical Significance and Martial Arts Relevance:

Injuries to the Elbow Joint

- **Supracondylar Fracture**

A supracondylar fracture is a fracture of the distal humerus which usually occurs due to a fall onto on outstretched, extended hand. It is typically a transverse fracture, spanning between the medial and lateral epicondyles in the relatively weak epicondylar region. The epicondylar region is formed by the olecranon fossa (posteriorly) and coronoid fossa (anteriorly) which lie opposite to each other in the distal humerus.

Direct trauma or swelling as a result of the fracture may disrupt the blood supply of the forearm via the brachial artery. The resulting ischemia can cause Volkmann's ischemic contracture – uncontrolled flexion of the hand, as the flexor muscles become fibrotic and shortened. Supracondylar fractures may also injure the medial, radial, or ulnar nerves.

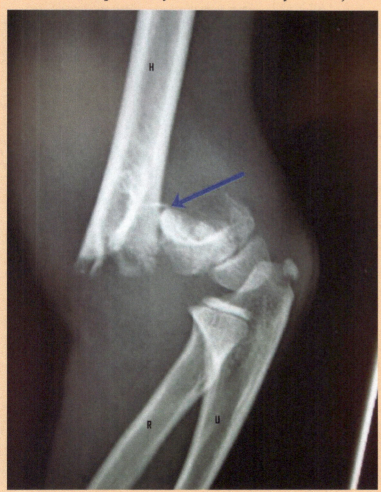

Fig. 4.63 – An elbow X-ray showing a supracondylar fracture in a young child (H= Humerus, R= Radius, U= Ulna, Fracture is marked by an arrow) Image Credit: James Heilman, MD, [CC BY-SA 3.0], via Wikimedia Commons

▪ Elbow Dislocation

An elbow dislocation most frequently occurs during sporting activities when a person falls on an outstretched hand. The distal end of the humerus is driven through the anterior side of the joint capsule, the weakest part. Additionally, the ulnar collateral ligament is usually torn and there may also be associated fractures of the radial head or coracoid process, or injury to ulnar nerve.

Elbow dislocations are one of the most common major joint dislocations, second to the shoulder joint. Ninety percent of all elbow dislocations are posterior dislocations. Elbow dislocations are named by the position of the dislocated ulna and radius, not the humerus.

The most common mechanism of injury for a posterior elbow dislocation is a combination of axial loading of the forearm with a bent elbow, supination (external rotation), and valgus posterolateral force from the weight of the fall. This scenario may occur during martial arts training with an improperly executed dive roll or breakfall from a high throw.

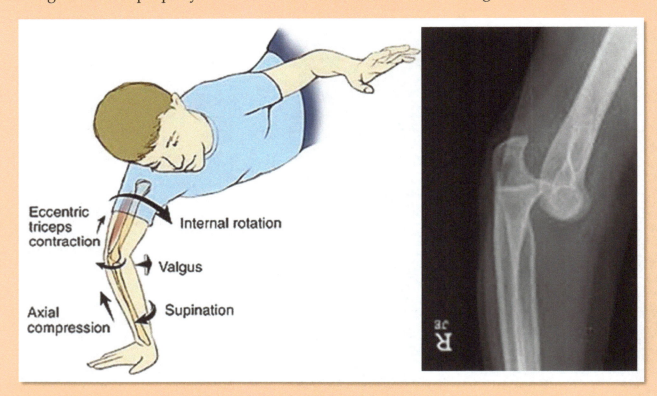

Fig. 4.64 – Left Image: Illustration of the common mechanism of injury resulting in a right posterior elbow dislocation: a FOOSH (Fall On Out-Stretched Hand) produces axial loading along the forearm with forced external rotation (supination) and valgus force stress. Image Credit: musculoskeletalkey.com/surgical-treatment-of-posterolateral-instability-of-the-elbow

Fig. 4.65 – Right Image: X-ray of a posterior dislocation of the elbow. Image Credit: orthobullets.com/trauma/1018/elbow-dislocation

Martial Arts Relevance:

Straight Armbar

With the growth and popularity of jujitsu and grappling related arts, the straight armbar has become one of the most utilized submissions, yet it is often misunderstood.

There are a variety of types, names, and applications of the straight armbar. These variations depend largely on the application (self-defense vs. sport), the plane in which it is applied (standing vs. ground), and the origins of the system in which it is being taught. Some of the misconceptions occur from not fully appreciating the anatomy of the elbow, and therefore discounting certain applications because of the inappropriate (actual or perceived) application of directions of force. Bear in mind that not every armbar is attempting to cause an isolated hyperextension injury of the ulnohumeral joint. Some may be directed at attacking the medial and lateral structures as well, especially if the intent is a quick "tap" (for compliance or otherwise), and not for a full dislocation or fracture.

The common denominators in every armbar that effect the elbow joint are the need to control of the wrist, elbow, and shoulder (directly or indirectly). Therefore, for ease of understanding (in this section), a joint locking technique that attacks the elbow with the upper extremity in extension will be referred to as a straight armbar.

The straight armbar involves applying force to one or more of the three joints of the elbow, which includes the ulnohumeral, radiohumeral, and proximal radioulnar joints.

There are numerous static structures and dynamic constraints that help to stabilize the elbow joint. The ulnohumeral articulation, the anterior band of the medial collateral ligament (MCL), and the lateral (radial) collateral ligament (LCL) are the primary static stabilizers. The radiohumeral articulation, the common flexor and common extensor tendons, and the capsule are the secondary stabilizers of the elbow. Muscles crossing the elbow joint that provide joint compressive forces also provide dynamic stability.

The primary stabilizing articulation of the elbow is formed by the humerus and the ulna. The proximal ulna forms a highly congruent joint with the trochlea of the distal humerus. The saddle shaped, semilunar (trochlear) notch of the ulna is formed by the olecranon process proximally, and the coronoid process distally. The trochlea of the distal humerus inserts into to the trochlear notch of the ulna. At full extension of the elbow, the olecranon process of the ulnar sits in the olecranon fossa of the posterior distal humerus, blocking further extension. While executing the straight armbar, the olecranon may compress the soft tissue of the posterior elbow within the fossa, causing significant pain without tearing the stabilizing structures of the joint.

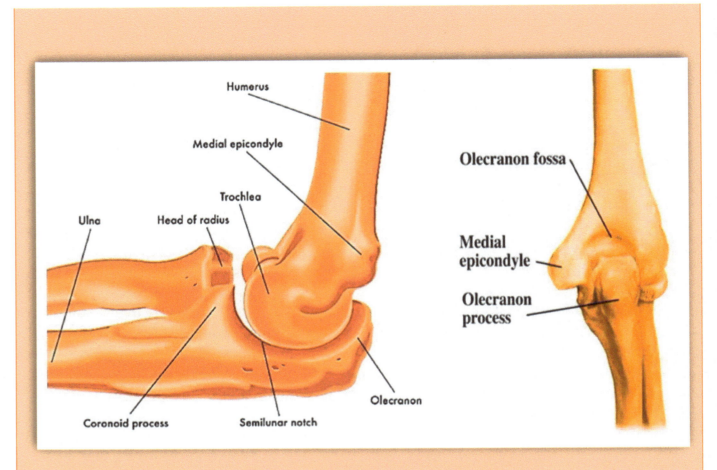

Fig. 4.66 - Left Image: Medial view of elbow trochlear (semilunar) notch formed by the olecranon and coronoid process. Right Image: Posterior view of elbow with olecranon process of ulna seated in the olecranon fossa of the humerus.

    The joint capsule, along with the medial and lateral collateral ligaments of the elbow (MCL and LCL are also present in the knee), are the passive soft tissue stabilizers of the elbow joint. The capsule of the elbow is attached to the articular margins of the joint. The fibrous connective tissue wraps around all three of the associated elbow joints and is supported by ligamentous structures. The capsule becomes taut anteriorly when the elbow is extended and is taut posteriorly when the elbow is flexed.

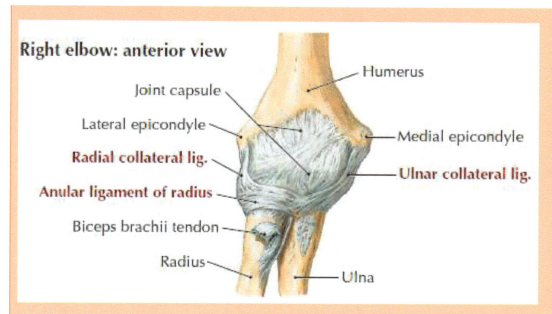

Fig. 4.67 - Right Elbow joint capsule with bony and soft tissue landmarks. Image Credit: Hansen, J. T., Netter, F. H. 1., & MD Consult LLC. (2010). Netter's clinical anatomy (2nd ed.), pg. 426. Philadelphia: Saunders/Elsevier.

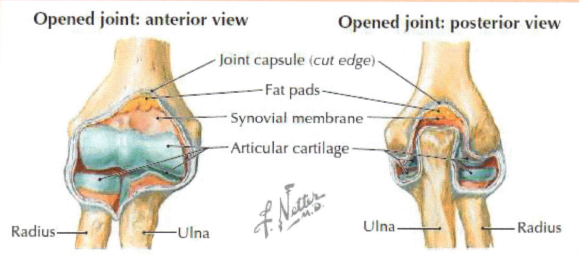

Fig. 4.68 - Right Elbow with opened joint capsule. Image Credit: Hansen, J. T., Netter, F. H. 1., & MD Consult LLC. (2010). Netter's clinical anatomy (2nd ed.), pg. 426. Philadelphia: Saunders/Elsevier.

The medial collateral ligament (MCL) of the elbow originates from the anteroinferior aspect of the medial epicondyle of the distal humerus (see Fig. 4.67 above). The MCL complex consists of three components: the anterior bundle, the posterior bundle, and the transverse segment. The anterior bundle is further subdivided into anterior, central, and posterior bands. The anterior bundle is taut throughout the arc of motion; the anterior bands are most taut in extension and the posterior bands become tightened in flexion.

The lateral collateral ligament (LCL) complex consists of the lateral ulnar collateral ligament, the radial collateral ligament, the annular ligament, and the accessory collateral ligament (see Fig. 4.67 above). The LCL originates at the lateral epicondyle near the axis of rotation of the elbow, allowing it to remain taut throughout flexion and extension. The lateral ulnar collateral ligament (LUCL) inserts at the tubercle of the supinator crest of the ulna providing varus and posterolateral stability. The radial collateral ligament inserts into the annular ligament, stabilizing the radial head. The annular ligament originates and inserts on the anterior and posterior margins of the radial notch of the ulna, keeping the radial head in contact with the ulna. The anterior insertion becomes taut during supination, and the posterior insertion become taut during pronation. The accessory collateral ligament attaches at the annular ligament and the supinator crest of the ulna, stabilizing the annular ligament during varus stress at the elbow.

Ulnohumeral hyperextension, or extreme varus or valgus stress to the elbow joint often leads to ligament sprain or rupture. If excessive force is continued, dislocation or fractures may occur. The capsuloligamentous anatomy of the elbow is highly innervated. The mechanoreceptors within the LCL and MCL, and articular sensory receptors in the joint capsule help to detect early passive tension. These nerve receptors allow for more response time in defending against an elbow lock in comparison to the defending against a heel hook or kneebar.

As presented in the next chapter of this text, the musculotendinous structures which cross the elbow joint provide dynamic stability to the elbow. These muscles include biceps brachii, brachioradialis, brachialis, flexor carpi radialis, flexor carpi ulnaris, palmaris longus, and pronator teres. See the *Introduction to the Muscular System* chapter for more details.

Controlling the position of the forearm while executing variations of the straight armbar will greatly improve the efficiency and efficacy of the technique. The "thumb up" position that is often taught during a straight armbar is meant (most often unwittingly) to control rotation of the forearm at the distal and proximal radioulnar joints. The position of the thumb, or more accurately (with a lax wrist joint), the distal radius dictates to the practitioner the alignment of the forearm bones. When the forearm is supinated (palm up) the radius sits lateral to the ulna. When the forearm is pronated (palm down) the radius crosses over the ulna; the radial head remains lateral to the ulna. When the hand and forearm are in a neutral (i.e., thumbs up) position the distal radius aligns on top of the ulna; again, the radial head remains lateral to the ulna proximally. Understanding these dynamics allows the practitioner to be more precise in the direction of force that is applied distally, while applying proper counter leverage at the fulcrum proximally. The result is a more deliberate attack on specific structures of the elbow joint.

If the hand and forearm remain in a neutral position, the direction of force applied on the distal extremity is towards the small finger and ulna, while the counter force at the fulcrum is posterior-to-anterior (in the direction of the thumb) through the distal humerus and elbow.

If the hand and forearm are supinated, the distally applied direction of force is again towards the small finger and ulna, while the counter force at the fulcrum is medial-to-lateral (in the direction of the thumb) through the distal humerus and elbow.

If the hand and forearm are pronated, the direction of force applied distally is still towards the small finger and ulna, while the counter force at the fulcrum is lateral-to-medial (in the direction of the thumb) through the distal humerus and elbow.

COMPREHENSIVE ANATOMY FOR MARTIAL ARTS

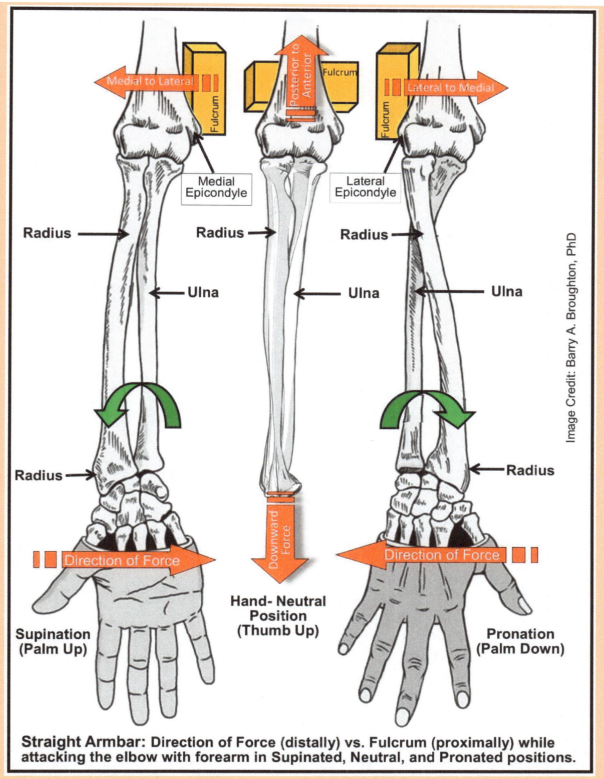

Fig. 4.69 - Straight Armbar direction of force distally and proximally will change based on the position of the forearm and the fulcrum.

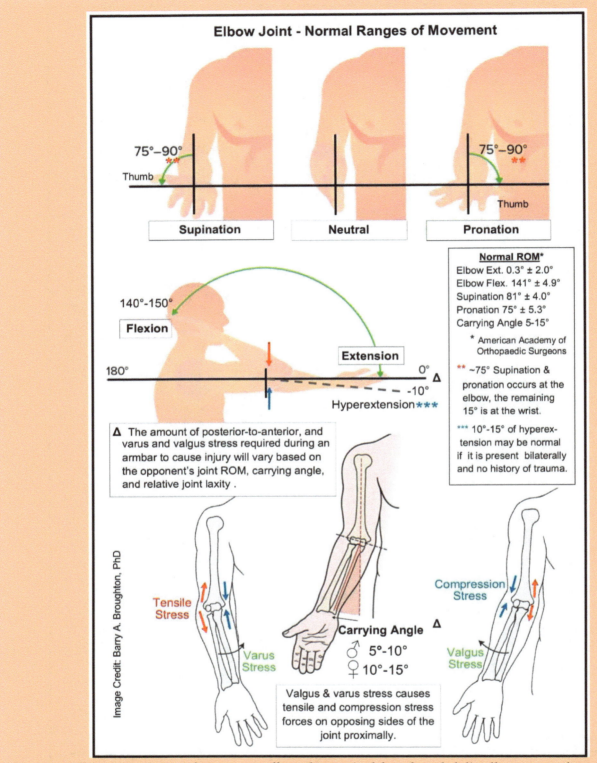

Fig. 4.70 - *Elbow joint ranges of movement effects the required forced needed distally to stress the anatomical structures of the elbow proximally.*

> The amount of force required prior to injury occurring, or to the opponent tapping, is dependent upon several factors such as the opponent's elbow flexibility, their normal range of motion (ROM) in all planes, and the carrying angle of the elbow. Understanding the elbow anatomy, and the directions of force required to affect them, allows the practitioner to seamlessly adjust the armbar technique based on the opponent's variations of what is considered to be normal ranges of motions.
>
> ▪ **Bent Elbow Locks**
>
> Though less common than bent armbar *shoulder* locks (see the *Clinical Significance and Martial Arts Relevance - Bent Armbar* section in the *Introduction to the Muscular System chapter*), bent *elbow* locks are similar in their set-up and acquisition. While the Americana, bent armbar, ude garami, etc., attack the structures of the shoulder - the bent elbow locks such as the Americana Elbow and Kimura Elbow Locks attack the anatomy surrounding the elbow joint.
>
> Understanding biomechanics, the functions of a fulcrum and lever, and human anatomy allows the martial artist to attack a different joint with minor adjustments. By changing the fulcrum more distally on the arm (near the elbow), and as well as the direction of force applies more stress to the distal humerus, proximal radioulnar, and surrounding soft tissue structures (see discussion above).

Forearm

The bones of the forearm include the radius and the ulna. Articulating with each other at both ends, they form the proximal and distal radioulnar (RU) joints. As pivot joints, the radioulnar joints allow for forearm pronation and supination of the hand and forearm. The proximal ends of the radius and ulna articulate with the distal humerus to form the elbow joint, while distally they articulate with the carpal bones of the wrist.

PLEASE REFER to the diagrams on the next page.

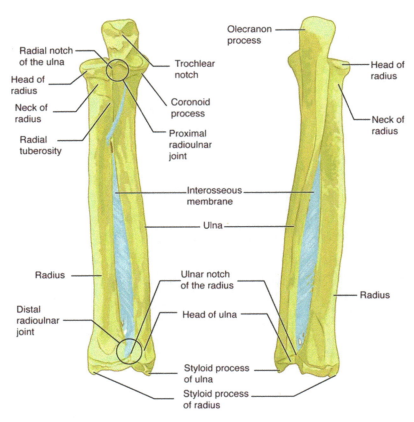

Fig. 4.71 - Radius and Ulna: Right Anterior (on Left) and Posterior (on Right) Views. The ulna is located on the medial side of the forearm (Remember, this is based on the anatomical position.), and the radius is on the lateral side. These bones are attached to each other by an interosseous membrane forming the middle radioulnar joint. Image Credit: Public Domain

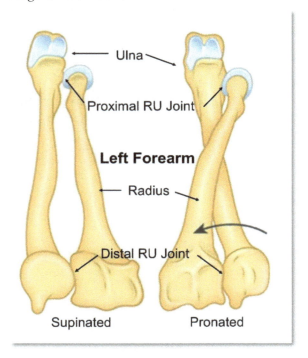

Fig. 4.72 - Left Forearm: Proximal and Distal Radioulnar Joints in supination and pronation.

- **Radius**

The radius is a long bone in the forearm that lies lateral and parallel to the ulna, the second bone of the forearm. The radius pivots around the ulna to produce movement at both the proximal and distal radioulnar joints.

The proximal end of the radius (radial head) articulates in both the elbow joint with the humerus, and the proximal radioulnar joint with the ulna. The annular ligament encircles the radial head and keeps it in contact with the radial notch of the ulna.

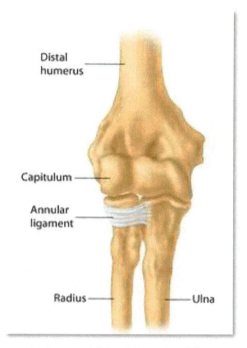

Fig. 4.73 - The radius articulates with both the distal humerus and proximal ulna.

Important bony landmarks include the head, neck and radial tuberosity:

- **Radial head** is disk-shaped structure with a concave articulating surface. It is thicker medially where it articulates in the proximal RU joint.
- **Neck** is the narrow area of bone which lies just distal the radial head and proximal to radial tuberosity.
- **Radial tuberosity** is the bony projection that serves as the place of attachment of the biceps brachii muscle.

The shaft of the radius expands in diameter as it moves distally and expands to form a rectangular end where it articulates with the carpals of the wrist. The lateral side projects distally to form the radial styloid. There is a concavity in the medial surface which articulates with the head of the ulna, called the ulnar notch, forming the distal radioulnar joint.

The distal surface of the radius has two facets that articulate with the scaphoid and lunate carpal bones of the wrist joint.

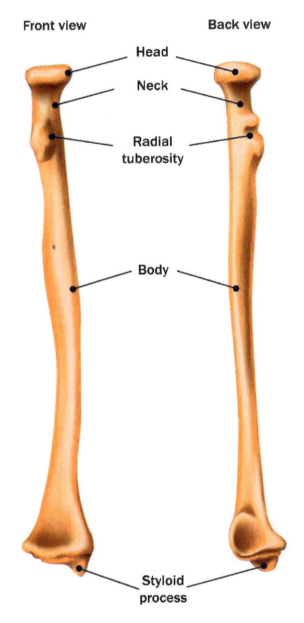

Fig. 4.74 - Radius Bone with bony landmarks.

- **Ulna**

The ulna is a long bone in the forearm that lies medially and parallel to the radius, the second bone of the forearm. The ulna functions as the stabilizing bone, with the radius pivoting over it to produce movement.

Proximally, the ulna articulates with the trochlea of the humerus at the elbow joint. Distally it articulates with the radius, forming the distal radioulnar joint.

Important landmarks of the proximal ulna are the trochlear notch, radial notch, olecranon, coronoid process, and the tuberosity of ulna:

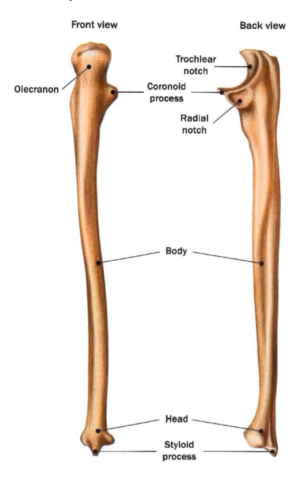

Fig. 4.75 - Posterior and lateral view of ulna bone.

- **Olecranon** – is a large bony projection that extends proximally, forming part of trochlear notch. The triceps muscle attaches to its superior surface. The olecranon can be palpated as the *tip* of the elbow.
- **Coronoid process** – is a ridge of bone that projects anteriorly, forming part of the trochlear notch.
- **Trochlear notch** – is formed by the olecranon and coronoid process. It is wrench-shaped and articulates with the trochlea of the humerus.
- **Radial notch** – is located on the lateral surface of the trochlear notch. This area articulates with the head of the radius forming the proximal RU joint.
- **Tuberosity of ulna** – is a roughened area just distal to the coronoid process where the brachialis muscle attaches.

Distal Radioulnar Joint

Formed by the articulation between the ulnar head and the ulnar notch on the distal radius, the distal RU joint is located just proximal to the wrist joint.

In addition to anterior (volar) and posterior (dorsal) ligaments strengthening the joint, there is also a fibrocartilaginous ligament called the articular disc. The articular disc provides two functions:

- Binds the radius and ulna together during movement at the joint.
- Separates the distal radioulnar joint from the wrist (carpal) joint.

The ulnar notch of the radius slides anteriorly over the head of the ulna allowing for pronation and supination of the forearm.

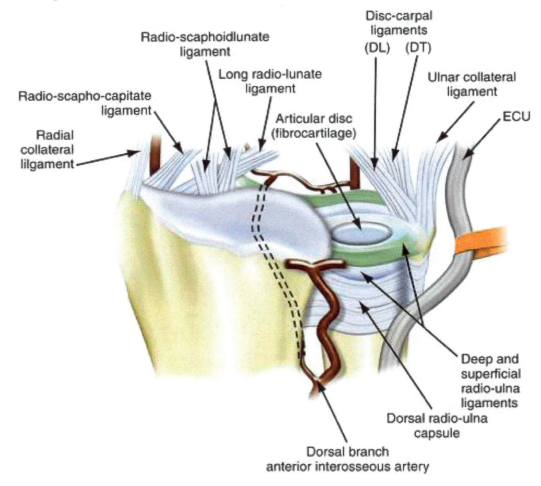

Fig. 4.76 - *The primary stabilizer of the distal RU joint is the triangular fibrocartilage (TFC). The TFC complex consists of superficial (green) and deep (blue) radioulnar fibers, the two disc-carpal ligaments (disc-lunate and disc-triquetral), and the central articular disc (white). The articular disc is responsible for transferring load from the medial carpus to the pole of the distal ulna. Image Credit: Kane Anderson, Thomas Trumble; Injuries to the Triangular Fibrocartilage Complex, clinicalgate.com*

Clinical Significance and Martial Arts Relevance:

▪ **Common Fractures of the Radius**

The forearm is a common site for bone fractures.

- **Fractures of the radial head** – This is characteristically due to falling on an outstretched hand. The radial head is forced into the capitulum of the humerus, causing it to fracture.

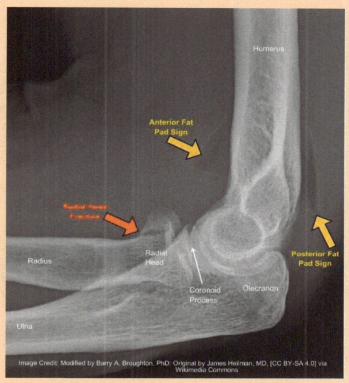

Fig. 4.77 - Fracture of the radial head with anterior and posterior fat pad sign, also known as positive sail sign, is indicative of elbow joint effusion. Image Credit: Modified by Barry A. Broughton, PhD: Original by James Heilman, MD, [CC BY-SA 4.0] via Wikimedia Commons.

- **Colles fracture** – The most common type of radius fracture. A fall onto an outstretched hand causing a fracture of the distal radius. The structures distal to the fracture (wrist and hand) are displaced posteriorly. It produces what is known as the *"dinner fork deformity"*.

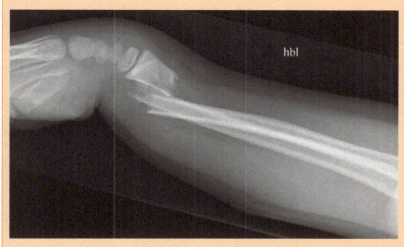

Fig. 4.78 – Colles fracture of the wrist. Note the "dinner fork deformity", produced by the posterior displacement of the radius.

- **Smith's fracture** – A fracture caused by falling onto the back of the hand. It is the opposite of a Colles fracture, as the distal fragment is displaced anteriorly.

The radius and the ulna are attached by the interosseous membrane. The force of a trauma to one bone can be transmitted to the other via this membrane. Thus, fractures of both the forearm bones are not uncommon.

There are two classical fractures:
- **Monteggia** – usually caused by a force from behind the ulna. The proximal shaft of ulna is fractured, and the head of the radius dislocates anteriorly at the elbow.

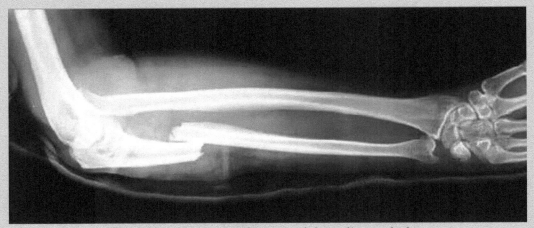

Fig. 4.79 – Monteggia fracture of the radius and ulna.

- **Galeazzi** – a fracture to the distal radius, with the ulna head dislocating at the distal radio-ulnar joint.

Mid Shaft Ulna Fracture

The "nightstick fracture" is a common eponym in orthopedic surgery used to describe an isolated fracture of the middle third of the ulnar shaft. The injury is termed for a fracture resulting from a defensive position when being struck with a police baton, causing a fracture of the ulnar diaphysis. This often occurs when one defends against an attacker wielding a stick (club, baseball bat, crowbar, truncheon, knobkerry, etc.) as they tend to protect their head by bringing up an arm(s) with their thumb pointing towards them (radial aspect) and their ulna presented to block the oncoming stick or club.

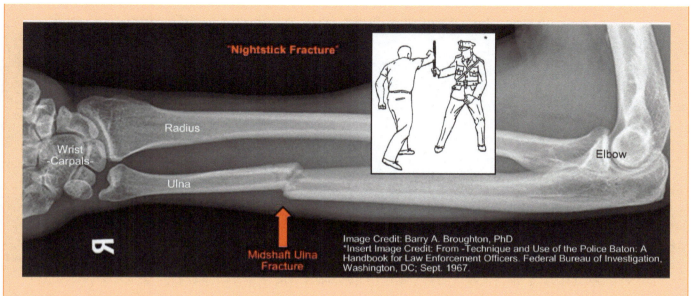

Fig. 4.80 - Nightstick Fracture. Image Credit: Barry A. Broughton, PhD
Insert Image Credit: From -Technique and Use of the Police Baton: A Handbook for Law Enforcement Officers. Federal Bureau of Investigation, Washington, DC; Sept. 1967.

Martial Arts Relevance:

- Learning proper breakfalls and avoiding FOOSH (Fall On Out-Stretched Hand) type injuries can assist in preventing injuries such as fractures and dislocations of the upper extremity.

- Do not step back and block with the ulna (radius/thumb facing you). Instead, move in and rotate the blocking forearm with thumb/radius pointing down, blocking the attacker's arm (not the weapon).

Wrist

The wrist is a complex joint between the radius and ulna of the forearm, and the five metacarpals of the hand. The wrist is composed of eight small, irregular bones (carpals) arranged roughly in to two rows.

The numerous bones of the wrist and their complex articulations give the wrist its flexibility and wide range of motion. Joints of the wrist include:

- **Distal radioulnar joint** - acts as a pivot for the forearm bones.
- **Radiocarpal joint** - consists of the radius and the first row of carpal bones (scaphoid, lunate, triquetrum), allowing for wrist flexion and extension.
- **Midcarpal joint** – between the two rows of carpal bones.
- **Intercarpal joints** - between adjacent carpal bones within each row.

▪ Carpals

The eight carpal bones are organized roughly into two rows, the proximal row, and the distal row. The carpal bones form an arch in the coronal plane. The transverse carpal ligament, a membranous band spans between the lateral and medial edges of the arch, forming the carpal tunnel.

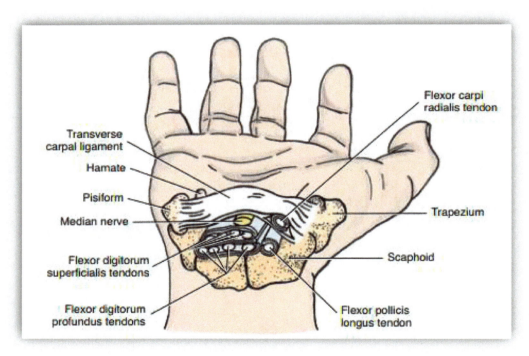

Fig. 4.81 - The carpal tunnel is formed by the arch of carpal bones and the transverse carpal ligament. Image Credit: epomedicine.com/wp-content/uploads/2014/05/carpal-tunnel

The proximal carpal row contains the scaphoid and lunate, which articulate with the radius to form the radiocarpal wrist joint. The carpals of the distal row articulate with the metacarpals.

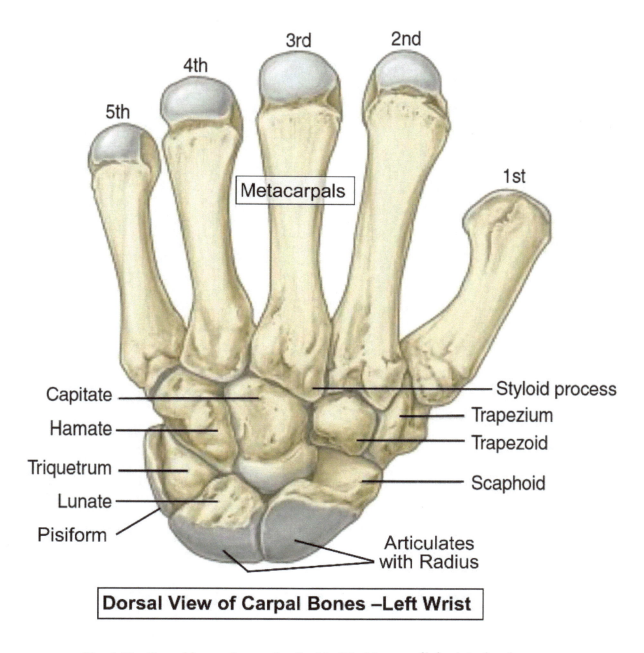

Fig. 4.82 - Carpal bones. Image Credit: Modified from radiologictechnology.org

Stability of the articulations between each of the neighboring carpals, the carpals and the bones of the forearm, and the carpals and the metacarpals, are provided by a host of ligaments.

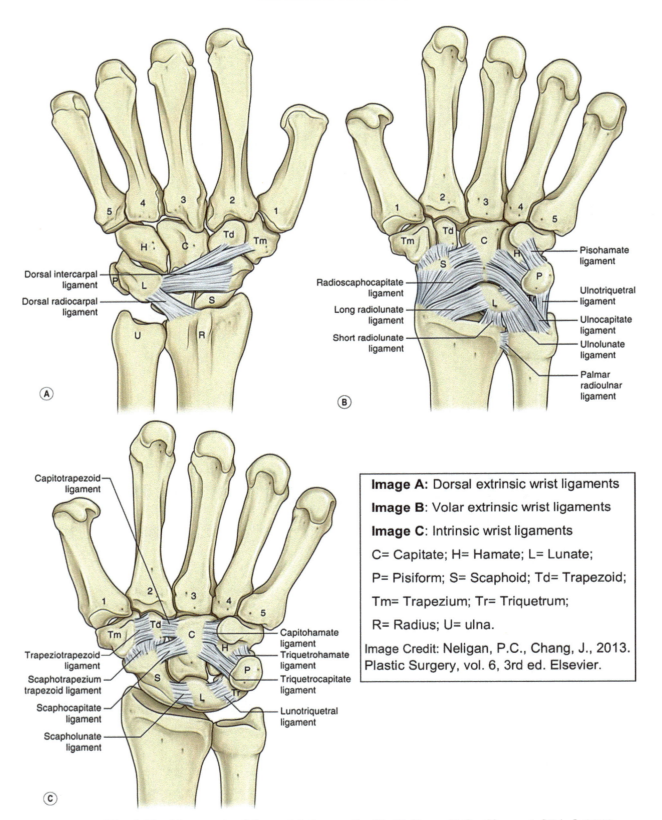

Fig. 4.83 - Ligaments of the wrist. Image Credit: Neligan, P.C., Chang, J. [Eds.], 2013. Plastic Surgery, vol. 6, 3rd ed. Elsevier.

Clinical Significance and Martial Arts Relevance:

Most wrist injuries that occur during martial arts training, or real-world self-defense, are from a fall on an outstretched hand or by a deliberate attack that isolates the wrist. FOOSH (Fall On Out-Stretched Hand) injuries often cause hyperextension of the wrist, while wrist locks also involve a forced flexion and simultaneous rotation. In any case, most ligament injuries (sprains/tears) of the wrist are caused by low energy force, while most fractures and dislocations involving the proximity of the wrist are high energy injuries. Low energy ligamentous injuries are caused by wrist locks forcing extremes in the ranges of motion. High energy injuries occur from throws, falls, takedowns, and sweeps. Sprains and other soft tissue injuries may also occur in the presence of a fracture.

- **Scaphoid Fracture**

The scaphoid bone is the most fractured carpal bone, accounting for 60% of all carpal fractures. Scaphoid fractures are typically caused by a fall that causes radial compression and hyperextension of the wrist. The characteristic clinical feature of a fractured scaphoid is pain and tenderness in the anatomical snuffbox. Because fractures of the scaphoid may not be seen on the initial radiographic imaging, it is often wise to initially treat the injury as a fracture and repeat x-ray imaging at a later date.

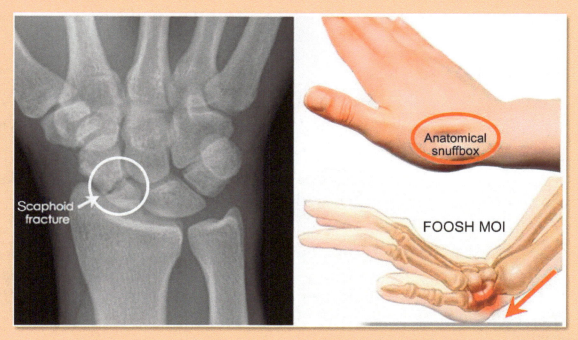

Fig. 4.84 – Left: Radiograph of a scaphoid fracture. Top Right: Anatomical snuffbox landmark for underlying scaphoid bone. Bottom Right: Mechanism of Injury for Scaphoid Fracture. Image Credit: medicoapps.org

There is risk of avascular necrosis (death of bone tissue) after a scaphoid fracture because the blood supply enters at its distal end. This means that a fracture to the middle (or "waist") of the scaphoid may disrupt the blood supply to the proximal end causing the bone to die. Martial artists with an untreated scaphoid fracture are likely to develop osteoarthritis of the wrist later in life.

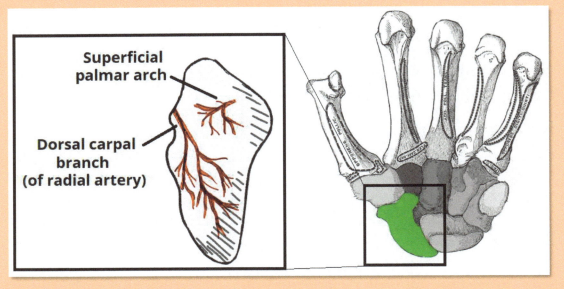

Fig. 4.85 – The blood supply to the scaphoid bone runs from distal to proximal. Image Credit: Adapted from work by Iiibalesiii [CC BY-SA 4.0] via Wikimedia Commons.

- **Anterior Dislocation of the Lunate**

A dislocation of the lunate may occur by falling on a hyperextended wrist. Should this occur, the lunate is forced anteriorly into the carpal tunnel, causing the symptoms of carpal tunnel syndrome.

Symptoms usually occur as paresthesia in the sensory distribution of the median nerve (see *Introduction the Nervous System* for details) and weakness of thenar muscles after history of a FOOSH injury. The lunate dislocation may also cause avascular necrosis, therefore immediate medical attention is required.

Triangular Fibrocartilage Complex Tear

The Triangular Fibrocartilage Complex (TFCC) aids in the stability of ulnar side of the wrist. The TFCC is made of tough fibrous tissue and cartilage that supports the joints between the distal ends of the radius and ulna and helps connect the forearm with the carpals in the ulnar side of the wrist.

The TFCC also acts as a cushion between the end of the ulna and the lunate and triquetrum of the wrist.

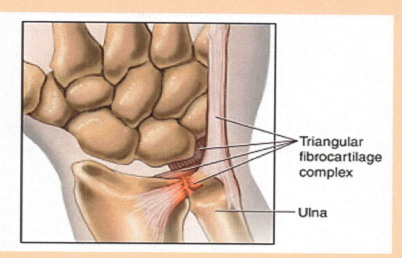

Fig. 4.86 - Triangular Fibrocartilage Complex injury.

There are two types of TFCC tears: degenerative and traumatic. Martial artists are susceptible to both. Traumatic tears typically result from falling on an outstretched hand, excessive wrist and forearm rotation, or a direct blow to the wrist. A distal radius fracture may also contribute to a tear of the TFCC.

Degenerative tears occur over time as the cartilage in the wrist wears down. Repetitive pronation and gripping can also accelerate this condition. Tears may occur with minimal force or trauma.

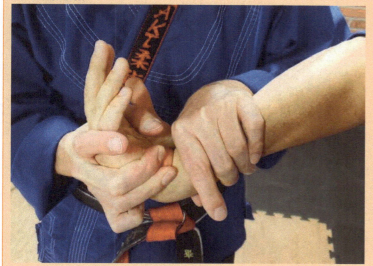

Fig. 4.87 - Wrist lock attacking the TFCC.

▪ **Wrist Locks**

There are a multitude of variations of wrist locks utilized in martial arts, combat sports, self-defense, and Police Defensive Tactics. The bulk of wrist lock techniques are either hyperextension, hyperflexion, radial or ulnar deviation, rotational, or a combination thereof.

The ligaments of the radiocarpal joint, the articular disc, and the TFCC are the structures most often injured during wrist locks.

Hyperextension wrist locks may injure the volar radiocarpal ligaments, while hyperflexion wristlocks affect the dorsal radiocarpal ligaments. Additional compression stress forces can also cause injury on the concave side of the locked wrist. Depending on the variation, introducing radial or ulnar deviation with a shearing rotational force may accentuate the efficacy of the wrist lock; especially if the elbow is stabilized or locked proximally.

Hand

With its ability to perform gross and fine motor movements the human hand is a highly complex structure. In addition to the metacarpal bones, ligaments, and subsequent joints, it is also composed of nerves, blood vessels, muscles, and tendons all working together to provide maximum dexterity.

• **Metacarpals** - Articulating proximally with the distal carpal row of the wrist are the five metacarpal bones which form the palm of the hand. The metacarpals also articulate distally with the proximal phalanges of the fingers. The metacarpals are numbered and are associated with a digit:

- Metacarpal I – Thumb.
- Metacarpal II – Index finger.
- Metacarpal III – Middle finger.
- Metacarpal IV – Ring finger.
- Metacarpal V – Little (Small) finger.

As with all long bones, metacarpal consists of a shaft with a base, and a head on either end. The medial and lateral surfaces of the metacarpals are concaved, allowing for the attachment of the interossei muscles.

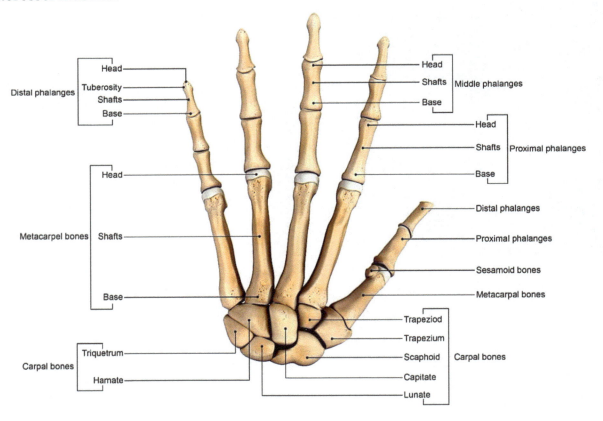

Fig. 4.88 - Left Hand: posterior (dorsal) view.

Clinical Significance and Martial Arts Relevance:

- **Boxer's Fracture**

A fracture of the *distal* 5th metacarpal (at the metacarpal neck) is often referred to as a Boxer's Fracture. It gets its name because the injury is common in inexperienced boxers, or from striking a hard surface with the smaller metacarpals with a clenched fist. The striking force fractures the neck of the 5th metacarpal bone of the little (pinky or small) finger. The neck of the metacarpal bone is where the shaft of the bone starts to widen outwards towards the knuckle, making it the weakest part of the bone. Therefore, Boxer's Fractures are the most common of all hand fractures and can often be treated conservatively with casting or splinting.

Not all 5th metacarpal fractures are Boxer's Fractures. A break at the mid-shaft of the metacarpal, or more proximally will require different treatment. The more proximal the fracture is on the metacarpal shaft; the less volar angulation of the fracture is accepted in treatment. In other words, if the break is closer to the wrist than the knuckle, and the broken fragment is angled towards the palm of the hand, it may require reduction and possibly surgery.

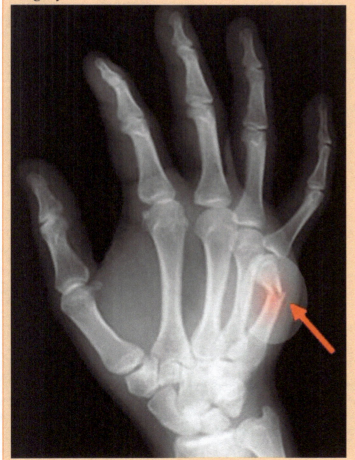

Due to the high incidence of a Boxer's Fracture in inexperienced fighters, avoid punching the assailant in the face or head with an ungloved punch. Palm Strikes are viable options for striking the head or face. A punch is an effective strike to the midsection, ribcage, solar plexus, side of the neck or throat.

Fig. 4.89 - A Boxer's Fracture is a fracture of the distal end on the 5th metacarpal caused by punching a hard object (i.e., a head or face), with the wrong part of the fist. Image Credit: Barry A. Broughton, PhD

- **Phalanges** – The 14 small bones of the fingers and thumb are called phalanges. The thumb has a proximal and distal phalanx, while the remaining fingers have proximal, middle, and distal phalanges.

The metacarpophalangeal (MCP) joint is formed by the metacarpal and the proximal phalange bones. The joints between each of the phalanges are called interphalangeal joints. The interphalangeal (IP) joint of the thumb is formed by the proximal and distal phalanges. The remaining fingers have proximal interphalangeal (PIP) joints at the articulation of the proximal and middle phalanges; as well as distal interphalangeal (DIP) joints at the middle and distal phalange articulations.

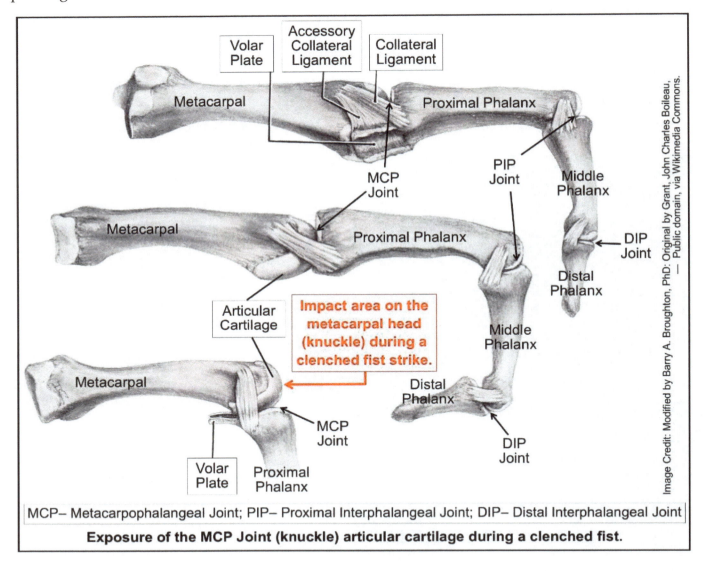

Fig. 4.90 - Vulnerability of MCP Joint articular cartilage during a closed fist strike. Image Credit: Modified by Barry A. Broughton, PhD: Original by Grant, John Charles Boileau, Public domain, via Wikimedia Commons.

Martial Arts Relevance:

▪ Knuckles

For those unfamiliar with anatomy of the hand, the knuckles are often imagined as round marble-like structures. Knuckles are formed by the MCP, PIP, and DIP joints. When the extrinsic muscles of the hand (located in the forearm — see next chapter *Introduction to the Muscular System*) contract in sequence, the fingers bend, forming a fist. Flexion of the DIP joint, followed respectively by the PIP and MCP joints causes the distal phalanx to flex on the distal end of middle phalanx; the middle phalanx to flex on the distal end of proximal phalanx; and the proximal phalanx to flex on the distal aspect of the metacarpal.

▪ Fight Bite

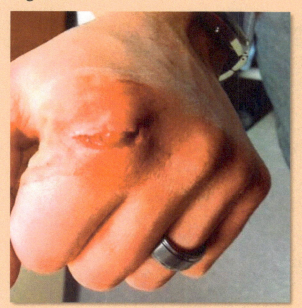

Fight bites are caused by the assailant's tooth cutting and puncturing the skin and joint capsule around the metacarpophalangeal (MCP) joint — the large knuckles of the hand that are formed by the metacarpal bones of the hand and the proximal phalanx of the finger. Because of the potential for a severe infection and damage to the cartilage in the joint, such an injury usually requires immediate surgery to wash out the joint and repair the joint capsule, followed by a course of intravenous antibiotics. I have had patients in which a piece of the assailant's tooth was broken off and imbedded in the in the joint! It is a nasty injury.

Fig. 4.91 - Fight bite involving the 2nd metacarpophalangeal joint.

Due to the severe clinical significance of Fight Bites, avoid punching the assailant in the mouth with an ungloved punch. Palm Strikes are viable options for striking the head or face.

▪ Arthritis of the Hand

Within the joint capsule, the flexed phalanx exposes the cartilage covered end of the more proximal bone (see Fig. 4.90). Therefore, the concept of "knuckle conditioning", as opposed to hand conditioning, is a misnomer. The repeated punching of the fist against different densities of materials actually injures the articular cartilage of the joints, causing osteoarthritis, not "knuckle conditioning". Note the difference between "knuckle conditioning" and hand conditioning. The centuries-old act of hand conditioning, done correctly, does indeed cause microfractures of the bones, increasing bone density over time.

However, the vast majority of people who attempt to "condition" their knuckles are in reality causing more harm than good. Bear in mind that when hand conditioning was popularized, gloves, training equipment, and modern weapons were not the norm. The majority of martial artists who train today do not need to routinely smash the small bones of their hands into the hard craniums of an enemy for survival on a daily basis. A large percentage do however need their hands for fine motor movements such as performing surgery, computer keyboarding, playing musical instruments, placing small objects into small holes, etc., in order to maintain their livelihood. Therefore, a risk-reward analysis must be considered when deciding to undergo the process of activities like hand conditioning. Does the potential need to have more dense hand bones outweigh the potential for the chronic pain and limited hand dexterity caused by arthritis?

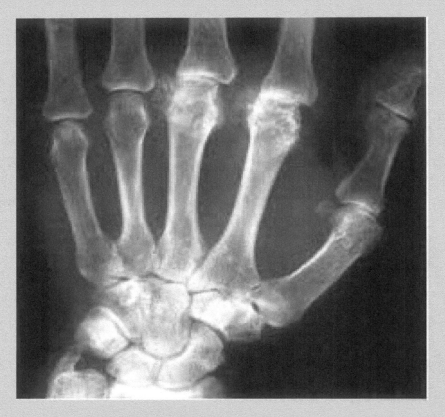

Fig. 4.92 - Radiograph of the left hand, showing severe osteoarthritis of the second and third metacarpophalangeal joints. Image Credit: Fam, A., Kolin., A., Arthritis and Rheumatism, Vol. 29, No. 10 Pg. 1285.

▪ **Finger Injuries**

Finger injuries are extremely common in martial arts, especially those involving throwing and grappling where vying for control is of utmost importance. Injuries to the fingers may occur when breaking a grip off of the opponent's uniform or extremity, by getting fingers caught in clothing during a maneuver, jamming them while blocking or striking, or during intentional finger attacks in self-defense scenarios.

The PIP and DIP are the joints most often effected with grip related injuries. Most finger injuries involve the collateral ligaments and/or the volar plate. Sprains result from stretching or partial tears of the ligaments. Frequently the ligament may cause an avulsion fracture, breaking off a piece of bone at its insertion site. If the ligament ruptures, joint dislocations can also occur.

Contrary to popular thinking, finger injuries should not be thought of as "just a finger injury". Instructors, coaches, and the martial athlete should take all finger fractures and dislocations seriously. Without an x-ray or proper physical exam, what may appear as a "simple dislocation" can also accompany fractures or significant soft tissue injuries. Therefore, self-reduced dislocations and improperly treated finger injuries in the dojo, academy, or gym can frequently contribute to complications and long-term sequelae.

Note: Fingers injuries involving the flexor and extensor tendons are addressed in the *Introduction to the Muscular System* chapter.

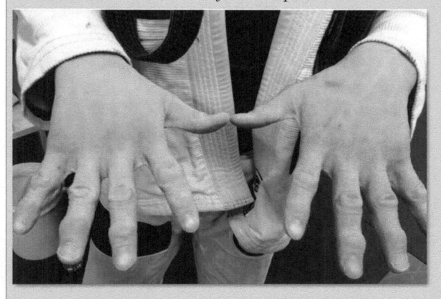

Unfortunately, many martial artists wear their gnarly malformed fingers and knuckles proudly. However, the long-term chronic pain and loss of dexterity later in life usually outweighs the neglect and mistreatment. Having a basic understanding of finger anatomy and knowing common mechanisms of injury (MOI) can help to prevent long-term disability.

Fig. 4.93 - Osteoarthritis after repetitive injury to the finger joints.
Image Credit: https://imgur.com/pzmQTJR

▪ Finger Collateral Ligament Injuries

The collateral ligaments (see Fig. 4.90) provide side-to-side stability to the joint throughout flexion and extension. Frequently referred to as a "jammed" finger, collateral ligament injuries are a result of a radial or ulnar directed forced applied to the distal finger. The rapid digital deviation may stress the collateral ligaments at any of the interphalangeal joints. Collateral ligament injuries present as pain and swelling at the affected ligament, most often the around PIP joint.

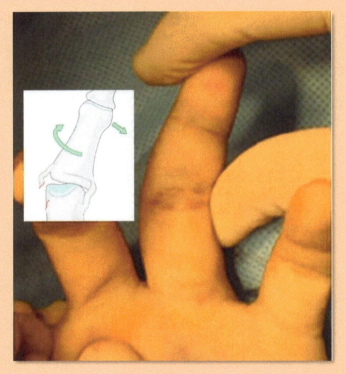

Fig. 4.94 - PIP joint collateral ligament tear.

▪ Volar Plate Injury and Fracture

The volar plate is the thick ligament that spans the palmar aspect of the PIP joint connecting the proximal and middle phalanx, preventing the finger from bending backwards and helping to stabilize the joint. Mild volar plate injuries stretch or partially tear the ligament and are frequently diminished as a "jammed" finger. More severe injuries may cause the volar plate to rupture or tear away from the bone, causing an avulsion fracture.

    Volar plate injuries commonly result from a forced, sudden hyperextension of the finger - causing pain, swelling, and bruising around the PIP joint. Severe volar plate injuries may cause joint instability or dislocation.

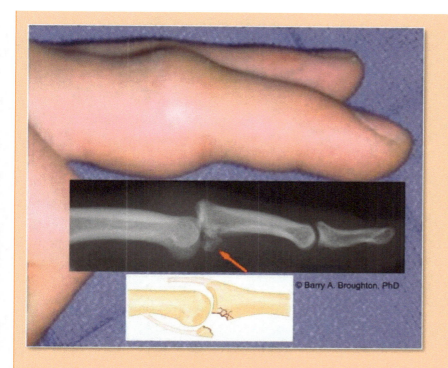

Because of the potential for long term complications, progressive static or dynamic splinting should be applied by a qualified healthcare provider. Prolonged static splinting can cause the volar plate to heal down onto itself and limit full extension of the PIP joint.

Fig. 4.95 - "Jammed finger" with volar plate fracture.

Swan Neck Deformity may result from an untreated volar plate injury. The chronic volar laxity causes hyperextension at the PIP joint and flexion at the DIP joint.

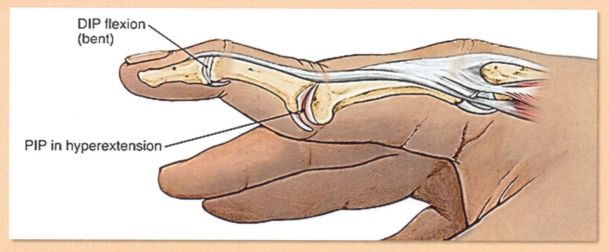

Fig. 4.96 - Swan neck deformity of the index finger PIP joint.
Image Credit: modified from Lex Medicus Pathologies.

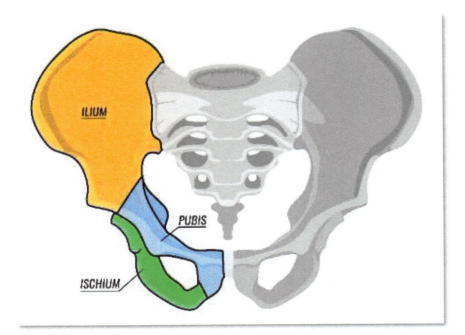

Pelvic Girdle

The pelvic girdle is a bony ring-like structure, located in the lower part of the torso. It connects the axial skeleton to the lower extremities and protects the internal pelvic organs. The pelvis supports the weight of the upper body while sitting, and transfers the weight to the lower extremities when standing. Additionally, the pelvic girdle serves as an attachment point for muscles of the torso and lower extremities.

Fig. 4.97 - Pelvic girdle.

The adult pelvic girdle consists of three regions: the ilium, ischium, and pubis. The three bones fuse together to form the socket (acetabulum) for the hip joint.

The ilium is the large, fan-shaped superior portion of the pelvis that attaches posteriorly to either side of sacrum, forming the sacroiliac (SI) joints. The ischium forms the posteroinferior portion of the pelvis, sitting inferior to the ilium and posterior the pubis. The pubis forms the anteromedial portion of the pelvic girdle.

The pubis bones are joined by a cartilaginous joint in the median plane called the symphysis pubis. In conjunction with the SI joints posteriorly, and the symphysis pubis anteriorly a stable pelvic ring is formed. Within the bony pelvis is the pelvic cavity, which primarily contains the reproductive organs and the rectum.

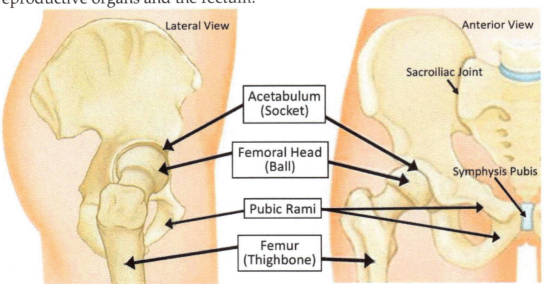

Fig. 4.98 - Lateral and anterior views of the pelvis.

Clinical Significance and Martial Arts Relevance:

- **Pubic Symphysis Injury**

Pubic symphysis diastasis is a separation of the pubic joint without a fracture. Traumatic causes of this separation may be due to high velocity falls from being thrown, kicks to the pubic bone area, or motor vehicle accidents.

- **Pubic Rami Fractures**

Each pubis is comprised of two smaller bones: the superior ramus and the inferior ramus. Located at the front of each side of the pelvis, the superior and inferior rami are referred to as the "pubic bones." The pubic rami can fracture from repetitive stress (known as a stress fracture) or from direct trauma.

Pubic rami fractures in martial artists are most commonly stress fractures that occur due to repetitive hip movements such as kicking, and repetitive loads on the pelvis during training. Traumatic fractures may also occur due to a direct blow from a kick or knee strike, or during a collision caused by an opponent falling on the pubis during a throw or takedown.

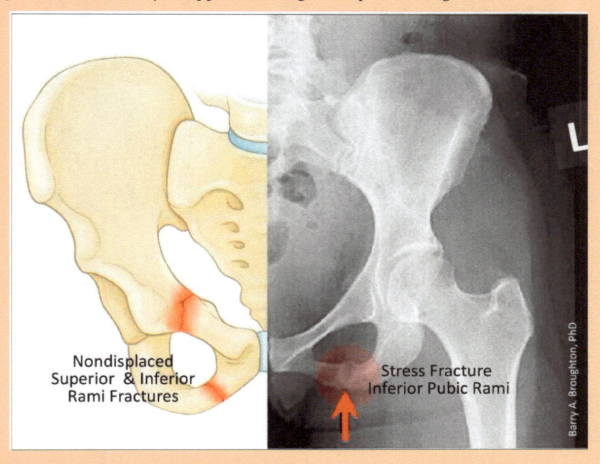

Fig. 4.99 - Left: Illustration representing pubic rami fractures. Right: Pelvic x-ray of a 40 year old male athlete with a stress fracture of the left inferior pubic rami.

- **Acetabulum Fractures**

    Isolated fractures to the socket (acetabulum) side of the hip (acetabulofemoral) joint are rare, however can occur as a result of direct trauma. A heavy fall onto the lateral hip or a forceful lunging activity can jam the head of the femur into the acetabulum causing a fracture.

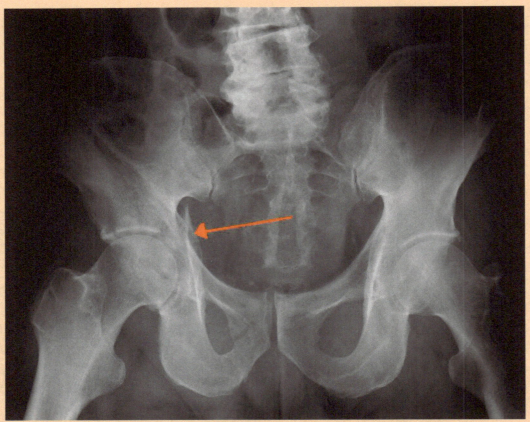

Fig. 4.100 - X-Ray demonstrating an acetabular fracture (arrow).
Image Credit: James Heilman, MD [CC-BY-SA-3.0], via Wikimedia Commons

Lower Extremity

The skeleton of the lower extremity includes 60 bones that are divided into three separate regions. The thigh is located between the hip and knee joints; the leg is located between the knee and ankle joints, while the foot is located distal to the ankle. The uppermost long bone of the thigh is the femur. The patella (kneecap) is a sesamoid bone in the anterior knee joint between the thigh and leg. The two bones of the leg are the fibula (laterally) and the tibia (medially). There are seven tarsal bones in each ankle. Both feet include 5 metatarsal bones, while there are 14 phalanges in the toes of each foot.

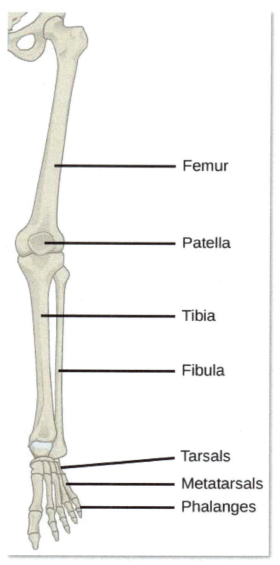

Fig. 4.101 - Bones of the left lower extremity.

Thigh

The thigh extends proximally from the acetabulofemoral (hip) joint to the knee joint distally.

- **Femur**

The femur (thigh bone) is the only bone in the thigh, and the longest and strongest bone in the human body. It supports the weight of the body while standing, walking and running. Its bony architecture makes it capable of carrying up to thirty times the weight of the body. Because of its involvement in human locomotion, numerous muscles and ligaments have their origin or attachments along the femur. The medullary cavity of the femur contains red bone marrow, which is involved in the production of red blood cells.

The femur is divided into three regions: proximal, shaft and distal.

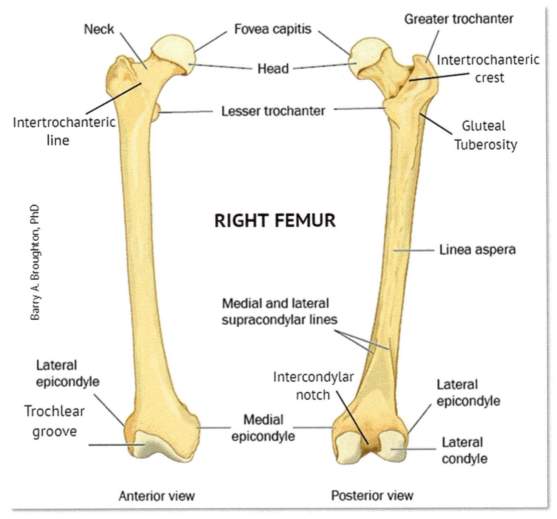

Fig. 4.102 - Anterior and Posterior views of Right Femur with bony landmarks.

The bony landmarks of the proximal femur consist of the femoral head, femoral neck, and two bony processes – the greater and lesser trochanters. Running between the two trochanters are also two ridges: the intertrochanteric line anteriorly and the trochanteric crest posteriorly.

Covered with articular cartilage, the femoral head articulates with the acetabulum of the pelvis forming the ball-and-socket acetabulofemoral (hip) joint. The fovea is a small oval depression on the surface of the head where the ligamentum teres attaches. Although not fully understood, the ligamentum teres provides stability to the hip joint and blood supply to the femoral head during childhood.

The femoral neck connects the head of the femur with the femoral shaft. Its cylindrical shape projects superior and medially from the shaft at an approximate angle of 125 degrees. The angled femoral neck allows for an increased range of motion at the acetabulofemoral joint making it more efficient for walking.

The palpable bony prominence on the lateral hip is the greater trochanter, and not the true hip joint as is often thought. The greater trochanter is lateral to the femoral neck and is the site of attachment for the muscles in the gluteal region.

The lesser trochanter projects from the posteromedial side of the femur, just inferior to the junction of the femoral neck and the shaft acting as the site of attachment for the iliopsoas muscle. Ligaments and muscles also attach to the intertrochanteric line and the trochanteric crest.

The femoral shaft descends in a slight medial direction bringing the knees closer to the midline, increasing the body's stability. The posterior surface of the femoral shaft flattens and contains longitudinally oriented ridges, called the linea aspera (Latin for rough line). The lines split distally to form the medial and lateral supracondylar lines.

The prominent rounded medial and lateral condyles of the distal femur articulate with the tibia and patella to form the knee joint. Between the distal posterior surfaces of the two condyles is a deep notch called the intercondylar fossa (or intercondylar notch).

Acetabulofemoral Joint

The hip (acetabulofemoral) joint is a ball and socket synovial joint that lies deep in the groin area. It is formed by an articulation between the femoral head and acetabulum of the pelvis. It forms a connection between the lower extremity and the pelvic girdle, with the primary function of stability and weight-bearing rather than an extensive range of movement like the glenohumeral joint of the shoulder.

Stability of the hip joint is increased due to several factors. The depth of the acetabulum surrounds nearly all the femoral head which decreases the potential for dislocation of the joint. Further improving the stability and depth of the joint is the acetabular labrum, a fibrocartilaginous horseshoe shaped ring, around the acetabulum that provides a larger articular surface for the head of the femur.

The capsule of the hip joint is formed by three ligaments: iliofemoral, pubofemoral, and ischiofemoral ligaments. Providing a large degree of stability, these ligaments run in a spiral orientation; allowing them to become tighter when the joint is extended.

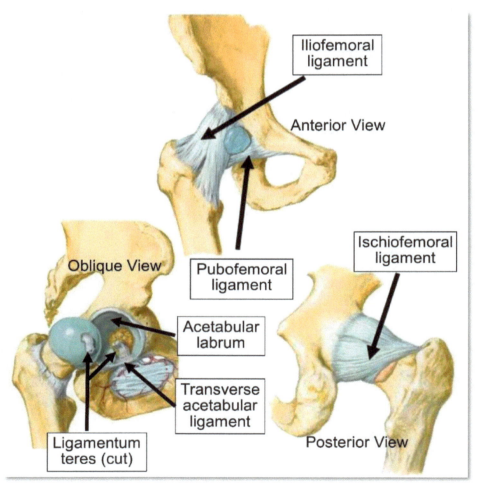

Fig. 4.103 - Ligaments of the hip joint.

Knee Joint

The distal aspect of the thigh joins with the proximal leg to form the knee joint, making it the largest and one of the most complex joints in the human body. It is formed by articulations between the femur, patella (kneecap), and tibia. As a synovial hinge joint, the knee allows for extension and flexion of the leg. There is some medial and lateral rotation that only occur when the knee is flexed, making it vulnerable to injury. If the knee is not flexed, the medial and lateral rotation occurs at the hip joint.

▪ Articulating Surfaces

The knee joint consists of two articulations: the patellofemoral and tibiofemoral joints. Hyaline cartilage covers each of the joint surfaces enclosed within a single joint capsule.

The patellofemoral joint is formed by the posterior aspect of the patella, and the trochlear groove of the anterior distal femur. The patella is embedded within the quadriceps femoris tendon (See *Introduction to the Muscular System*), glides within the trochlear grooves, and functions as a fulcrum for the knee extensor. It also serves as a stabilizing structure that reduces friction that is placed on the femoral condyles.

The tibiofemoral joint surface is formed by the articulation between the medial and lateral condyles of the femur, and the tibial plateau. Because it is a weightbearing surface, the medial femoral condyle is wider and has a larger articulating surface than the lateral condyle. The posterior and inferior surfaces of the condyles articulate with the tibia and menisci within the knee joint.

The more prominent lateral condyle helps to prevent the natural lateral tracking of the patella within the trochlear groove. A flatter lateral condyle is more likely to result in patellar dislocation.

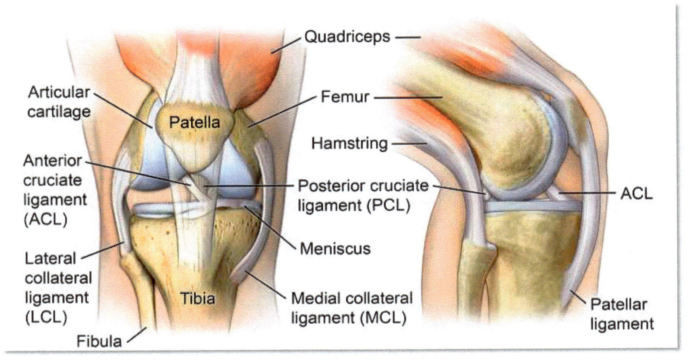

Fig. 4.104 - Anatomical structures of the right knee.

- **Ligaments**

The major ligaments in the knee joint include:

> **Patellar ligament** – frequently called the patella tendon, is a continuation of the quadriceps femoris tendon (in which the patella is embedded) that runs distally from the patella and attaches to the tibial tuberosity.
>
> **Collateral ligaments** (medial and lateral) – act to stabilize the knee by preventing excessive medial or lateral movement during extension and flexion.
>
>> The medial (tibial) collateral ligament (MCL) is a wide and flat ligament on the medial side of the joint. Its proximal origin of the MCL is the medial epicondyle of the femur and inserts distally several centimeters below the joint line directly into edge of medial tibial plateau.
>>
>> The lateral (fibular) collateral ligament (LCL) is thinner and rounder than the medial collateral. The origin of the LCL is the lateral epicondyle of the femur, distally it inserts in a depression on the lateral surface of the fibular head.

Cruciate Ligaments (anterior and posterior) – the two cruciate ligaments connect the femur and the tibia, preventing anterior and posterior translation of the tibia on the femur, as well as rotational stability. In doing so, the two ligaments cross each other, hence the term "*cruciate*" (Latin for *cross*).

> The anterior cruciate ligament (ACL) prevents anterior displacement of the tibia onto the femur. The ACL arises from the posteromedial aspect of lateral femoral condyle in the intercondylar notch, crosses anterior to the posterior cruciate ligaments, and inserts in the anteromedial aspect of the tibial plateau.

> The posterior cruciate ligament (PCL) prevents posterior displacement of the tibia on the femur. The PCL arises from the anterolateral aspect of the medial femoral condyle within the intercondylar notch and inserts along the posterior aspect of the tibial plateau.

- **Menisci**

The medial and lateral menisci are C-shaped wedge-formed fibrocartilage structures in the knee that serve two primary functions: The first, to deepen the articular surface of the tibia, thereby increasing stability of the joint. Secondly, to act as shock absorbers by increasing surface area and further dissipate impact forces.

The menisci are attached at both ends to the intercondylar area of the tibia. Additionally, the medial meniscus is attached to the medial collateral ligament and the joint capsule. Injury to the medial collateral ligament often results in a tear of the medial meniscus as well.

The lateral meniscus is smaller and does not have the additional attachments, making it more mobile and less prone to injury.

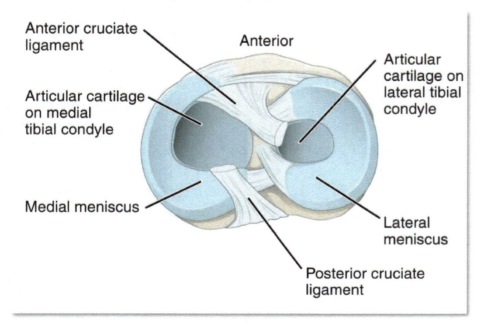

Fig. 4.105 - Top view of the of a disarticulated right knee with the femur removed, revealing the medial and lateral menisci on the tibial plateau.

Clinical Significance and Martial Arts Relevance:

- **Patellar Dislocation**

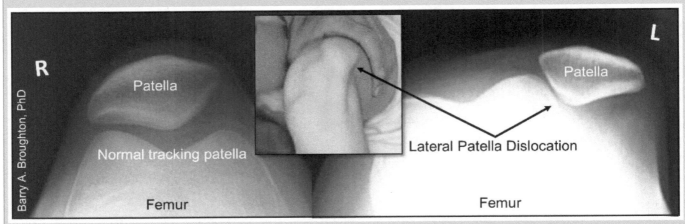

Fig. 4.106 - X-ray (Sunrise View) and image insert showing left lateral patella dislocation.

Patellar dislocations occur when the patella (kneecap) is displaced out of the patellofemoral groove of the distal femur. Most patella dislocations occur laterally (approximately 93% of the time) and are caused by a high force impact on the patella, or from a forceful sudden twisting of the knee. These mechanisms of injury make patellar dislocation more common in individuals participating in contact sports and martial arts where collisions and strikes occur.

Even though patella dislocations are relatively easy to reduce, and oftentimes are reduced in the field, individuals should still seek medical attention for proper treatment after a dislocation. Because knee ligaments can be injured during a dislocation, the patella is often unstable after the injury. This frequently results in further dislocations, often requiring less force than the initial dislocation. The recurrence rate after a first-time patella dislocation varies between 15-60% depending on appropriate treatment of the initial injury.

- **Patellar Fracture**

Patellar fractures usually result from direct trauma to the anterior knee, or sudden contraction of the quadriceps muscle. Patella fractures are more common in males in the 20–50-year age range. If the patella fractures into fragments, the fragments will usually become displaced. Because of the pull of the quadriceps tendon and patellar tendon (ligament), the proximal fragment becomes displaced superiorly and the distal fragment is pulled inferiorly.

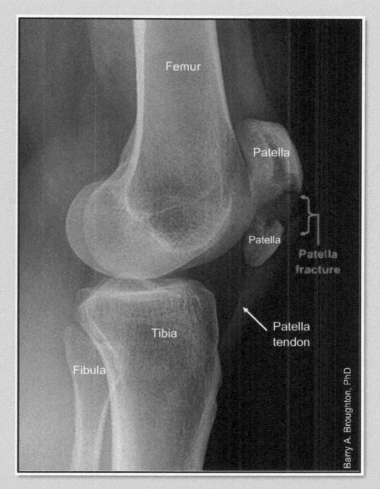

Fig. 4.107 - X-ray of patella fracture. Note the displacement of the proximal and distal fragments.

▪ Medial Collateral Ligament Tear

Injury to the medial collateral ligament (MCL) is the most common pathology affecting the knee joint. The mechanism of injury is usually the result of valgus stress applied to the lateral side of the knee while the foot is planted on the ground. A direct blow to the lateral knee from a kick, strike, or from someone falling onto it is frequently sufficient force to tear the MCL. The MCL may also be injured during an excessive outward torsional twist while the foot is planted on the ground. A resisted inward reap to knee while grappling will also cause a similar valgus stress force.

Isolated injuries to the MCL may occur, however medial meniscus tears often accompany MCL injures because of the proximity of their attachments.

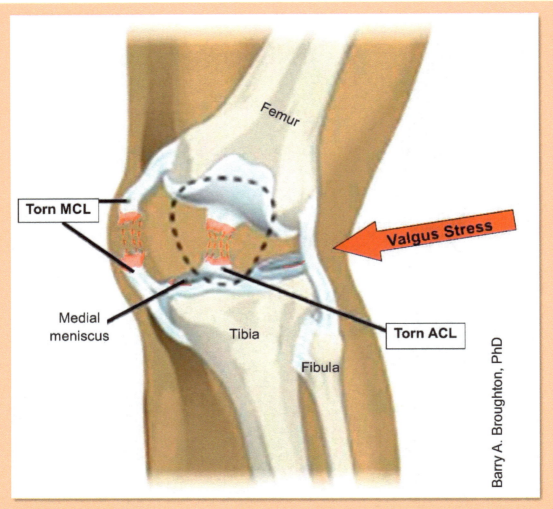

Fig. 4.108 - Valgus stress and rotational forces to the knee may cause tears to the menisci, collateral and cruciate ligaments.

▪ Anterior Cruciate Ligament Tear

As the main stabilizer for the knee joint, an anterior cruciate ligament injury can be a devastating and career-ending injury for many martial artists. When the ACL ligament is torn, it can lead to general instability of the knee with buckling and giving way, especially during activities. Depending on the severity of the injury, returning to full training after an ACL tear can take up to one year.

The ACL can be torn with or without contact from another competitor. The mechanism of injury usually involves a significant force to the back of the knee with the joint partly flexed, or hyperextension of the knee joint. The ACL can be injured in several ways including: cutting and changing angles rapidly, stopping suddenly on a planted foot, landing incorrectly after a jumping (jump spinning kicks), hyperextension, from direct contact (i.e., kick to the leg), or from a collision during a takedown.

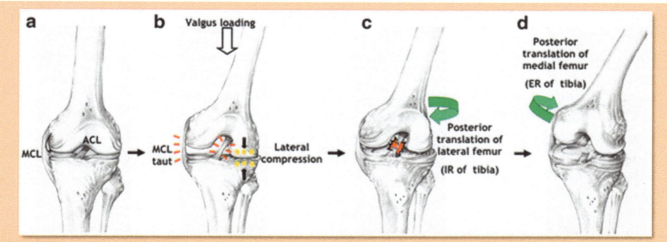

*Fig. 4.109 - The mechanism of injury for non-contact ACL injury includes the following: (**a**) An unloaded knee. (**b**) When valgus loading is applied, the MCL becomes taut and lateral compression occurs. (**c**) This compressive load causes a lateral femoral posterior displacement, probably due to the posterior slope of lateral tibial plateau, and the tibia translates anteriorly and rotates internally, resulting in ACL rupture. (**d**) After the ACL is torn, the primary restraint to anterior translation of the tibia is gone, causing the medial femoral condyle to also be displaced posteriorly, resulting in external rotation of the tibia. Image Credit: Sports Injuries and Prevention; Chapter 9.4. Springer, Tokyo.*

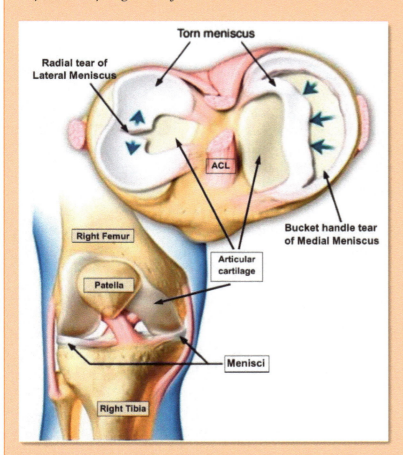

Fig. 4.110 - Illustration of radial tear of the lateral meniscus and bucket handle tear of the medial meniscus.

- **Meniscus Tear**

There are two basic types of meniscal tears: traumatic and degenerative tears. A traumatic meniscal tear often involves twisting of the knee, i.e., when an athlete quickly turns their body, pivoting on the knee while the foot is planted firmly on the ground or mat. A degenerative meniscal tear is caused by repetitive wear over time, with or with a previous knee injury.

Treatment for a torn meniscus depends greatly on the type, size, and location of the tear. If the knee is not locked, due to a buckle handle tear of the meniscus that is flipped into the intercondylar notch, treatment most often *begins* conservatively with rest, ice, and therapy. Degenerative tears that are aggravated by activity often improve over time.

Attacks to the Knee: Low Kicks, Kneebars, Reaps, and Heel Hooks!

As the largest joint in the body, the knee is the most injured joint among athletes- accounting for nearly 55% of all sports injuries. Because of its susceptibility to injury, especially in contact and combat sports, there are often restrictive rulesets in place to protect the knee.

A low roundhouse kick, oblique kick, or low side kick to the knee can all have obvious damaging effects on the ligaments in the knee; especially if it is delivered directly to the lateral, anterior, or medial aspect of the joint itself, and not just the lateral mid-thigh. The real-world application of such techniques is to create maximal stress to the knee joint, causing damage to any of the soft tissue stabilizing architecture, or bony anatomy.

In combat sports, the problem usually arises however when addressing joint locks that affect the knee. The attacks can be insidious, and the injuries can be devastating. The prevalence of knee injuries is not necessarily because of competitor malice, especially in grappling related sports where leg entanglement is commonplace. Oftentimes knee injuries occur because the defender lacks an understanding of the anatomy and biomechanics of the knee joint. Therefore, they do not know how to properly protect it. Unfortunately, for those who do not fully appreciate the idiosyncrasies of the knee, by the time they attempt to protect it, it is too late.

Understanding the nuances of knee biomechanics are not only important for maintaining safety during sport, but it also provides the opportunity to exploit vulnerabilities for real-world personal protection. In addition to the obvious, restrictive rulesets protecting the knee are in place for several reasons. First, ligament tears do not heal as easily as other soft tissue injuries, and frequently need surgical repair and subsequent rehabilitation. Second, because of a lack of understanding, many athletes (and coaches/instructors) do not know how to properly defend against a knee attack and inadvertently cause further injury. Third, and probably most important, ligaments do not have the same pain and sensory receptors that muscles and tendons do. By the time tension or pain is felt within the knee joint, the opportunity to adequately defend and tap has passed.

Martial arts instructors and coaches have an obligation to teach their athletes and students how to protect themselves. Not only from violent physical assaults, but also from themselves, by avoiding injury while training. Having a foundational understanding of anatomy, and the concepts and principles of biomechanics will prolong their training lifecycle by diminishing unintended training injuries. Hence the phrase "tap early, tap often". Not doing so will only leave a wake of injured former students who are no longer able to train.

Understanding how a joint lock affects the vulnerable anatomy will aid in injury prevention, as well as improving the effectiveness of the technique. A kneebar has a different mechanism of injury than a knee reap and an ankle hook, although they can each injure the same anatomical structures. There are multiple variations in the execution of a kneebar, just as there are in executing an inside or outside knee reap, or inside and outside heel hooks. This text is not intended to give step-by-step instructions in the execution of various techniques; however, in general, a kneebar causes hyperextension of the extended knee, while knee reaping and heel hook techniques cause rotation and torsion to occur during varying degrees of knee flexion.

While the kneebar can tear the posterior capsular ligaments; like reaps and heel hooks, it can also injury the cruciate and collateral ligaments, as well as the menisci.

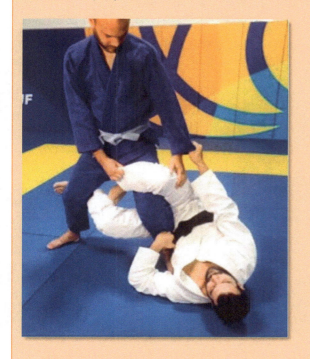

Fig. 4.111 – Example of a knee reap that could potentially injure the blue player's left knee. Valgus stress is being placed on his bent knee while the foot is planted. Image Credit: IBJJF Rules Book General Competition Guidelines. January 2021

When teaching seminars, coaching, or refereeing at sport jujitsu and grappling tournaments, I am often surprised by those who are not aware of the potential severity of injury that can occur with these techniques — especially with heel hooks and knee reaping on a planted foot. Contrary to many, I am not an advocate for banning these highly effective techniques. I am, however, an advocate for those who do use them to understand not only how to execute the specific technique, but also what joint is being attacked during its execution. As a case in point, I am astonished by those who get offended and angered when a referee stops a bout due to a potential knee injury while a competitor is executing an inside heel hook. In outrage they usually exclaim that they were "just doing a heel hook", seemingly unaware that the rotation at the tibiofemoral (knee) joint is going to tear the menisci or knee ligaments before injuring the substantial (strong) deltoid ligament of the medial ankle (See the Medial Ligaments of the Ankle later in this chapter).

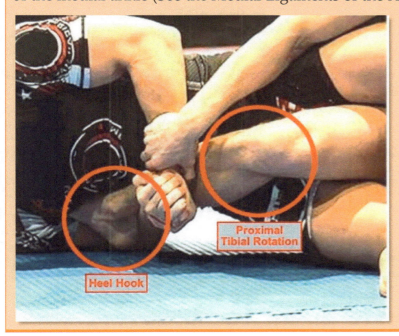

Fig. 4.112 - Heel Hook distally causing tibial rotation at the knee proximally.

Leg

The portion of the lower extremity that extends proximally from the knee joint to the ankle joint distally is known as the leg. The leg contains two very strong long bones, the tibia and the fibula. The tibia (shinbone) is located medial to the fibula and is the thicker and stronger of the two bones. The fibula is notably smaller and is situated lateral to the tibia.

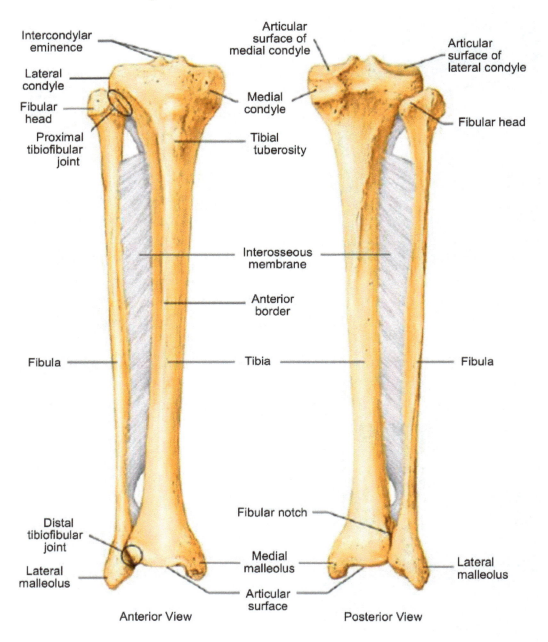

Fig. 4.113 - Anterior and posterior views of the bones of the right leg. Image credit: OpenStax College, [CC BY 3.0], via Wikimedia Commons.

The tibia and fibula are connected by three junctions; the proximal and distal tibiofibular joints, and via the interosseous membrane that connects their shafts, forming the middle tibiofibular joint.

The proximal tibiofibular joint is a plane type synovial joint, while the distal joint is a syndesmosis (fibrous joint). These joints have minimal function in terms of movement but play a significant role in stability and weight-bearing. The interosseous ligament is a fibrous structure that spans between the shafts of tibia and fibula providing stability to the distal tibiofibular joint.

- Tibia

The tibia is the main bone of the leg, forming what is commonly referred to as the shin. It flares out at its proximal and distal ends, articulating with the knee and ankle joints, respectively. As the second largest bone in the body, the tibia is a key weight-bearing structure.

Proximal Tibia

The proximal tibia is widened, forming the medial and lateral condyles known as the tibial plateau. This relatively flat surface articulates with the femoral condyles to form the articulation of the knee joint.

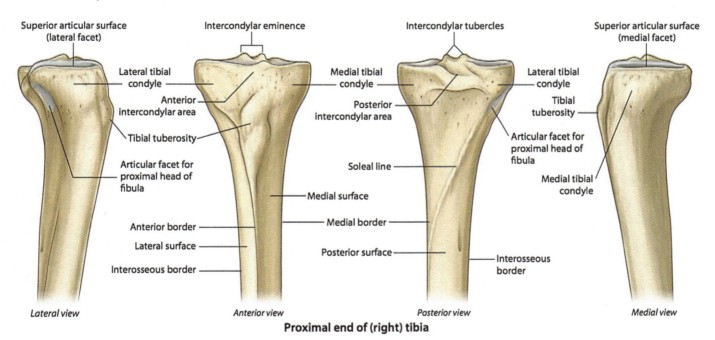

Fig. 4.114 - Lateral, anterior, posterior, and medial views of the right proximal tibia landmarks.

Located between the condyles on the tibial plateau is a region called the intercondylar eminence. The medial intercondylar tubercle is a protrusion on the medial condyle, while the lateral intercondylar tubercle is a protrusion on the lateral condyle. The tubercles provide sites for attachments of the cruciate ligaments and the menisci of the knee joint. The intercondylar tubercles of the tibia articulate with the intercondylar notch of the distal femur.

Tibial Shaft

The prism-shaped tibial shaft is divided into three surfaces: anterior/medial, posterior and lateral.

The anterior/medial surface of the shaft is palpable down the length of the leg. Proximally it contains the tibial tuberosity, the bony protrusion where the patellar ligament inserts.

The lateral surface serves as the attachment of the interosseous membrane which connects the tibia and fibula.

The posterior surface contains the soleal line that serves as the origin for the soleus, flexor digitorum longus, and tibialis posterior muscles.

Dividing the anterior/medial and lateral surfaces is the anterior crest, the palpable edge of the tibia. This "sharp" edge makes an ideal surface to use for striking, blocking kicks, or dragging across and opponent's extremity while grappling!

Distal Tibia

The distal portion of the tibia widens into box-like shape to assist with weight-bearing. Because of its mass, it too is ideal to use as a striking surface during kicks.

The medial malleolus is an inferior projecting bony prominence on the medial aspect of the tibia. The inferior surface, also known as the tibial plafond, of the distal tibia articulates with the talus (a tarsal bone) to form the ankle joint. There is a groove on the posterior surface of the tibia through which the tendon of tibialis posterior passes.

Laterally is the fibular notch where the fibula is bound to the tibia, via the tibiofibular ligaments, forming the distal tibiofibular joint.

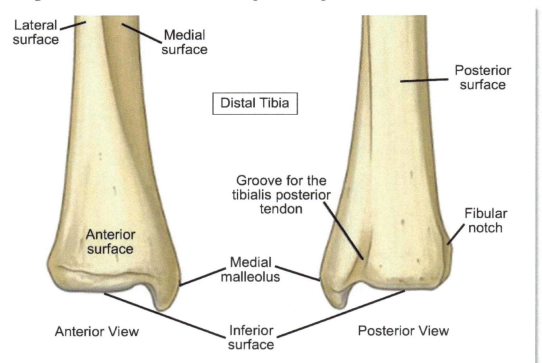

Fig. 4.115 - Anterior and posterior views of the distal tibia landmarks.

▪ Fibula

The fibula is a long bone of the leg that is located lateral to the tibia. The main function of the fibula is to act as an attachment for muscles of the lower extremity. Unlike the tibia, it is not a weight-bearing bone, however, it does provide for some stability to the ankle joint.

The fibula has three main articulations:

- Proximal tibiofibular joint – articulates with the posterolateral aspect of lateral condyle of the proximal tibia.
- Distal tibiofibular joint – articulates with the fibular notch on the lateral aspect of the distal tibia.
- Ankle joint – articulates with the talus bone of the foot.

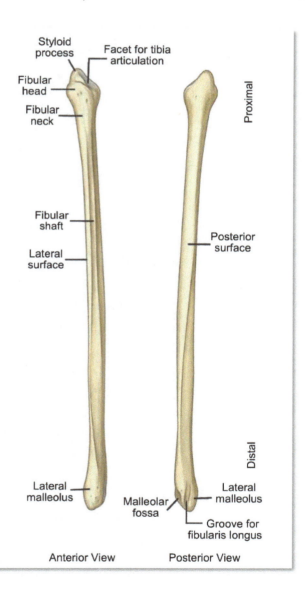

Fibular Shaft

There are three surfaces along the shaft of the fibula: the anterior, lateral, and posterior surfaces. There are nine different muscles (see *Introduction to the Muscular System*) that attach along the surfaces of the fibula to aid in movement and stability.

Proximal Fibula

The proximal end of the fibula has an enlarged head that contains a facet which articulates with the posterolateral aspect of lateral condyle of the tibia. A fibrous capsule between the fibula and tibia secures the proximal tibiofibular joint in place.

Fig. 4.116 - Anterior and proximal view of fibula bony landmarks.

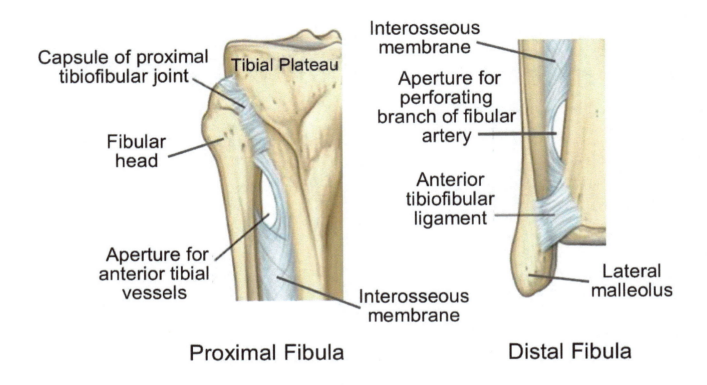

Fig. 4.117 - Anterior views of the right proximal and distal fibula landmarks.

Distal Fibula

The anterior tibiofibular ligament inserts on the distal fibula and tibia at the distal tibiofibular joint. The posterior talofibular ligament attaches to the malleolar fossa, a rough depression on the posterior aspect of the distal fibula. The lateral malleolus is the palpable lateral prominence of the distal fibula. It extends inferiorly below the inferior surface of the tibia and provides some lateral stability to the ankle joint.

Clinical Significance and Martial Arts Relevance:

- **Fractures of the Tibia**

The tibia is the most frequently fractured long bone in the body. Being vulnerable to injury from direct and indirect high-energy trauma, the severity and subsequent treatment depend on multiple factors, including the location of the fracture. Tibial *shaft* fractures are divided into thirds: proximal, middle, and distal.

Depending on the mechanism of the injury; in addition to fractures of the tibial shaft, fractures can also occur proximally at the tibial plateau, and distally at the ankle. Injuries to the menisci and ligaments of the knee are common in tibial plateau fractures. Distally at the ankle, the medial malleolus may be fractured. This is frequently caused by the ankle being twisted inwards (over-inverted), forcing the talus against the medial malleolus, causing a spiral-type fracture. This rarely happens in isolation, often the lateral malleolus is also fractured; potentially causing an unstable fracture that requires surgical management.

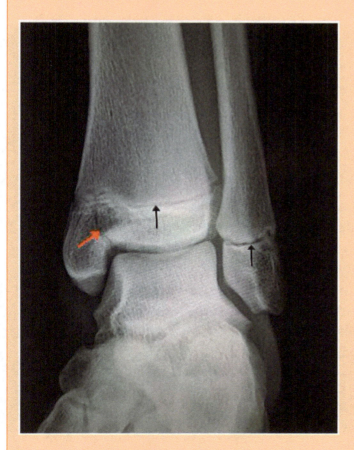

Fig. 4.118 – Fracture (Salter Harris type III) of the medial malleolus (red arrow) in a child. The black arrows identify normal growth plates of the tibia and fibula. Image Credit: By James Heilman, MD [CC-BY-SA-3.0], via Wikimedia Commons. Modified by Barry A. Broughton, PhD

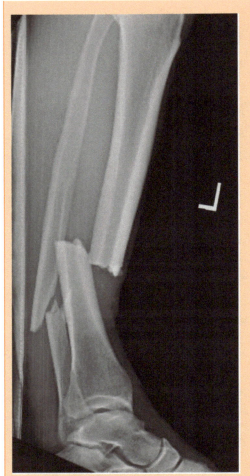

The location of any associated fibula fracture has been shown to correlate with the amount of energy involved with the mechanism of injury. Trauma involving higher levels of energy are more likely to result in a fibula fracture at the same level as the tibia fracture. Lower energy mechanisms of injury may result in a fibula fracture at a different level (i.e., more proximal) to the tibia fracture.

Fig. 4.119 - X-ray lateral view of left middle third tibia and fibula fracture that was sustained from a low kick that was blocked by the opponent's tibial plafond.

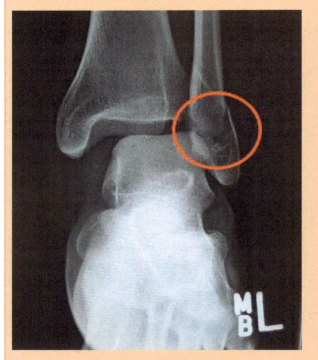

- **Fractures of the Distal Fibula**

Isolated distal fibula fractures involving the lateral malleolus represent the majority of ankle fractures. They are frequently caused by low-energy injuries resulting from external rotation and supination of the ankle. Depending on the mechanism of injury, the forced talus against the lateral malleolus can cause a spiral fracture or a transverse fracture of the distal fibula.

Fig. 4.120 – Fracture of the lateral malleolus. Image Credit: By James Heilman, MD [CC-BY-SA-3.0], via Wikimedia Commons

Ankle Joint

The ankle joint (or talocrural joint) is a synovial joint that connects the foot to the distal lower extremity. It is formed by the distal leg bones (tibia and fibula) and the talus, a tarsal bone of the foot. The ankle functions as a hinge type joint, permitting dorsiflexion and plantar flexion of the foot.

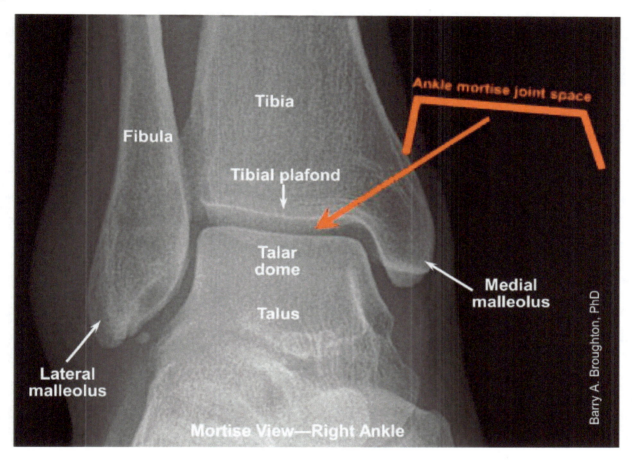

Fig. 4.121 - X-ray of a normal ankle joint. Notice the mortise shaped joint formed by the tibia, fibula, and talus.

    The distal tibia and fibula are secured together by the strong tibiofibular ligaments. Together, they form a square shaped socket, covered in hyaline cartilage. This bony socket is known as a mortise, much like in woodworking. The body of the talus fits snugly into the mortise formed by the lateral malleolus, tibial plafond, and medial malleolus. The talar dome of the talus articulates within the mortise joint.

    The body of the talus is wider anteriorly and narrower posteriorly. The wedge-shaped configuration of the talus provides more ankle stability with the foot in dorsiflexion. Because the posterior portion of the talus within the mortise is narrower, the ankle is less stable, making it susceptible to injury while in plantar flexion. This is a crucial point to understand in order to effectively apply straight ankle locks in martial arts.

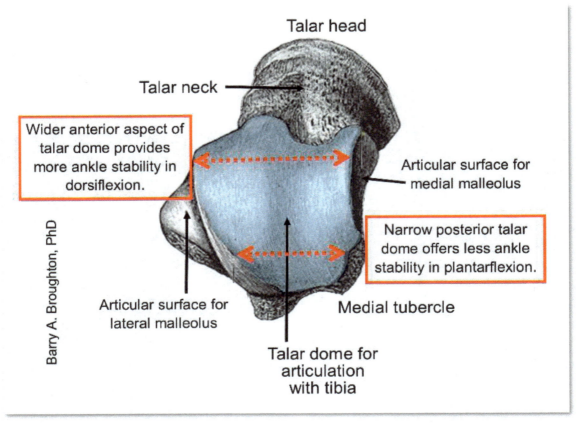

Fig. 4.122 - Superior view of the left talus. The talar dome is wider anteriorly, providing more joint stability during dorsiflexion.

- **Ligaments**

In addition to the anterior and posterior tibiofibular ligaments, there are four primary ligaments of the ankle. The main stabilizing ligaments laterally are the anterior and posterior talofibular ligaments, and the calcaneofibular ligament; medially is the deltoid ligament.

- Lateral Ligaments

Lateral stabilization of the ankle is achieved by three separate ligaments: the anterior and posterior talofibular ligaments, and the calcaneofibular ligament. The lateral ligaments stabilize the resistance against inversion and internal rotation stress of the ankle. By attaching the lateral malleolus to the tarsal bones below the ankle joint, they also serve as a guide to direct ankle motion.

The anterior talofibular ligament (ATFL) connects the lateral aspect of the talus to the lateral malleolus of the fibula. As the weakest of the three lateral ligaments, the ATFL is the most frequently injured ankle ligament.

The posterior talofibular ligament connects the posterior aspect of the talus to the lateral malleolus.

The calcaneofibular ligament connects the distal fibula to the calcaneus inferiorly.

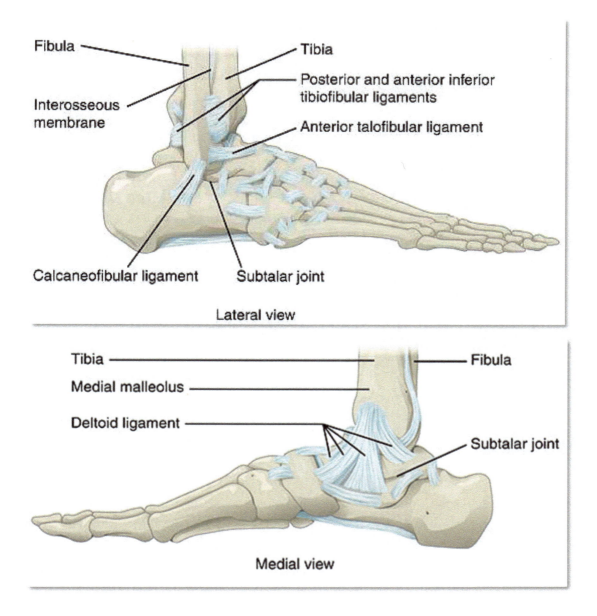

Fig. 4.123 - Ligaments of the ankle joint. Image credit: OpenStax College [CC BY 3.0], via Wikimedia Commons.

▪ Medial Ligament

The deltoid ligament complex (or medial ligament) consists of four ligaments that form a triangle connecting the tibia to the inferior tarsal bones. The deltoid ligament fans out from the medial malleolus and attaches to the navicular, calcaneus, and talus bones. It stabilizes the ankle joint during eversion (outward turning) of the foot and prevents subluxation of the ankle joint.

The anterior and posterior tibiotalar ligaments connect the tibia to the talus.

The tibionavicular ligament which attaches to the navicular anteriorly and the tibiocalcaneal ligament which attaches to the calcaneus inferiorly.

Clinical Significance and Martial Arts Relevance:

Ankle Movement and Stability

The movement of the ankle joint is dictated by the convex trochlear surface of the talus within the fixed concave mortise formed by the distal tibia and fibula. While walking, the concaved mortise moves over the convex articular surface of the talus.

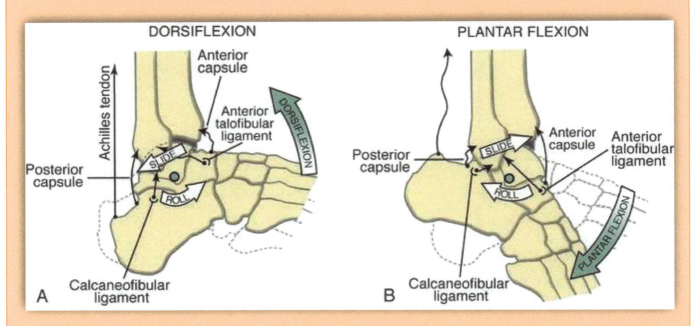

Fig. 4.124 - *Lateral view of the ankle and foot showing articular surface movement within the ankle joint during dorsiflexion (A- Left image) and plantar flexion (B- Right image). Stretched structures are shown as thin elongated arrows; slackened structures are shown as wavy arrows. Image Credit: Neumann DA: Kinesiology of the musculoskeletal system: foundations for physical rehabilitation, ed 2, St Louis, 2010, Mosby*

    The ankle joint is most stable during maximal dorsiflexion because the collateral ligaments and plantar flexor muscles are all taut in this position. Additionally, the ankle is stabilized further in dorsiflexion because the superior articulating surface of the talus is wider anteriorly than it is posteriorly. Full dorsiflexion of the ankle results in a wedging effect within the joint as the wide anterior portion of the talus is pressed into the mortise formed by the tibia and fibula.

    This maximum stability is required in preparation for the contraction of the strongly activated plantar flexor muscles (see next chapter) during jumping or the push-off phase of fast walking and running.

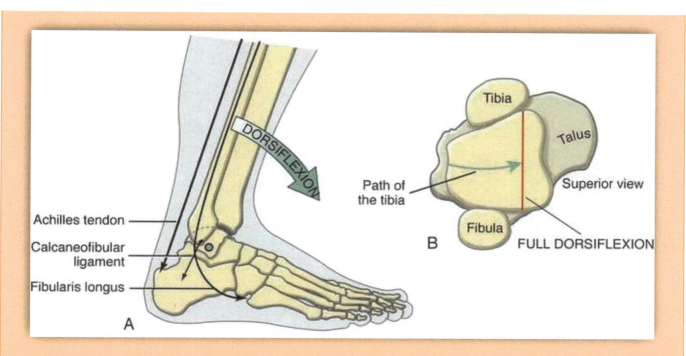

Fig. 4.125 - Factors that increase the mechanical stability of the fully dorsiflexed ankle joint. Image A (on left): In dorsiflexion there is increased tension of the soft tissue structures, indicated by thin black arrows. Image B (on right): The superior articulating surface of the talus is wider anteriorly than it is posteriorly. Image Credit: Neumann DA: Kinesiology of the musculoskeletal system: foundations for physical rehabilitation, ed 2, St Louis, 2010, Mosby

The ankle joint is least stable when placed in a full plantar flexed position. Plantar flexion moves the narrower posterior articulating aspect of the talus within the mortise, releasing the wedged tension between the medial and lateral malleoli. Plantar flexion also loosens most of the collateral ligaments and soft tissue stabilizers.

Weight-bearing on a fully plantar flexed ankle places the joint at a relatively unstable position, making it suspectable to injury. Landing from a jump in a plantar flexed, and often inverted, position increases the likelihood of tearing the lateral ankle ligaments.

• **Ankle Locks**

A Straight ankle lock primarily attacks the talocrural (ankle) joint. Because the ankle joint only moves in dorsiflexion and plantar flexion, a straight ankle locks forces excessive plantar flexion of the joint. Soft tissue structures that resist excessive plantar flexion include the anterior talofibular ligament (ATFL) on the lateral ankle, the deltoid ligament medially (see Fig. 4.123), the joint capsule, and the tibialis anterior muscle (see next chapter). As demonstrated previously in Fig. 4.122 (Superior view of the left talus), the talar dome is narrower posteriorly, providing less joint stability during plantar flexion.

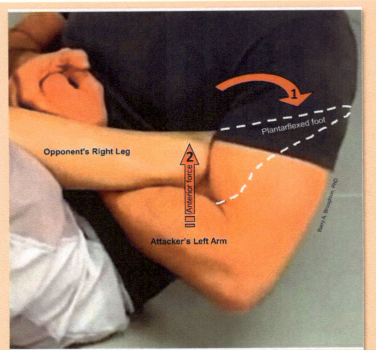

Fig. 4.126 - Straight ankle lock. Begin by bringing the ankle and foot to its least stable position in full plantar flexion, followed by anterior force applied to the posterior talus.

Variations of a straight ankle lock include the attacker using their distal radius and radial styloid to gouge into the opponent's highly innervated Achilles tendon. Those not familiar with the ankle locks and anatomy will oftentimes attempt to lean back and stretch the foot and ankle in an attempt to finish the technique. However, if the objective is to inflict maximal injury and dysfunction, the ankle must be forced to the endpoint of plantar flexion first; then apply anterior force to the posterior talus with the attacker's radius to dislocate the talocrural joint.

Fig. 4.127 - Figure four ankle lock (toe hold).

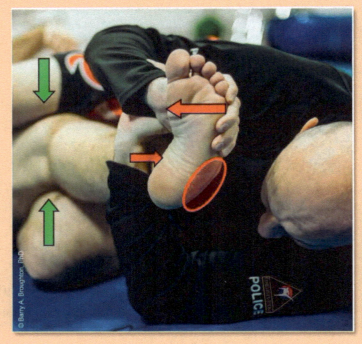

Toe holds and Figure-4 ankle locks attack the ankle joint, the subtalar joint, and the surrounding soft tissues. The variations of these submissions cause a torque force of plantar flexion and inversion of the ankle and hind foot. Significant force applied during ankle locks can cause an ankle sprain, rupture the ligaments, or even dislocation of the ankle.

The two primary ligaments that are affected during a Figure-4 ankle lock are the ATFL and the calcaneofibular ligament (CFL). The anterior talofibular ligament is the most commonly sprained ligament and is generally the first to tear during an ankle lock, followed by the calcaneofibular ligament. Subsequently, the peroneal retinacula, the fibrous bands that restrain the peroneus longus and brevis tendons (see next chapter) along the lateral side of the ankle, may also be torn. When these soft tissue structures become inadequate, the talus may dislocate from within the mortise.

Bimalleolar Fracture-Dislocation

A bimalleolar fracture, also known as a Pott's fracture, is an injury that involves a fracture of both the medial and lateral malleoli. Because both sides of the mortise joint are injured, the ankle joint becomes unstable due to disruption of the structural integrity. Left untreated, an unstable talocrural joint is susceptible to further damage and premature arthritis of the ankle. Therefore, surgical treatment is common in repairing the fractures to stabilize the ankle joint.

Bimalleolar fractures often occur by forced eversion of the foot. The forced eversion pulls on the deltoid ligaments of the medial ankle, producing a fracture of the medial malleolus. The talus then moves laterally, breaking off the lateral malleolus. In trimalleolar fractures, the tibia is then forced anteriorly, shearing off the distal and posterior aspect against the talus.

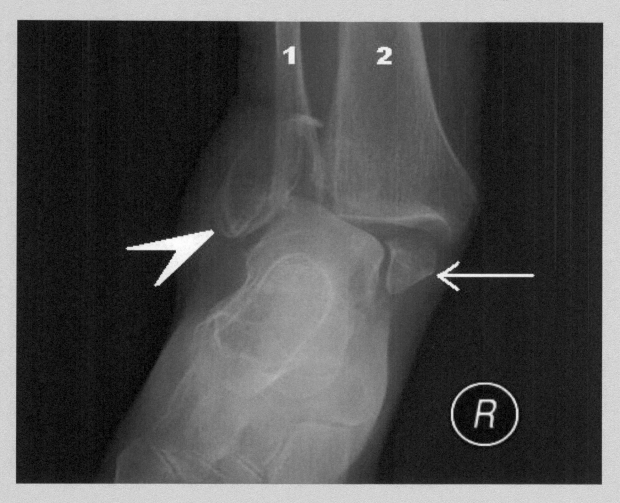

Fig. 4.128 – Bimalleolar fracture of the ankle. 1. Fibula - Large arrowhead reveals lateral malleolus fracture. 2. Tibia- Narrow arrow reveals medial malleolus fracture. Image Credit: By Steven Fruitsmaak [CC by-SA 3.0], from Wikimedia Commons

Ankle Sprains

An ankle sprain refers to a partial or complete tear in the ligaments of the ankle joint. Ankle sprains usually occur from excessive inversion to a plantarflexed and weight-bearing foot. Eight-five percent of all ankle sprains occurs laterally, most often injuring the anterior talofibular ligament. Because the deltoid ligament of the medial ankle is much stronger, it is less likely to be injured than the lateral ligaments.

Avulsion Fractures

Avulsion fractures occur when a small fragment of bone attached to a ligament or tendon gets pulled away from the main part of the bone. Because of the insertion of the anterior talofibular and calcaneofibular ligaments on the distal fibula, avulsion fractures frequently occur concomitantly with lateral ankle sprains. Avulsion fractures of the distal fibula occur with an incidence as high as 60 to 70% of children with ankle sprains. Of note, individuals with avulsion fractures have a higher risk of recurrent ankle sprain occurring within 2 years than those without avulsion fractures.

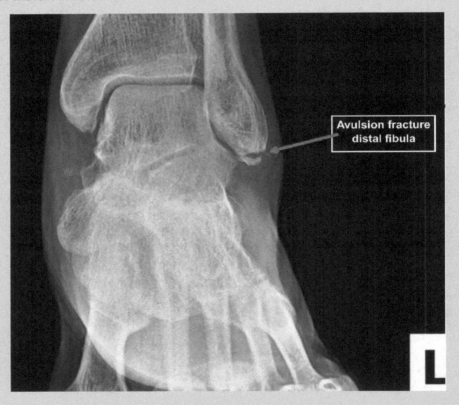

Fig. 4.129 - Lateral malleolus avulsion fracture. Image Credit: Modified by Barry A. Broughton, PhD. Original by Timdwilliamson, [CC BY-SA 4.0], via Wikimedia Commons.

Foot

Extending from the ankle as the terminal end of the lower extremity, the foot consists of 26 bones and 33 joints. The foot is a flexible structure of bones and soft tissue that allows humans to stand upright and perform activities like walking, running, and jumping. The bony architecture of the foot provides support for the soft tissues; helping it to withstand the weight of the body while standing and in motion.

The foot is divided into three distinct sections:

- The hindfoot is formed by the ankle and heel. The talus (a tarsal bone) supports the tibia and fibula of the leg, forming the ankle. The talus articulates with the calcaneus (heel bone), the largest bone in the foot.

- The midfoot is a pyramid-like row of the remaining tarsal bones that forms the arch of the foot. These include the three cuneiform bones, the cuboid bone, and the navicular bone.

- The forefoot contains the five longer bones (metatarsals) and the five toes (phalanges).

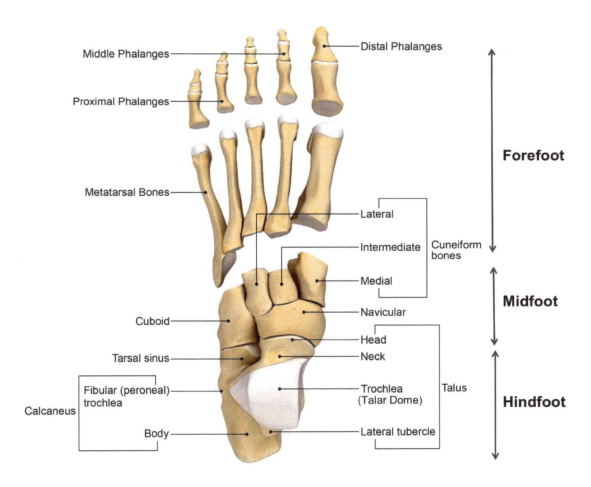

Fig. 4.130 - Bones of the left foot.

▪ Tarsals

The seven tarsal bones are organized into three rows (proximal, intermediate, and distal) which form the hindfoot and midfoot sections of the foot. The tarsal bones include the talus, calcaneus, navicular, cuboid, and the three cuneiforms (lateral, intermediate, medial).

- The talus, or ankle bone, is the most superior of the tarsal bones. The talar dome is wider anteriorly than it is posteriorly. Superiorly it articulates with the tibia and fibula of the lower leg to form the ankle joint. Anteriorly it articulates with the navicular bone as the talonavicular joint. Inferiorly the joint formed via the talus and the calcaneus is called the subtalar joint.

    The main function of the talus is to transmit the weight of the entire body to the calcaneus (heel bone) and foot.

- The calcaneus, or heel bone, is largest of the seven tarsal bones. It is positioned below the talus and plays an essential role in supporting body weight as the heel strikes the ground while walking. The posterior protrusion of the calcaneus forms the calcaneal tuberosity to which the Achilles tendon attaches.
- The remaining five tarsal bones form the arch of the midfoot. They include the navicular, cuboid, and the lateral, intermediate, and medial cuneiforms.

PLEASE REFER to Fig. 4.131 - Tarsal bones of the foot on next page.

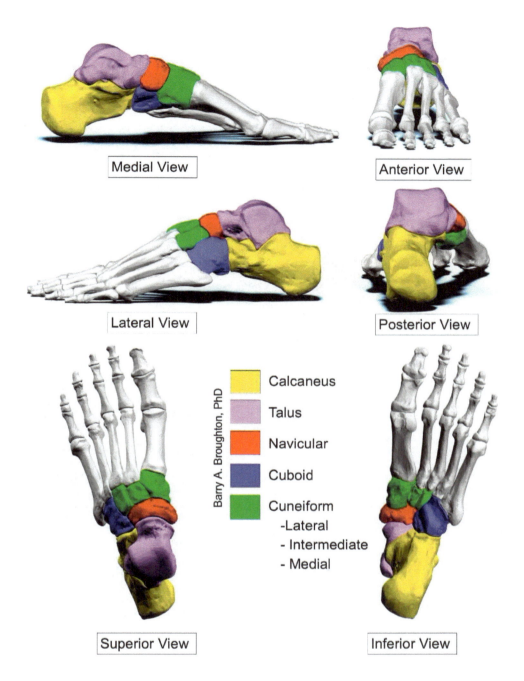

Fig. 4.131 - Six views of tarsal bones forming the arch of the left hindfoot and midfoot. Image Credits: Modified by Barry A. Broughton, PhD, Original by BodyParts3D is made by DBCLS., [CC BY-SA 2.1 JP] via Wikimedia Commons.

Subtalar Joint

The anatomical subtalar (talocalcaneal) joint is a synovial joint formed by the articulation between talus and the calcaneus. More specifically, between the posterior calcaneal articular facet of the talus, and the convex posterior articular facet of the calcaneus. These two bones are held together by the fibrous capsule, as well as the medial, lateral, and interosseous talocalcaneal ligaments, and the cervical ligament.

The primary movements that occur at the subtalar joint is supination and pronation.

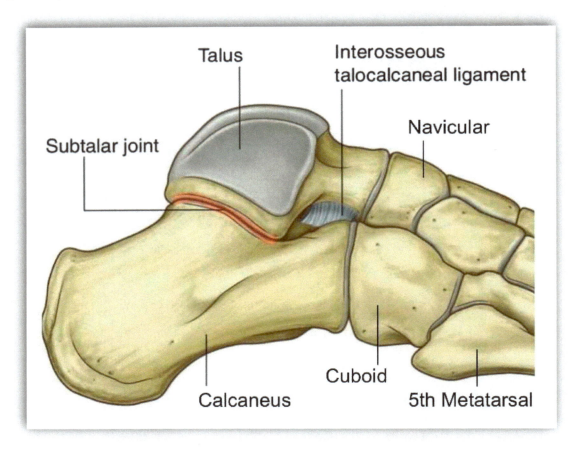

Fig. 4.132 - Lateral view of subtalar joint.

Clinically, the subtalar joint is considered as a functional unit formed by the anatomical (talocalcaneal) subtalar joint posteriorly, and its articulation with the navicular bone anteriorly (talocalcaneonavicular joints). In the middle of this functional unit is the cone-shaped interosseous tunnel forming the tarsal canal and tarsal sinus.

- **Metatarsals**

The metatarsal bones are the long bones in the forefoot, between the tarsals and phalanges, helping to maintain balance while standing and walking. There are five metatarsal bones, numbered one through five from the hallux (great toe) medially to the small toe laterally.

Each of the metatarsal consist of a proximal base, a shaft, a neck, and a head. The metatarsal base articulates proximally with the tarsal bones forming the tarsometatarsal joints. They also articulate with the adjacent metatarsal to form the intermetatarsal joints. Distally, the metatarsal heads form the metatarsophalangeal (MTP) joints with the proximal phalanx of each toe.

- **Phalanges**

Like the fingers, there are 14 small bones in the toes of each foot called phalanges.

The hallux (great toe) has a proximal and distal phalanx, while the remaining toes have proximal, middle, and distal phalanges.

The metatarsophalangeal (MTP) joint is formed by the metatarsal head and the proximal phalange bones. These joints form the ball of the foot. The joints between each of the phalanges are called interphalangeal joints. The interphalangeal (IP) joint of the hallux is formed by the proximal and distal phalanges. The remaining toes have proximal interphalangeal (PIP) joints at the articulation of the proximal and middle phalanges; as well as distal interphalangeal (DIP) joints at the middle and distal phalange articulations.

Clinical Significance and Martial Arts

- **Fractures of the Talus and Calcaneus**

Forming the bony architecture of the hindfoot, the talus and calcaneus transmits forces from the body to the ground. Therefore, they are the most frequently fractured of all the tarsal bones.

Talus

Fifty percent of all fractures of the talus occur in the talar neck. While fractures can also occur in the talar body or lateral process, talar head fractures are the least common.

Talar neck fractures typically occur from high-energy injuries caused by excessive dorsiflexion of the foot. The neck of the talus is forcefully pushed against the distal tibia causing the neck to fracture. The blood supply to the talus may be disturbed with talar neck fractures, leading to avascular necrosis of the bone.

Fractures to the body of the talus usually occur from jumping from a height.

Calcaneus

The calcaneus is often fractured as a result of falling from a great height, causing axial loading on the heel of the foot. Fractures to the calcaneus can also occur from improper breakfalls and striking the posterior heel on the ground or hard surface.

Even after appropriate treatment, calcaneal fractures can cause long-term problems. The fracture of the calcaneus extending into sub-talar joint frequently causes the joint to become arthritic in the future.

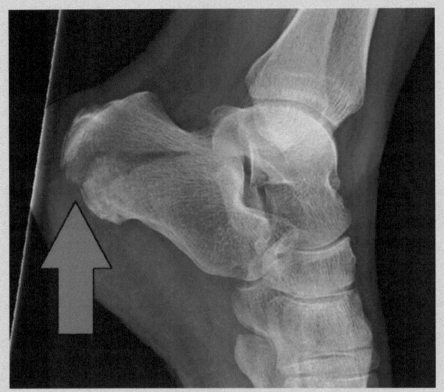

Fig. 4.133 - Lateral X-ray of calcaneus fracture. Image Credit: James Heilman, MD, [CC BY-SA 4.0] via Wikimedia Commons

▪ Fractures of the Metatarsal Bones

Metatarsal fractures occur most often from a direct blow to the foot. The metatarsals are vulnerable to being stomped on by someone else, a heavy object being dropping onto the foot, or from striking an opponent's elbow, knee, or head while executing a kick.

Excessive inversion of the foot can also cause the metatarsals to be fractured. If the foot is violently inverted, the tendon of the peroneus brevis (see next chapter) can cause an avulsion fracture at the base of the fifth metatarsal.

A transverse fracture at the proximal metaphysis of the fifth metatarsal, commonly referred to as a Jones fracture, is one of the most common fractures of the foot. Because of the poor blood supply at the base of the metatarsal, a Jones fracture may take longer to heal than most other fractures. In some cases, a Jones fracture may not heal at all, causing a nonunion that requires surgical intervention.

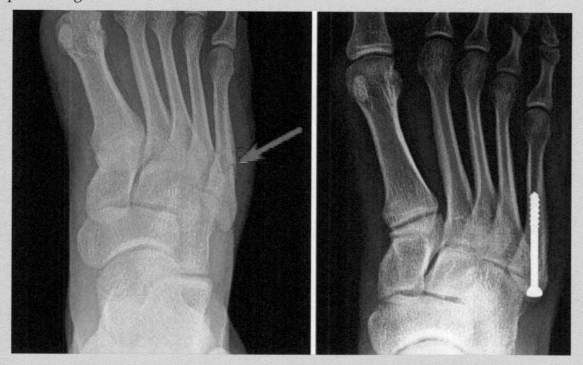

Fig. 4.134 - (Left) Red arrow shows a Jones fracture at the base of the fifth metatarsal. (Right) An intramedullary screw has been used to hold the bone in place while it heals.

Stress fractures of the metatarsals are also common in athletes. A stress fracture is an incomplete fracture that is caused by repeated stress to the bone. Metatarsal stress fractures occur most frequently at the necks of the second and third metatarsals and the proximal fifth metatarsal.

- **Plantar Fasciitis**

Plantar fasciitis (fashee-EYE-tiss) is the most common cause of heel pain. The plantar fascia is a long thin ligament that lies directly beneath the skin on the plantar aspect of the foot. The strong fibrous band connects the calcaneus to the metatarsal heads, providing support to the arch of the foot.
The plantar fascia absorbs the high stresses and strains placed on the feet during daily activities. Too much pressure on the fascia causes stress and micro-tears of the tissue. The body's natural response to these stressors is inflammation; resulting in the heel pain and the stiffness associated with plantar fasciitis.

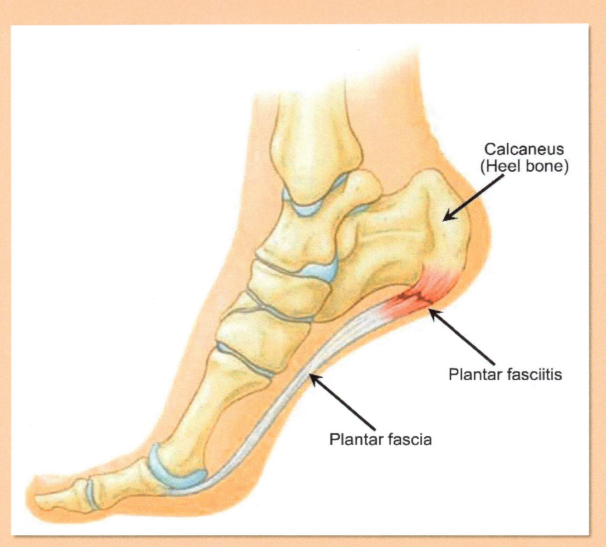

Fig. 4.135 - Too much pressure on the plantar fascia can damage or tear the tissues, causing heel pain.

The symptoms of plantar fasciitis include:

- Pain and tenderness on the bottom of the foot near the heel.

- Pain with the first few steps after getting out of bed in the morning, or after sitting for a prolonged period; the pain then diminishes after a few minutes of walking.

- Increased pain after (not necessarily during) exercise, activity, or prolonged standing.

Plantar fasciitis most often occurs without a specific identifiable cause. However, there are numerous factors that can contribute to the condition in martial artists:

- Tight calf muscles that limit dorsiflexion of the foot (bringing the toes up toward the shin). Repetitive impact activities, to include running and jumping.

- New or increased activities causing stress to the deconditioned foot.

- A change in footwear; or not wearing shoes when the foot is used to walking with a heel wedge.

- Obesity or a very high arch of the foot.

Although many people with plantar fasciitis do have heel spurs; heel spurs are *not* the cause of plantar fasciitis pain. Heel spurs can happen as a reaction to the stress and inflammation caused by plantar fasciitis. Over time the body responds to the stress by building extra bone tissue, forming a heel spur.

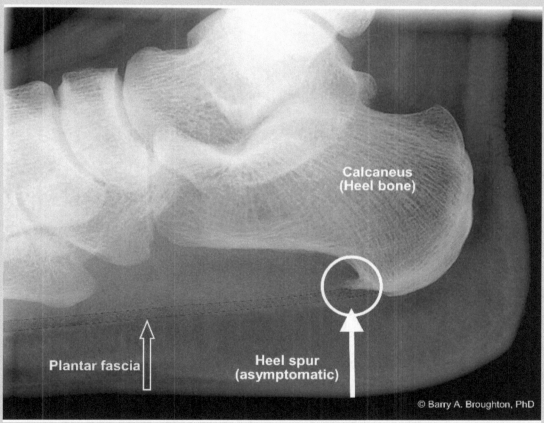

Fig. 4.136 - Heel spurs do not cause plantar fasciitis pain.

Because heel spurs are not the cause of plantar fasciitis but rather the result, the associated pain of plantar fasciitis can be treated without removing the spur (if one is present).

More than 90% of patients with plantar fasciitis improve with conservative treatment options to include:
- Stretching: Because plantar fasciitis is aggravated by tight muscles in the feet and calves, a diligent stretching regime addressing both areas is the most effective way to relieve the pain.
- Rest: Temporarily decreasing, or even stopping, the activities that make the pain worse may be of benefit while beginning a stretching program.
- Ice: Rolling the affected foot over ice or a cold-water bottle for 15-20 minutes several times a day is effective.
- Orthotics or cushioned shoe inserts while implementing daily stretching.
- Nonsteroidal anti-inflammatory medications.

Chapter 5

Introduction to the Muscular System

The muscular system contains three types of muscles: smooth, cardiac, and skeletal, that are responsible for movement within the human body. Consisting of approximately 700 different muscles, the muscular system makes up 40 to 50 percent of a person's body weight. Muscles are attached to bones, internal organs, and blood vessels.

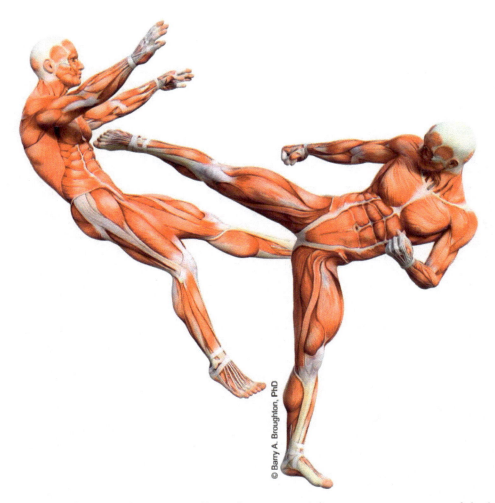

Fig. 5.1 - The muscular system allows for gross and fine motor movements of the human body.

The coordinated action of skeletal muscles upon bones and joints produces complex movements such as running, jumping, and kicking. Skeletal muscles are also responsible for more subtle movements such as respiration, facial expressions, and eye movement.

In addition to bodily movement, muscle contraction also aids in other crucial functions such as joint stability, posture, and the production of heat. The tendons of many muscles extend across joints contributing to their stability. This is especially evident in the shoulder joint, where muscle tendons are a major factor in its stability. Posture, such as standing is maintained because of muscle contraction. Skeletal muscles are continually making fine adjustments that maintain the body in stationary positions. An important by-product of muscle contraction is the production of heat. Muscle metabolism produces nearly 85 percent of the heat produced in the human body, providing a crucial role in maintaining body temperature.

Types of Muscle Tissue

Muscle tissue can be divided functionally as voluntarily or involuntarily controlled; and morphologically as striated or non-striated. Some involuntary muscle functions include heart beating, breathing, digestion, and eye reflexes; however, some of these actions also have voluntary control to a certain extent, i.e., breathing, salivation, swallowing, defecation, urination, and eye blinking.

The three types of muscle in the human body include: smooth, cardiac, and skeletal.

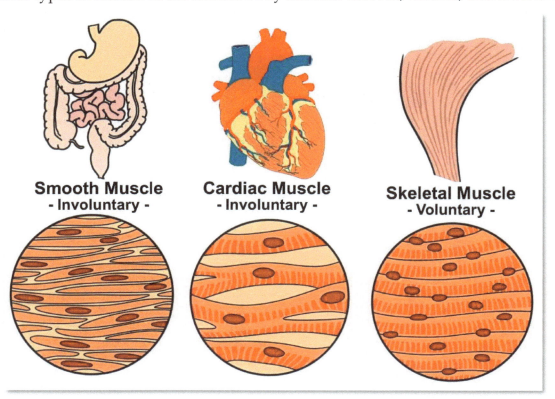

Fig. 5.2 - Type of muscle tissue include smooth, cardiac and skeletal.

Smooth Muscle

Smooth (non-striated) muscle is located the in the gastrointestinal tract, the walls of hollow internal organs such as the bladder, uterus, blood vessels, and throughout the body, including the eyes. Controlled by the autonomic nervous system (see next chapter), smooth muscle cannot be controlled consciously, and is therefore considered involuntarily muscle. The cell of smooth muscle is spindle-shaped and has one central nucleus.

Cardiac Muscle

Found in the walls of the heart, cardiac muscle is also considered involuntary muscle. The strong, rhythmical contractions of cardiac muscle is also controlled by the autonomic nervous system. Like smooth muscle, the cell of cardiac muscle has one central nucleus, but it also is striated like skeletal muscle.

Smooth and cardiac muscle will be discussed in greater detail in the chapters of their respective systems. Because of the physical nature of movement in martial arts and combat sports, this chapter will primarily focus on the skeletal muscle.

Skeletal Muscle

Skeletal muscle, also referred to as striated muscle, attaches to bones and is responsible for skeletal movement. Skeletal muscle is controlled consciously and is therefore considered voluntary muscle. The motor cortex (see next chapter) region of the brain is involved in planning, control, and execution of voluntary movements. The brain sends signals down the central nervous system to the peripheral nervous system to stimulate muscular movement.

The basic unit of skeletal muscle is the muscle fiber which contains transverse streaks called striations. Containing many nuclei, each muscle fiber acts independently of neighboring muscle fibers.

Structure of Skeletal Muscle

As with other organ systems, the muscular system contains a unique set of organs with distinct responsibilities. The specific organs of the muscular system are the individual skeletal muscles. Each muscle (organ) contains skeletal muscle tissue, connective tissue, vascular tissue, and nerve tissue.

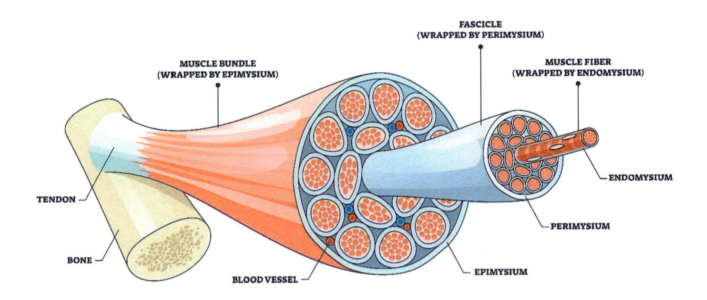

Fig. 5.3 - Structure of Skeletal Muscle.

Each individual skeletal muscle is composed of hundreds to thousands of muscle fibers (a single cylindrical muscle cell) bundled together and wrapped in a connective tissue sheath called the epimysium. The epimysium divides the muscle into compartments which contains a bundle of muscle fibers. Each bundle, called a fascicle, is surrounded by a layer of connective tissue called the perimysium. Within the fascicle, each muscle fiber is surrounded by connective tissue called the endomysium.

Because, like other cells in the body, skeletal muscle cells (fibers) are delicate, the connective tissue covering provides protection and support which allows them to withstand the forces of contraction. The connective tissue coverings also provide pathways for nerves and blood vessels. Separating individual muscles from each other, and from overlying skin are fibrous connective tissue sheets called fascia.

The endomysium, perimysium, and epimysium extend beyond the muscle belly to form either a tough, high-tensile-strength, cord-like tendon, or a broad, flat sheet-like aponeurosis. The tendon and aponeurosis form attachments to the periosteum of bones, or to the connective tissue of other muscles or organs (such as the eyeball). Typically, a muscle crosses a joint and is attached to bones at both its origin and insertion by tendons. One of the bones usually remains stable, while the other end moves as a result of muscle contraction.

Because the primary function of skeletal muscle is contraction, each muscle contains an abundant supply of nerves and blood vessels. For a skeletal muscle fiber to contract, it must first receive an impulse from a nerve cell. An artery and at least one vein accompany each nerve that penetrates the epimysium of a skeletal muscle.

Understanding Muscle Names

Individual muscles and muscle groups often have complex names that can be difficult to remember. Understanding how muscles are named will not only assist in recalling their names but also in knowing their purpose. Most skeletal muscles have names that are associated with its characteristics, location, and/or function.

The following list of terms relates to muscle features that are used in naming muscles.

- **Action:** flexor (to flex); extensor (to extend); abductor (to abduct); adductor (to adduct); levator (to lift or elevate); masseter (chew).

- **Location:** medialis (medial); lateralis (lateral); pectoralis (chest); brachii (arm); digitorum (digits, fingers, toes); gluteus (buttock); supra- (above); infra- (below); sub- (under or beneath), external (outer), internal (inner).

- **Size:** major (larger); minor (smaller); vastus (huge); maximus (large); longus (long); minimus (small); brevis (short).

- **Shape:** deltoid (triangular); rhomboid (like a rhombus with equal and parallel sides); latissimus (wide); teres (round); trapezius (like a trapezoid, a four-sided figure with two sides parallel).

- **Number of origins:** biceps (two heads); triceps (three heads); quadriceps (four heads).

- **Direction of fibers:** rectus (straight); transverse (across); oblique (diagonally); orbicularis (circular).

- **Origin and insertion:** brachioradialis (origin on the brachium or arm, insertion on the radius); sternocleidomastoid (origin on the sternum and clavicle, insertion on the mastoid process).

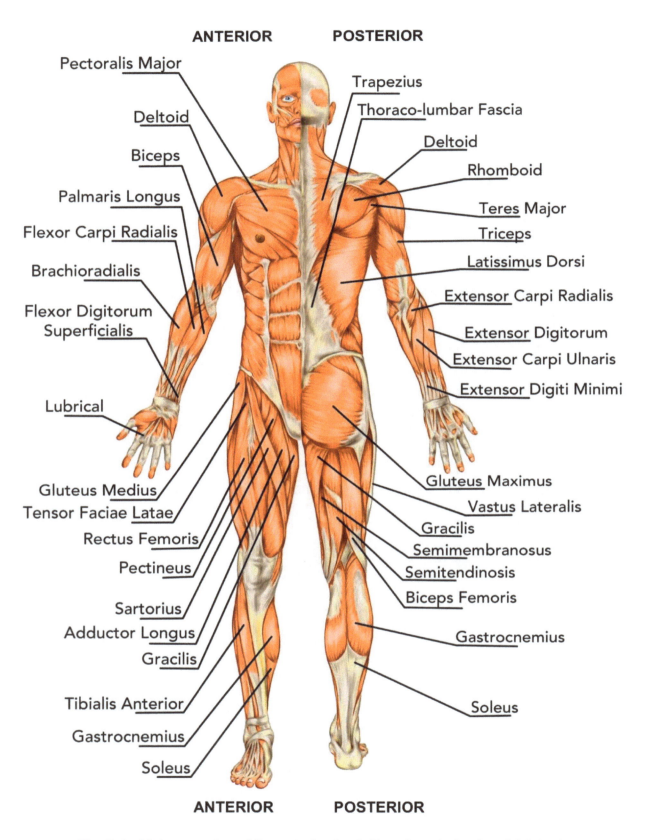

Fig. 5.4 - Major muscles of the anterior (on left) and posterior (on right) body.

Muscles by Region

Major muscles and muscle groups will be discussed briefly by region in the section.

Note: Please reference the Skeletal Muscles charts at the end of this chapter for specific muscles, their origin, insertion, and actions.

Muscles of the Head and Neck

Facial expressions are of crucial importance in nonverbal communication. Humans have well-developed facial muscles that allows for the expression of emotions such as excitement, fear, anger, surprise, disgust, and more. Controlling those facial expressions despite true emotions is of great benefit in self-defense and combat sports. Muscles that allow for facial expression include the *orbicularis oculi, frontalis, orbicularis oris, zygomaticus,* and *buccinator*.

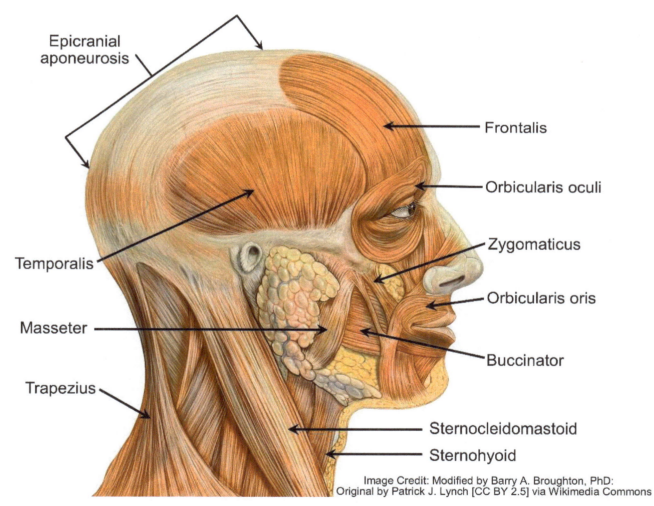

Fig. 5.5 - *Muscles of the head and neck.*

There are four pairs of muscles connected to the mandible that are responsible for chewing (or mastication). As some of the strongest muscles in the body, they include the *temporalis, masseter, medial pterygoid,* and *lateral pterygoid* muscles.

More than 20 neck muscles extend from the base of the skull and jaw inferiorly to the scapulae and clavicles. Providing stability and support to the head, neck, and cervical spine, they also assist in moving the head in different directions and aid in swallowing and breathing.

Muscles of the Torso

The muscles of the torso include those that form the thoracic and abdominal walls, those that move the vertebral column, and those that cover the pelvic outlet.

▪ Anterior Torso

The anterior muscles of the torso (trunk) include the chest and abdominal muscles. Chest muscles function in respiration while abdominal muscles function in torso movement and in maintenance of posture of and balance.

Muscles of the Chest

Pectoral Muscles

Pectoral muscles lie in the anterior chest and exert force through the shoulder to move the upper arm.

- *Pectoralis Major*: The pectoralis major is the most superficial muscle in the pectoral region. It is large and fan shaped, and is composed of a clavicular head and a sternal head:
    - Clavicular head – originates from the anterior surface of the medial clavicle.
    - Sternocostal head – originates from the anterior surface of the sternum, the superior six costal cartilages, and the aponeurosis of the external oblique muscle.
    - Insertion: The distal attachment of both heads is the greater tubercle of the humerus.
    - Action: Adducts and medially rotates the upper limb and draws the scapula anteroinferiorly. The clavicular head also acts individually to flex the upper limb.

- *Pectoralis Minor:* The pectoralis minor lies beneath the pectoralis major. Both muscles form part of the anterior wall of the axilla region.
    - Attachments: Originates from the third to fifth ribs and inserts into the coracoid process of the scapula.
    - Action: Stabilizes the scapula by drawing it anteroinferiorly against the posterior thoracic wall.

- *Serratus Anterior:* The serratus anterior is located in the lateral wall of the chest.
    - Attachments: The muscle is formed of several strips originating from the first to eighth ribs, each of which attaches to the scapula.
    - Action: Supports and rotates the scapula, allowing the arm to be raised over 90 degrees.

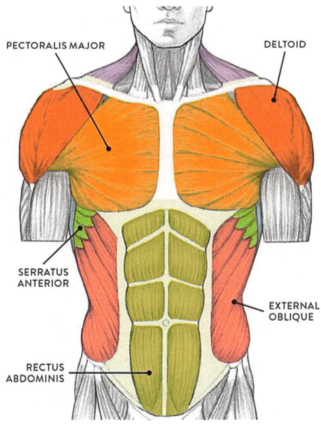

Fig. 5.6 - Superficial muscles of the anterior torso. Image Credit (modified): Medical Library, dorctorlib.info /anatomy/classic-human-anatomy-motion/6.html

Muscles of the Abdomen

The abdomen, unlike the thorax and pelvis, has no bony structures for reinforcement or protection. The skeletal muscles of the abdomen form the abdominal wall, which holds and protects the organs of the gastrointestinal system.

The five muscles forming the abdominal wall are divided into flat and vertical groups. The flat muscles act to flex, laterally bend, and rotate the trunk. The muscle fibers run in different directions and cross each other, strengthening the abdominal wall.

The vertical muscles aid in compressing the abdominal cavity, stabilizing the pelvis, and depressing the ribs while walking. The muscles form aponeuroses toward the midline, which merge into the linea alba.

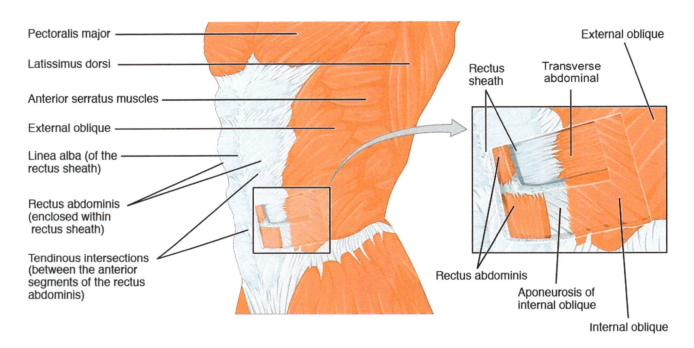

Fig. 5.7 - The anterior abdominal muscles include the medially located rectus abdominis, which is covered by connective tissue (rectus sheath). On the flanks of the body, lateral to the rectus abdominis, the abdominal wall is composed of three layers. The external oblique muscles form the superficial layer, while the internal oblique muscles form the middle layer, and the transverses abdominis forms the deepest layer. Image Credit: OpenStax College, [CC BY 3.0], via Wikimedia Commons

- *External Oblique*: The external oblique is the largest and most superficial of the flat muscles.
    - Attachments: Originates from the lower ribs and attaches to the pelvis, forming an aponeurosis toward the midline and linea alba.

- *Internal Oblique*: Lying deep to the external oblique, the internal oblique is smaller and thinner. Its muscle fibers run perpendicular to the external oblique, improving the strength of the abdominal wall.
    - Attachments: Originates from the iliac crest of the pelvis and thoracolumbar fascia. Attaches to the lower ribs and forms an aponeurosis toward the midline and linea alba.
- *Transverse Abdominal*: Consisting of transversely running muscle fibers, the transverse abdominal is the deepest of the flat muscles.
    - Attachments: Originates from the lower ribs, thoracolumbar fascia, and pelvis, forming an aponeurosis toward the midline and linea alba.
- *Rectus Abdominis*: A long vertical muscle that covers the length of the abdomen. Lying below the flat muscles, it is split through the midline by the linea alba formed from the aponeuroses of the abdominal muscles and separated by horizontal tendinous intersections giving the "six pack" appearance.
    - Attachments: Originates from the pubis and attaches to the lower edge of the rib cage and sternum.
- *Pyramidalis*: The pyramidalis is a small triangular vertical muscle that is superficial to the rectus abdominis.
    - Attachments: Originates from the pubis and attaches to the linea alba.
    - Action: Tenses the linea alba.

Clinical Significance and Martial Arts Relevance:

Abdomen vs Stomach

Frequently during instruction and training someone will use the misnomer of "punch the opponent in the stomach", or to "lie on your stomach". What they are actually referring to is the region of the abdomen; therefore, you would be striking the *abdomen* or be lying prone on the *abdomen*. The *stomach* is one of several organs within the abdominal cavity (See the *Introduction to the Digestive System* chapter).

▪ Intercostal Muscles

The muscles of the thoracic wall are involved primarily in the process of breathing. The *intercostal muscles* are located in spaces between the ribs. They contract during forced expiration. *External intercostal muscles* contract to elevate the ribs during the inspiration phase of breathing.

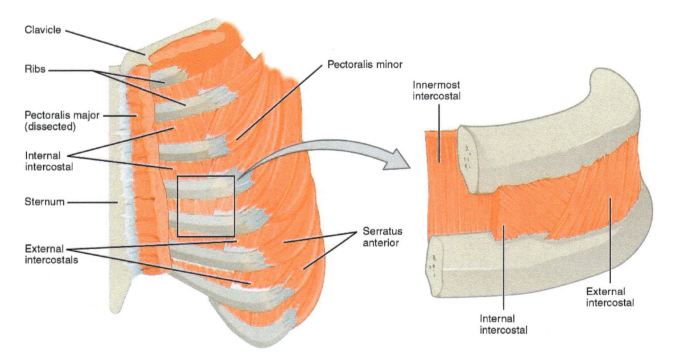

Fig. 5.8 - Intercostal muscles aid in the elevation and depression of the ribcage during respiration.

Image Credit: OpenStax, [CC BY 4.0], via Wikimedia Commons

▪ Diaphragm

The *diaphragm* is a dome-shaped muscle that forms a partition between the thorax and the abdomen. It has three openings in it for structures that have to pass from the thorax to the abdomen.

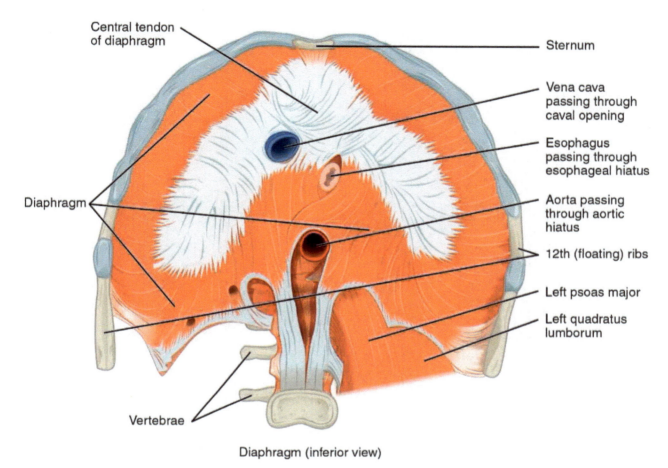

Diaphragm (inferior view)

Fig. 5.9 - Inferior view of the diaphragm separating the thoracic and abdominal cavities. Image Credit: OpenStax, [CC BY 4.0], via Wikimedia Commons

▪ Posterior Torso

Muscles providing movement and stability to the spine include flexors, obliques, and extensors.

- The **flexor muscles** attach to the anterior spine and enable flexing, bending forward, lifting, and arching the lumbar spine.
- The **oblique muscles** attach laterally on vertebra and helps rotate the spine and maintain proper posture.
- The **extensor muscles** attach to the posterior spine and are primarily responsible for extending the vertebral column to maintain an erect posture.

Muscles of the posterior torso can be divided into superficial, intermediate, and deep muscle groups.

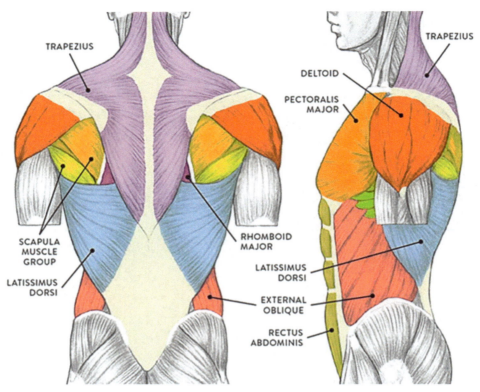

Fig. 5.10 - Superficial muscles of the posterior and lateral torso. Image Credit (modified): Medical Library, dorctorlib.info /anatomy/classic-human-anatomy-motion/6.html

The **superficial muscle group**, also known as the appendicular group, stabilizes and controls movements of the pectoral girdle. Arising from the vertebral column, they attach throughout the shoulder to assist in movement of the upper extremity.

Superficial muscles of the posterior torso include:

    A. Most superficial muscles include:

- *Trapezius:* The trapezius is a broad, flat, triangular shaped muscle. The muscles bilaterally form a trapezoid shape. It is the most superficial of all the back muscles.
    - Attachments: Originates from the skull, ligamentum nuchae and the spinous processes of C7-T12. The fibers attach to the clavicle, acromion, and the spine of the scapula.
    - Action: The upper fibers elevate the scapula and rotates it during abduction of the arm. The middle fibers of the trapezius adduct (retract) the scapula. The lower fibers depress and aid the upper fibers in upwardly rotating the scapula.

- *Latissimus dorsi*: The latissimus dorsi originates from the lower part of the back, where it covers a wide area.
    - Attachments: Has a broad origin – arising from the spinous processes of T6-T12, thoracolumbar fascia, iliac crest, and the inferior three ribs. The fibers converge into a tendon that attaches to the bicipital groove of the humerus.
    - Action: Extends, adducts, and medially rotates the upper extremity.

B. Covered by the trapezius are:

- *Levator scapulae*: The levator scapulae is a small strap-like muscle.
    - Attachments: Originates from the transverse processes of the C1-C4 vertebrae and attaches to the medial border of the scapula.
    - Action: Elevates the scapula.
- *Rhomboid minor*:
    - Attachments: Originates from the spinous processes of C7-T1 vertebrae. Attaches to the medial border of the scapula at the level of the spine of the scapula.
    - Action: Retracts and rotates the scapula.
- *Rhomboid major*:
    - Attachments: Originates from the spinous processes of T2-T5 vertebrae. Attaches to the medial border of the scapula, between the scapula spine and inferior angle.
    - Actions: Retracts and rotates the scapula.

The **intermediate muscle group** lies deep to the rhomboids and latissimus dorsi. With their origin arising from the vertebral column and inserting on the ribs, the following muscles assist in the respiratory effort:

- *Serratus posterior superior*: The serratus posterior superior is a thin, rectangular-shaped muscle.
    - Attachments: Originates from the lower part of the ligamentum nuchae and the cervical and thoracic spines (usually C7-T3). The fibers pass in an inferolateral direction, attaching to second to fifth ribs.
    - Action: Elevates second to fifth ribs.

- *Serratus posterior inferior*: The serratus posterior inferior is a strong broad muscle that lies beneath the latissimus dorsi.
    - Attachments: Originates from the thoracic and lumbar spines (usually T11 – L3). The fibers pass in a superolateral direction, attaching to the nineth – twelfth ribs.
    - Action: Depresses ribs 9-12.

The **deep muscle group**, also known as the **intrinsic back muscles**, lies deep to the thoracolumbar fascia. Associated with movements of the vertebral column the intrinsic back muscles are further divided into three layers:

1. Superficial (Spinotransversales) layer: The two muscles in this group are associated with movements of the head and neck.

- *Splenius capitis*:
    - Attachments: Originates from the lower aspect of the ligamentum nuchae, and the spinous processes of C7-T3/4 vertebrae. The fibers ascend, attaching to the mastoid process and the occipital bone of the skull.
    - Action: Rotates head to the same side.
- *Splenius cervicis*:
    - Attachments: Originates from the spinous processes of T3-T6 vertebrae. The fibers ascend, attaching to the transverse processes of C1-3/4.
    - Actions: Rotates head to the same side.

Note: Acting together, the splenius muscles can also extend the head and neck.

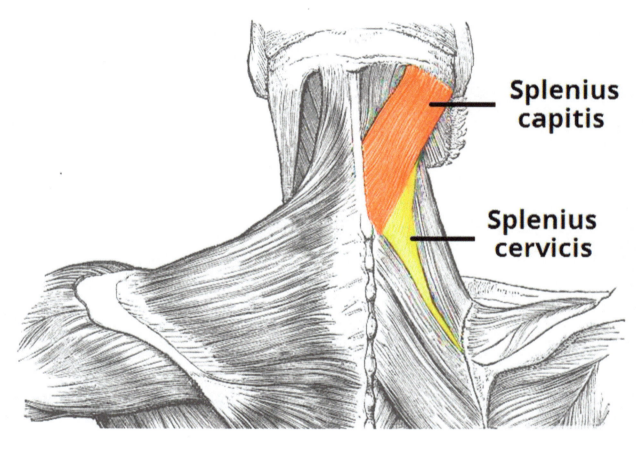

Fig. 5.11 - Spinotransversales layer of the deep muscle of the posterior torso.

2. Intermediate (Erector spinae) layer: These have a common tendinous origin from: Lumbar and lower Thoracic vertebrae, Sacrum, posterior aspect of Iliac crest, Sacroiliac and Sacrospinous ligament:

- *Spinalis* (*thoracis, cervicis and capitis*): attaches to spinous process of vertebrae and occipital bone of skull.
- *Longissimus* (*thoracis, cervicis and capitis*): attaches to transverse process of vertebrae and mastoid process of skull.
- *Iliocostalis* (*lumborum, thoracis and cervicis*): attaches to ribs and cervical transverse processes.

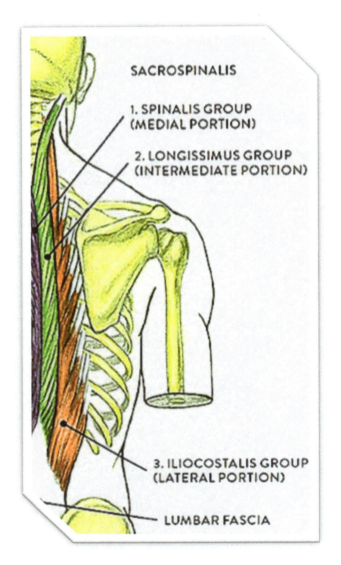

Fig. 5.12 - Intermediate muscles of the posterior torso. Image Credit (modified): Medical Library, dorctorlib.info/anatomy/classic-human-anatomy-motion/6.html

When contracted bilaterally, they function as the primary extensor of the back. Contracted unilaterally, they assist with lateral bending and rotation of the spine.

3. Deep (Transversospinales) layer: Originates from transverse process and inserts into spinous process:

- *Semispinalis* (*thoracis, cervicis, capitis*): From C4-T10 to C2-T4 and occipital bone (most superficial of deep muscle).
- *Multifidus:* Runs the entire length of the spine, traveling from Transverse Process to Spinous Process every 2-4 vertebrae (between *semispinalis* and *rotatores*).
- *Rotatores:* Runs from Transverse Process to Spinous Process every 1-2 vertebrae (deepest).

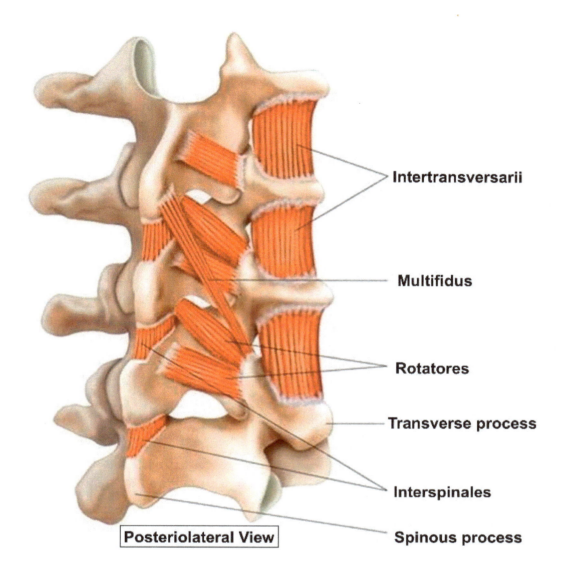

Fig. 5.13 - Transversospinales muscles.

These muscles assist in extending the back posteriorly when contracted bilaterally. When unilateral contraction occurs, they are responsible for assisting with lateral bending and rotation.

Muscles of the Upper Extremity

The muscles of the upper extremity can be divided into six different regions: pectoral, shoulder, arm, anterior forearm, posterior forearm, and the hand.

The muscles of the pectoral region (pectoralis major, pectoralis minor, and serratus anterior) are discussed in the Anterior Torso: Muscles of the Chest section of this chapter. Collectively, they are involved in the movement and stabilization of the scapula, as well as movements of the upper extremity.

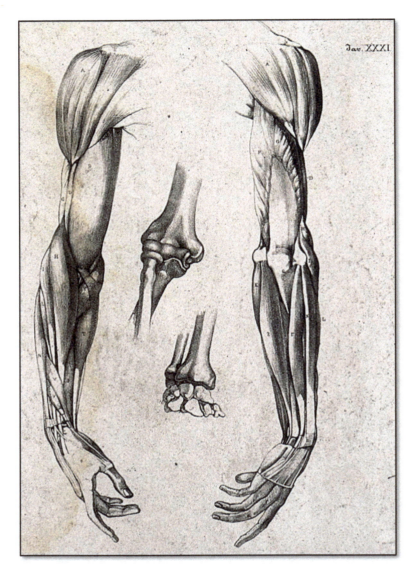

Fig. 5.14 - An 1839 lithograph by Battistelli of muscles and bones of the shoulder, arm and hand. Image Credit: Modified/cropped, Fæ, [CC BY 4.0], via Wikimedia Commons

The muscles of the shoulder are divided into extrinsic and intrinsic groups. The extrinsic muscles originate from the torso and attach to the bones of the shoulder. The intrinsic muscles of the shoulder originate from the bones of the shoulder girdle and attach the humerus. Collectively, they move the arm and stabilize the shoulder joint.

The arm, located between the shoulder and elbow joint, has anterior and posterior compartments. The muscles located in the anterior compartment are involved with flexion of the elbow and shoulder joint, whereas the muscle in the posterior compartment, the triceps brachii, extends the elbow joint.

Muscles of the forearm are divided into anterior and posterior compartments. The muscles of the anterior compartment are subdivided further into superficial, intermediate, and deep layers. Muscles of the anterior forearm act to pronate the forearm, and flex the wrist and digits of the hand.

The muscles of the posterior compartment of the forearm are subdivided into superficial and deep layers. These muscles are known as the extensors because of their general action of extending the wrist and fingers.

Hand muscles are also divided into extrinsic and intrinsic muscle groups. The extrinsic muscles originate from the forearm and attach to the bones of the hand. The extrinsic muscles are associated with more forceful movements of the hand such as making a closed fist. The intrinsic muscles both originate and attach within the hand itself and are involved with more delicate fine-tuned movements.

Muscles of the Shoulder

The muscles of the shoulder include intrinsic and extrinsic muscle groups that work together to provide movement of the arm and stabilize the shoulder.

The **extrinsic shoulder** muscles originate at the torso and attach to the clavicle, scapula, and humerus. These muscles include the trapezius, latissimus dorsi, levator scapulae, and the two rhomboids, which are discussed in the Muscles of the Posterior Torso section of this chapter.

The **intrinsic muscles** (scapulohumeral group) of the shoulder originate from the clavicle and scapula and insert on the humerus. The six scapulohumeral muscles include: the deltoid, teres major, and the four muscles of the rotator cuff (supraspinatus, infraspinatus, subscapularis, and teres minor).

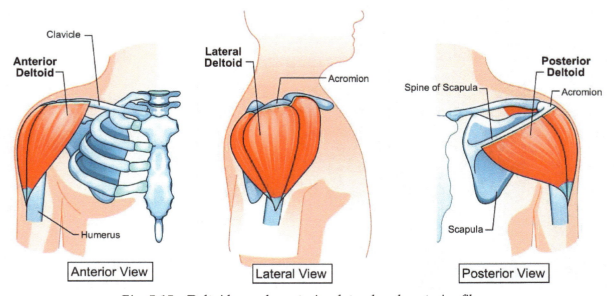

Fig. 5.15 - Deltoid muscle: anterior, lateral and posterior fibers.

- *Deltoid:* The deltoid muscle is shaped like an inverted triangle that provides the rounded contour to the shoulder. It can be divided into three distinct sections: anterior, lateral, and posterior.
    - Attachments: Originate from the lateral third of the clavicle, the acromion, and the spine of the scapula. It attaches to the deltoid tuberosity on the lateral aspect of the humerus.
    - Action:
    Anterior fibers – flexion and medial rotation.
    Lateral fibers – the major abductor of the arm (takes over from the supraspinatus, which abducts the first 15 degrees).
    Posterior fibers – extension and lateral rotation.

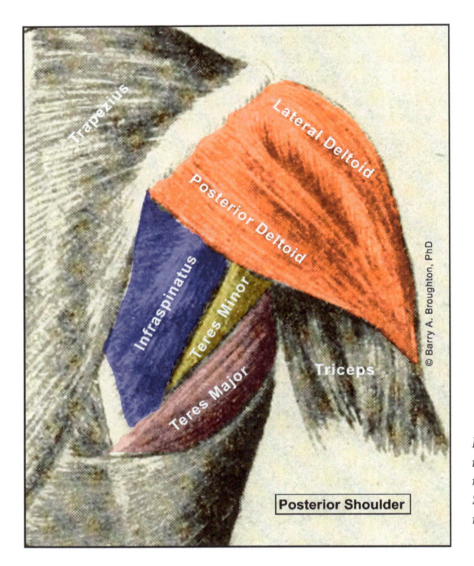

Fig. 5.16 - Poster shoulder intrinsic muscles: deltoid, teres major, teres minor, infraspinatus. Supraspinatus and subscapularis not shown.

- *Teres Major:* The teres major forms the inferior border of the quadrangular space – the "gap" that the axillary nerve and posterior circumflex humeral artery pass through to reach the posterior scapula region.
    - Attachments: Originates from the posterior surface of the inferior angle of the scapula. It attaches to the medial lip of the intertubercular groove of the humerus.
    - Actions: Adducts and extends at the shoulder, and medially rotates the arm.

▪ Rotator Cuff Muscles

The rotator cuff is a group of four muscles that provides movement and stability of the glenohumeral joint. Each of the four muscles have origins arising from the scapula and inserting on the humeral head. Collectively, they act to maintain the humeral head in the glenoid fossa, providing more stability than just the bony architecture while allowing for maximal range of motion.

In addition to the collective function of the rotator cuff, each of the individual muscles also have their own actions.

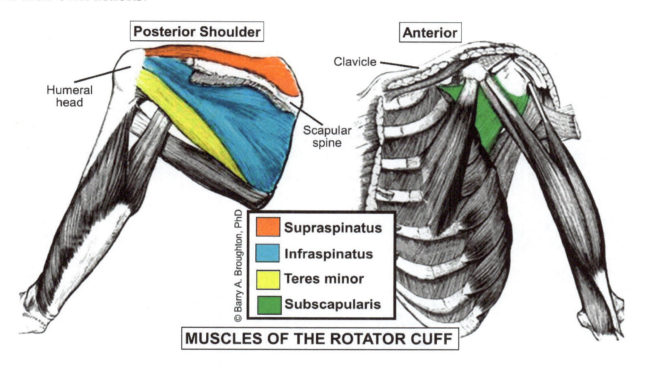

Fig. 5.17 – The muscle of the rotator cuff provides stability and mobility to shoulder joint.

- *Supraspinatus:*
    Attachments: Originates from the supraspinous fossa of the scapula, inserts on the greater tubercle of the humerus.
    Action: Abducts the arm 0-15°, and assists deltoid for 15-90°.
- *Infraspinatus:*
    Attachments: Originates from the infraspinous fossa of the scapula, inserts on the greater tubercle of the humerus.
    Action: Laterally rotates the arm.
- *Subscapularis:*
    Attachments: Originates from the subscapular fossa, on the costal (anterior) surface of the scapula. It inserts on the lesser tubercle of the humerus.
    Action: Medially rotates the arm.

- *Teres Minor:*
    Attachments: Originates from the posterior surface of the scapula, adjacent to its lateral border, and inserts on the greater tubercle of the humerus.
    Actions: Laterally rotates the arm.

Clinical Significance and Martial Arts Relevance:

▪ Rotator Cuff Tendonitis and Rotator Cuff Tear

Rotator cuff (not "cup") tendonitis refers to inflammation of one or more tendons of the rotator cuff muscles. The supraspinatus is most often affected. Rotator cuff injuries usually occurs secondary to repetitive use of the shoulder joint, most often overhead related type activities.

During abduction, the supraspinatus tendon rubs against the structures of the coracoacromial arch, which is formed by the inferior surface of the acromion, the coracoid process of the scapula, and the coracoacromial ligament which spans between them. Over time, the repetitive rubbing can cause inflammation and degenerative changes in the tendon itself.

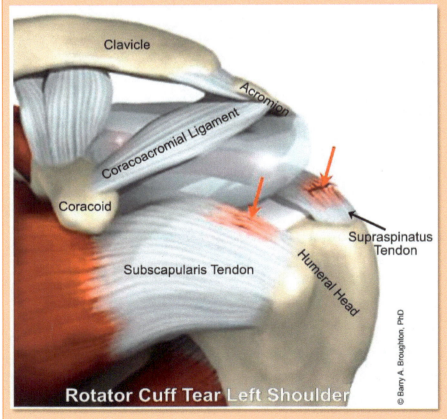

Conservative treatment of rotator cuff tendonitis usually involves rest, ice, anti-inflammatories, analgesic medications if needed, and physiotherapy. In more severe cases, steroid injections or surgery can be considered. Untreated chronic tendonitis can progress to a degenerative tear of the tendons of the rotator cuff. Partial or complete rotator cuff tears can also occur secondary to acute trauma involving a fall on the arm and shoulder or from heavy lifting.

Fig. 5.18 - Rotator cuff tears of the left shoulder.

▪ Bent Armbar

The bent armbar (also known as the Americana, figure four armlock, ude garami, keylock, top shoulder lock, chicken wing, paintbrush, and more) has as many variations for its application as it does names. Even though this type of shoulder lock can be applied from numerous positions, it has several key elements that remain the same.

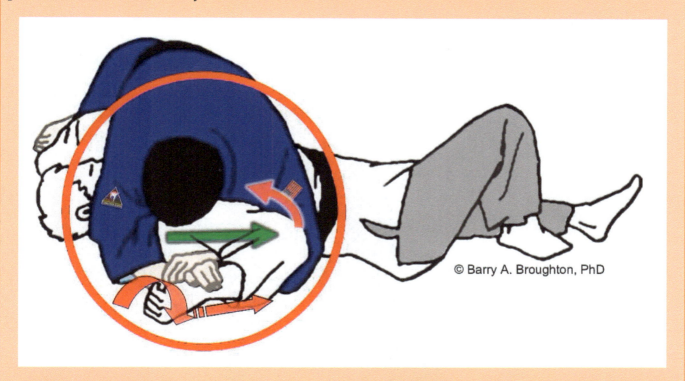

Fig. 5.19 - Bent Armbar from side control.

Execution of the bent arm bar is begun while the elbow of the attacked arm is bent (forearm flexed) and the arm (humerus) is abducted. While applying the bent armbar, the opponent's thorax must be stabilized to minimize movement of the scapula and clavicle.

Maximally pronating (rotating the palm outward) the forearm (with the elbow bent) rotates the radius over the ulna, which in turn helps to externally rotate the humeral head on the glenoid. External rotation of the humerus elongates the subscapularis. Adducting the attacked arm elongates the arm abductors, supraspinatus, and deltoid. With the resulting tightened glenohumeral joint, elbow/distal humerus range of motion is restricted; thereby shortening the height needed to lift the elbow/distal humerus (lever) before injury occurs.

Depending on the aggressiveness and variation of bent armbar being executed, anterior dislocation the glenohumeral joint may occur, as well as tears to the glenoid labrum, rotator cuff, and surrounding soft tissues.

Muscles of the Arm

The arm is located between the glenohumeral joint proximally and the elbow joint distally. Containing four muscles, the arm is divided into two compartments. There are three muscles in the anterior compartment (biceps brachii, brachialis, coracobrachialis), and one in the posterior compartment (triceps brachii) of the arm.

- **Anterior Compartment**

There are three muscles located in the anterior compartment of the arm: the biceps brachii (biceps), brachialis, and the coracobrachialis.

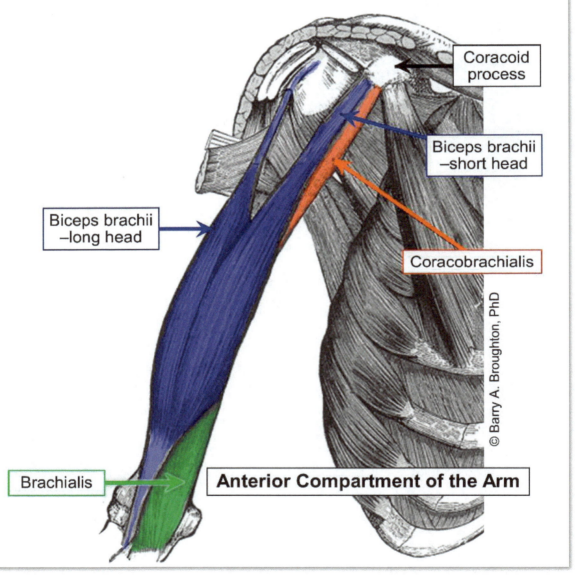

Fig. 5.20 - Muscle of the anterior compartment of the arm.

- *Biceps Brachii:* The biceps brachii is commonly referred to as the biceps. In Latin, the term brachii means arm. The biceps muscle is composed of two heads, a short head and a long head. The long head is located on the lateral side of the biceps, while the short head is located on the medial side. Although most of the muscle mass is located anterior to the humerus, the biceps is not attached to the humerus itself.
    - Attachments: The long head of the biceps originates from the supraglenoid tubercle (at the top glenoid) of the scapula, while the short head originates from the coracoid process. It inserts distally into the radial tuberosity, and the deep fascia of the forearm via the bicipital aponeurosis.
    - Action: Flexes the forearm at the elbow, and weakly assists flexion of the shoulder. Supination of the forearm.
- *Brachialis:* The brachialis muscle lies deep to the biceps brachii and is found more distally than the other muscles of the arm. It forms the floor of the cubital fossa.
    - Attachments: Originates from the medial and lateral surfaces of the humeral shaft and inserts into the ulnar tuberosity, just distal to the elbow joint.
    - Action: Flexion at the elbow.
- *Coracobrachialis:* The coracobrachialis muscle lies medial to the biceps brachii and the brachialis in the arm.
    - Attachments: Originates from the coracoid process of the scapula. The muscle passes through the axilla, and attaches the medial side of the humeral shaft, at the level of the deltoid tubercle.
    - Action: Flexion of the arm at the shoulder, and weak adduction.

Clinical Significance and Martial Arts Relevance:

Rupture of the Biceps Tendon

The two main causes of biceps tendon tears include injury and overuse. Falling hard on an outstretched arm, flexing the elbow against a resisted force (i.e., during grappling or throwing), or lifting something too heavy can cause a partial tear or complete rupture of the biceps tendon.

Many biceps tendon tears are also the result of overuse and fraying of the tendon that occurs slowly over time. This naturally occurs as we age, as well as with repetitive actives of the upper extremity.

The long head of the biceps tendon is more likely to be injured because it travels through the shoulder joint to its insertion into the superior aspect of the glenoid, making it more suspectable to rupture. The short head of the biceps rarely tears. Because of the attachment of *both* heads, most people can still use their biceps even after a complete tear of the long head.

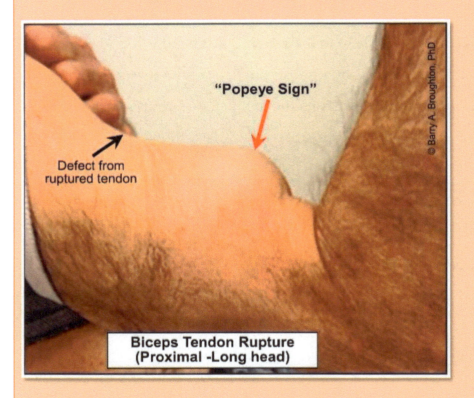

Fig. 5.21 - "Popeye Sign" resulting biceps tendon rupture.

A rupture of the long head of the biceps produces a characteristic bulge in the muscle belly upon flexing the elbow, often referred to as a "Popeye Sign". Those experiencing a biceps tendon rupture may feel and hear a popping sensation in the anterior arm and shoulder during injury. Initial severe pain may be also accompanied by swelling and ecchymosis (black and blue discoloration). After the initial symptoms subside, most people do not notice significant residual weakness in the upper extremity because of the action of the brachialis and supinator muscles.

Risk factors for rupturing the biceps tendon include age, smoking, obesity, use of corticosteroids, and overuse.

▪ **Posterior Compartment**

The posterior compartment of the arm contains the triceps brachii muscle. The triceps has three heads; the medial head lies deeper to the long head and lateral head, which cover it.

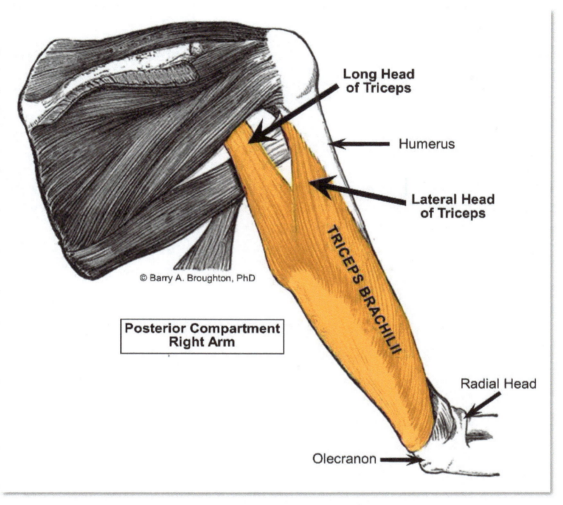

Fig. 5.22 - Posterior compartment of the arm contains the triceps brachii muscle.

- *Triceps Brachii*:
    - Attachments: Long head – originates from the infraglenoid tubercle (at the bottom of the glenoid) of the scapula. Lateral head – originates from the humerus superior to the radial groove. Medial head – originates from the humerus inferior to the radial groove. Distally the three heads converge onto one tendon and insert into the olecranon of the ulna.
    - Action: Extension of the arm at the elbow.

Muscles of the Forearm

The forearm is located between the elbow joint proximally and the wrist distally. Divided into two compartments (the anterior and posterior compartments), the twenty muscles located in the forearm provide movement of the forearm, wrist, and fingers.

▪ Anterior Compartment of the Forearm

The muscles in the anterior compartment of the forearm are subdivided into three layers: superficial, intermediate, and deep.

In general, muscles in the anterior compartment of the forearm perform flexion at the wrist and fingers, and pronation.

Superficial Layer

The superficial muscles in the anterior compartment are the flexor carpi ulnaris, palmaris longus, flexor carpi radialis, and pronator teres. They all originate from a common tendon, which arises from the medial epicondyle of the humerus.

- *Flexor Carpi Ulnaris:*
    - Attachments: Originates from the medial epicondyle with the other superficial flexors. It also has a long origin from the ulna. It passes into the wrist and attaches to the pisiform carpal bone.
    - Action: Flexion and adduction at the wrist.
- *Palmaris Longus:* The palmaris longus may be absent in about 15% of the population.
    - Attachments: Originates from the medial epicondyle, attaches to the flexor retinaculum of the wrist.
    - Actions: Flexion at the wrist.
- *Flexor Carpi Radialis:*
    - Attachments: Originates from the medial epicondyle, attaches to the base of metacarpals II and III.
    - Action: Flexion and abduction at the wrist.
- *Pronator Teres:* The lateral border of the pronator teres forms the medial border of the cubital fossa, an anatomical triangle located over the elbow.
    - Attachments: It has two origins, one from the medial epicondyle, and the other from the coronoid process of the ulna. It attaches laterally to the mid-shaft of the radius.
    - Action: Pronation of the forearm.

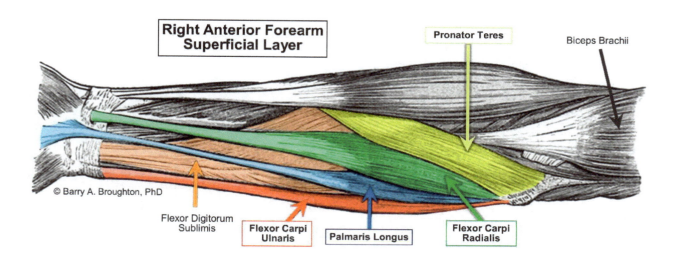

Fig. 5.23 – The superficial muscles of the anterior forearm.

Intermediate Layer

Lying between the superficial and deep layers, the flexor digitorum sublimis is the only muscle in the intermediate layer of the forearm. In some individuals, the flexor digitorum sublimis can sometimes be classified as a superficial muscle and is therefore also referred to as the flexor digitorum superficialis.

- *Flexor Digitorum Sublimis (FDS):* The FDS muscle is a good surgical landmark in the forearm because the median nerve and ulnar artery pass between its two heads, and then travels posteriorly.

    Attachments: Contains two heads proximally: one originates from the medial epicondyle of the humerus, while the other originates from the radius. The muscle splits into four tendons at the wrist, then travels through the carpal tunnel, and attaches to the middle phalanges of the four fingers.

    Action: Flexes the metacarpophalangeal joints and proximal interphalangeal joints at the four fingers, and flexes the wrist.

Deep Layer

There are three muscles in the deep layer of the forearm anterior compartment: flexor digitorum profundus, flexor pollicis longus, and pronator quadratus.

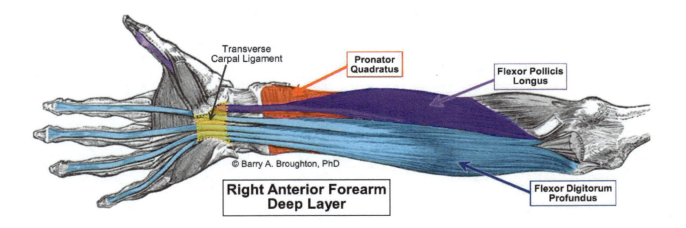

Fig. 5.24 – Deep flexor muscles of the anterior forearm.

- *Flexor Digitorum Profundus (FDP):*
    - Attachments: Originates from the ulna and associated interosseous membrane. As it progresses distally it splits into four tendons that pass through the carpal tunnel at the wrist. The tendons insert into the distal phalanges of the four fingers.
    - Action: The FDP is the only muscle that can flex the distal interphalangeal joints of the fingers. It also flexes at metacarpophalangeal joints and at the wrist.
- *Flexor Pollicis Longus:* The flexor pollicis longus (FPL) lies laterally to the FDP.
    - Attachments: Originates from the anterior surface of the radius and surrounding interosseous membrane and attaches to the base of the distal phalanx of the thumb.
    - Action: Flexes the interphalangeal joint and metacarpophalangeal joint of the thumb.
- *Pronator Quadratus:* A square shaped muscle found deep to the tendons of the FDP and FPL.
    - Attachments: Originates from the anterior surface of the ulna and attaches to the anterior surface of the radius.
    - Action: Pronates the forearm.

Clinical Significance and Martial Arts Relevance:

- **Epicondylitis**

Most of the wrist flexor and extensor muscles located in the forearm have a common tendinous origin. The flexor muscles originate from the medial epicondyle, while the extensor muscles originate from the lateral epicondyle.

The significant force exerted on the origins of the flexor and extensor muscles during sports related activities can cause athletes to develop overuse injuries of the elbow. Repeated grasping against a resisted force (of either flexion or extension) causes strain at the origin of the affected muscles on either condyle. Epicondylitis results in pain and inflammation around the area of the affected epicondyle.

Medial epicondylitis is caused by the excessive force used in wrist flexion, while lateral epicondylitis is caused by excessive force used in wrist extension.

Because of their prevalence among athletes, lateral epicondylitis is often referred to as Tennis Elbow, while medial epicondylitis is referred to as Golfer's Elbow or Baseball Elbow. These injuries can also occur in martial artists and combat sport athletes, however, it is more common among those participating in arts that include grappling and throwing techniques.

Making a Proper Fist

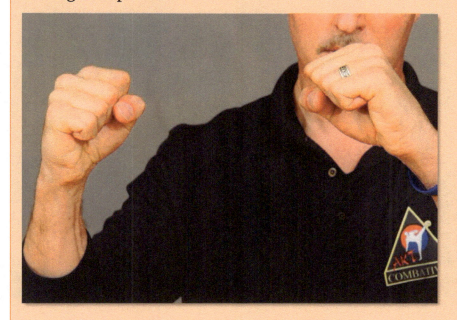

Fig. 5.25 - Making a proper fist. Image Credit: Beyond Self-Defense, Barry A. Broughton, 2016

In order to form a proper fist for actual striking, you must first understand that a fist is not just a closed hand. Even though punching is one of the first things taught in boxing and in most martial arts, surprisingly many people have never been taught how to correctly form a proper fist. Oftentimes they can close their hand in what appears to be a proper fist, yet it is ineffective for striking anything substantial. Additionally, striking a heavy bag or an assailant with an improperly formed bare fist (without tape or gloves) can cause a hyperextension or hyperflexion injury of the wrist, resulting in a wrist sprain.

Forming a proper fist is crucial in delivering an effective punch. I am not referring to only striking with the first two knuckles of the fist or aligning your hand, wrist, and forearm on the same plane as is often taught, though they are certainly important principles. I am referring to the true fundamentals of how to properly roll your fingers into the palm of your hand by contracting the forearm muscles — thereby making your fist, wrist, and forearm one solid unit that is used as weapon of personal protection.

The intrinsic muscles of the hand, located within the hand itself, are responsible for fine motor functions of the hand, not flexion of the fingers. It is the extrinsic muscles that are located in the anterior compartment of the forearm that are the primary muscles that aid in forming a proper fist. The extrinsic muscles control movement of the fingers and produce a forceful grip and fist. To flex your fingers and form a fist, your brain instructs your forearm muscles to contract. The contracted muscles pull and shorten the tendons that run across your wrist and insert into each of the bones of your fingers, pulling them sequentially into the palm of your hand. This might seem like a moot point, but, it is vitally important if your fist is intended to save your life.

To form a proper fist, start by fully extending your fingers. Keep the back of your hand, wrist, and forearm flat and in a straight line throughout the entire process of forming the fist. Using only the flexor digitorum profundus muscles of the forearm begin to flex only the most distal (DIP) joints of your fingers.

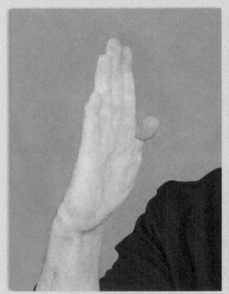
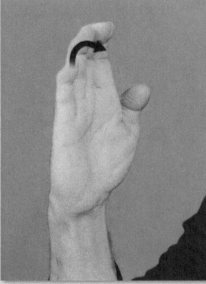

Fig. 5.26 and Fig. 5.27 - Keep dorsum of the hand, wrist, and forearm in a straight line. Contract the FDP to flex the distal (DIP) joints of the fingers. Image Credit: Beyond Self-Defense, Barry A. Broughton, 2016

Note: Do not form a fist with a bent wrist and *then* attempt to straighten and align the back of the fist with your forearm; in doing so you are weakening the wrist by keeping the tendons elongated, allowing your wrist to buckle and become injured when striking an actual target.

As the DIP joints become flexed, slowly allow the middle (PIP) joints of your finger to flex.

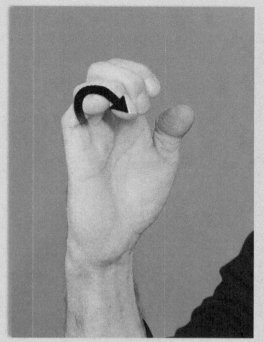 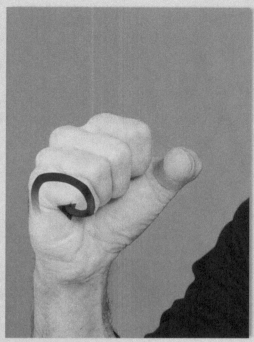

Fig. 5.28 and Fig. 5.29 - Continue to contract the muscles of the anterior forearm as the DIP, PIP, and MCP joints sequentially flex into the palm of your hand. Image Credit: Beyond Self-Defense, Barry A. Broughton, 2016

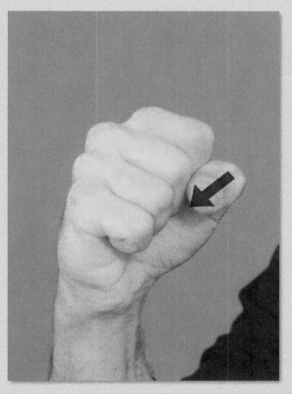

While keeping the hand, wrist, and forearm straight as you are flexing your fingers — envision the muscles and tendons of your anterior and posterior forearm pulling the metacarpal and carpal bones (of your hand and wrist) into the bones of your forearm. Continue to contract your forearm muscles, flexing and rolling your fingers into the palm of your hand.

Continue by contracting the flexor pollicis longus (FPL) and flexing the thumb into place over the middle phalanx of the index and middle finger.

Having maintained a straight hand, wrist, and forearm throughout the flexion of your fingers into the palm of your hand, you have now formed one solid stable unit that can be used as a weapon.

Fig. 5.30 - Contract the FPL to flex the thumb into proper position. Image Credit: Beyond Self-Defense, Barry A. Broughton, 2016

▪ Posterior Compartment of the Forearm

The muscles in the posterior compartment of the forearm produce extension of the wrist and fingers; and are therefore commonly referred to as the extensor muscles. The posterior compartment is divided into superficial and deep layers that are separated by a layer of fascia.

Superficial Layer

There are seven muscles in the superficial layer of the posterior forearm. Four of extensor muscles share a common tendinous origin at the lateral epicondyle: the extensor carpi radialis brevis, extensor digitorum, extensor carpi ulnaris and the extensor digiti minimi.

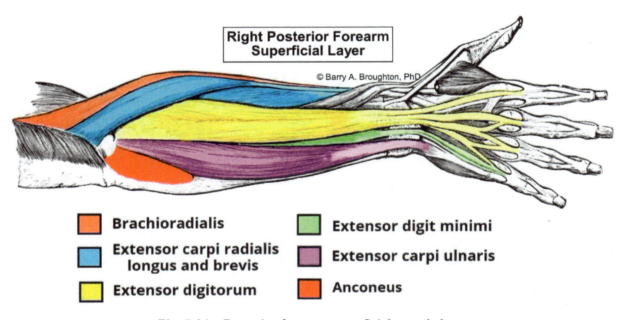

Fig. 5.31 - Posterior forearm superficial muscle layer.

- *Brachioradialis:* The brachioradialis is unique compared to other muscles in the human body because it originates from the distal end of one bone and inserts into the distal end of another bone. Its origin is characteristic of an extensor muscle, but it is actually a flexor at the elbow.
  The brachioradialis is most visible when the forearm is pronated and flexed at the elbow against resistance.
    - Attachments: Originates from the proximal aspect of the lateral supracondylar ridge of humerus, and attaches to the distal end of the radius, just proximal the radial styloid process.
    - Action: Flexes at the elbow, but also functions to supinate or pronate depending on the rotation of the forearm.

- *Extensor Carpi Radialis Longus (ECRL) and Brevis (ECRB):* The extensor carpi radialis muscles are positioned on the lateral aspect of the posterior forearm.
    - Attachments: The ECRL originates from the supracondylar ridge of the humerus, while the ECRB originates from the lateral epicondyle. Their tendons attach to second and third metacarpals.
    - Action: Extends and abducts the wrist.
- *Extensor Digitorum:* The extensor digitorum is the main extensor of the fingers.
    - Attachments: Originates from the lateral epicondyle of the humerus. In the distal aspect of the forearm the tendon splits into four tendons, inserting into the extensor hood of each finger.
    - Action: Extends the four fingers at the MCP and IP joints.
- *Extensor Digiti Minimi:* The extensor digiti minimi originates from the extensor digitorum muscle. The extensor digiti minimi lies medially to the extensor digitorum. In some people, the digitorum and minimi muscles are fused together.
    - Attachments: Originates from the lateral epicondyle of the humerus and inserts, along with the extensor digitorum tendon, into the extensor hood of the little finger.
    - Action: Extends the little finger and aids in extension at the wrist.
- *Extensor Carpi Ulnaris:* The extensor carpi ulnaris is located on the medial aspect of the posterior forearm.
    - Attachments: Originates from the lateral epicondyle of the humerus, and inserts into the base of the fifth metacarpal.
    - Action: Extension and adduction of wrist.
- *Anconeus:* The anconeus lies medially and superiorly in the extensor compartment of the forearm. It is blended with the fibers of the triceps; oftentimes the two muscles can be indistinguishable.
    - Attachments: Originates from the lateral epicondyle and inserts into the posterior and lateral part of the olecranon.
    - Action: Extends and stabilizes the elbow joint and abducts the ulna during pronation of the forearm.

Deep Layer

The deep layer of the posterior forearm contains five muscles: the supinator, abductor pollicis longus, extensor pollicis brevis, extensor pollicis longus, and extensor indicis. Excluding the supinator, the muscles of the deep layer act upon the thumb and the index finger.

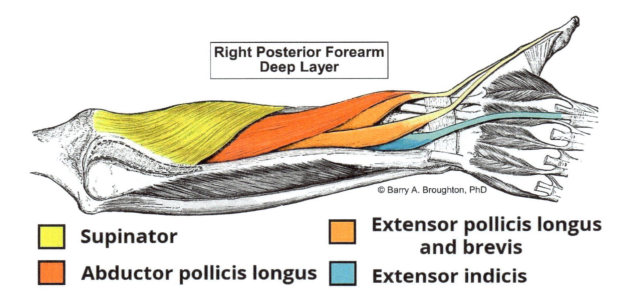

Fig. 5.32 - Posterior forearm deep muscle layer.

- *Supinator:* The supinator lies deep in the cubital fossa.
    Attachments: The supinator has two proximal heads: one originates from the lateral epicondyle of the humerus, while the second originates from the posterior surface of the ulna. They merge and insert together into the posterior surface of the radius.
    Action: Supination of the forearm.
- *Abductor Pollicis Longus:* The abductor pollicis longus lies just distal to the supinator muscle. Its tendon contributes to the lateral border of the anatomical snuffbox.
    Attachments: Originates from the interosseous membrane and the posterior surfaces of the radius and ulna. It inserts into the lateral side of the base of first metacarpal.
    Action: Abducts the thumb.

- *Extensor Pollicis Brevis (EPB):* The extensor pollicis brevis is found medial and deep to the abductor pollicis longus. Its tendon also contributes to the lateral border of the anatomical snuffbox.
    - Attachments: Originates from the posterior surface of the radius and interosseous membrane and inserts into the base of the proximal phalanx of the thumb.
    - Action: Extends at the metacarpophalangeal and carpometacarpal joints of the thumb.
- *Extensor Pollicis Longus (EPL):* The extensor pollicis longus muscle has a larger muscle belly than the EPB. The tendon of the EPL travels medial to the dorsal tubercle at the wrist, using it as a "pulley" to increase the force exerted.

  The tendon of the extensor pollicis longus forms the medial border of the anatomical snuffbox in the hand.
    - Attachments: Originates from the posterior surface of the ulna and interosseous membrane. It attaches to the distal phalanx of the thumb.
    - Action: Extends all joints of the thumb: carpometacarpal, metacarpophalangeal, and the interphalangeal.
- *Extensor Indicis Proprius:* The extensor indicis allows the index finger to be independent of the other fingers during extension.
    - Attachments: Originates from the posterior surface of the ulna and interosseous membrane distal to the extensor pollicis longus. Inserts into the extensor hood of the index finger.
    - Action: Extends the index finger.

Clinical Significance and Martial Arts Relevance:

- **Mallet Finger**

    Mallet Finger is an injury to the thin extensor tendon that extends the distal phalanx of a finger or thumb. Although it is also known as "baseball finger," this injury can occur anytime an unyielding object strikes the tip of a finger or thumb and forces hyperflexion of the DIP joint. The resulting injury prevents straightening (extension) the tip of the finger or thumb.

    The injury may rupture the tendon or pull the tendon away from its insertion on the distal phalanx. In some cases, a small piece of bone is pulled away along with the tendon, causing what is referred to as an avulsion injury.

    Mallet finger occurs most often in the long (middle), ring, and little fingers of the dominate hand. The distal finger is usually painful, swollen, and bruised over the DIP joint area. The fingertip will droop noticeably and will straighten only if you push it up with your other hand.

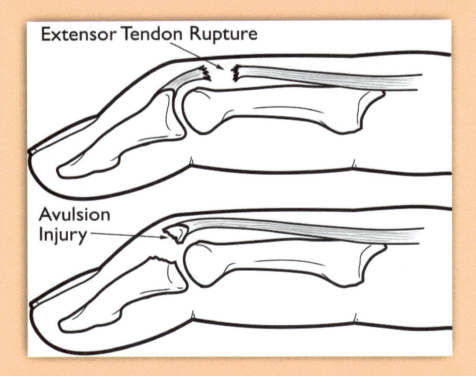

Fig. 5.33 - Top image: Mallet finger caused by a rupture of the extensor tendon. Bottom Image: Mallet finger caused by an avulsion fracture of the distal phalanx.

COMPREHENSIVE ANATOMY FOR MARTIAL ARTS

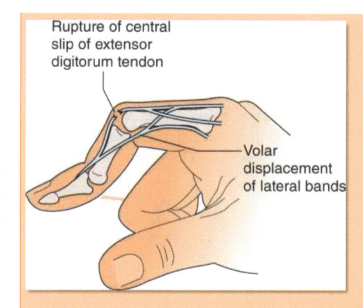

Fig. 5.34 - Boutonniere Deformity of the finger. Image Credit: Musculoskeletal Key

▪ A Boutonniere Deformity

A Boutonniere Deformity commonly occurs when the PIP joint is forcibly flexed while actively extended, or by a forceful blow to the top (dorsal) side of a flexed PIP joint. It also can be caused by a laceration over the PIP joint such as getting hit with an escrima stick. The resulting injury can sever the central slip of the extensor tendon from its attachment to the bone; allowing the lateral bands to slip below the axis of the PIP joint. The tear looks like a buttonhole ("boutonnière" in French). In some cases, the bone can pop through the opening. The deformity causes flexion of the PIP joint with hyperextension of the DIP joint, not allowing the finger to straighten. Unless this injury is treated promptly, the deformity may progress, resulting in permanent deformity and impaired functioning.

Jersey Finger

Jersey finger injury is a traumatic rupture of the flexor tendon (specifically the flexor digitorum profundus or FDP) from its point of attachment at the base of the distal phalanx.

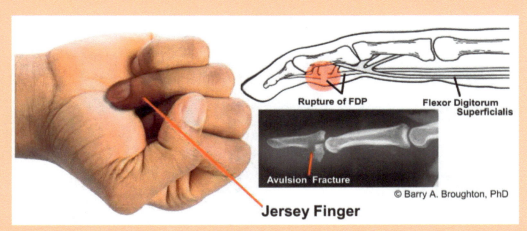

Fig. 5.35 - Jersey Finger right ring finger:
Top Right image via rupture of flexor digitorum profundus,
Bottom Right image via avulsion of the FDP from the distal phalanx.

The FDP tendon is responsible for flexing the distal interphalangeal (DIP) joint. Jersey finger occurs when there is a strong contraction of the FDP tendon that is resisted by a force into DIP hyperextension, such as occurs when a player grabs another player's jersey or gi top while the opponent is pulling away. Because the FDP is the only tendon that flexes the DIP joint, a jersey finger injury with a full rupture of the tendon causes loss of active flexion of the DIP joint. Approximately 75% of jersey finger injuries affect the ring finger.

Muscles of the Hand

Muscles that provide movement of the hand are divided into two groups: the extrinsic and intrinsic muscles.

As discussed in the previous section of this chapter, the extrinsic muscles of the hand are located in the anterior and posterior compartments of the forearm. The extrinsic muscles control the gross hand movements; as well as producing a forceful grip, and proper fist.

The intrinsic hand muscles are located within the hand itself and are responsible for its fine motor functions. This section addresses the anatomy of the intrinsic muscles of the hand.

- **Thenar Muscles**

The three short thenar muscles located at the base of the thumb are responsible for fine movements of the thumb. The three muscle bellies form the prominent bulge in the proximal lateral palm, known as the thenar eminence.

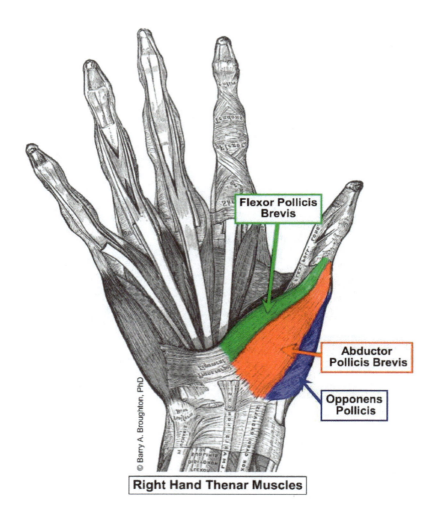

Fig. 5.36 - Thenar muscles produce the larger eminence in the lateral palm.

- *Opponens Pollicis:* The opponens pollicis is the largest of the three thenar muscles and lies beneath the other two.
    - Attachments: Originates from the tubercle of the trapezium and its associated flexor retinaculum. It inserts into the lateral margin of the metacarpal of the first metacarpal.
    - Action: Opposes the thumb by medially rotating and flexing the first metacarpal on the trapezium.
- *Abductor Pollicis Brevis:* The abductor pollicis brevis is located anteriorly to the opponens pollicis and proximal to the flexor pollicis brevis.
    - Attachments: Originates from the tubercles of the scaphoid and trapezium, and their associated flexor retinaculum. Inserts into the lateral side of the proximal phalanx of the thumb.
    - Action: Abducts the thumb.
- *Flexor Pollicis Brevis:* The flexor pollicis brevis is the most distal of the thenar muscles.
    - Attachments: Originates from the tubercle of the trapezium and from the associated flexor retinaculum. Attaches to the base of the proximal phalanx of the thumb.
    - Action: Flexes the metacarpophalangeal (MCP) joint of the thumb.

- **Hypothenar Muscles**

The three hypothenar muscles produce the smaller protrusion on the medial side of the palm, at the base of the little finger, known as the hypothenar eminence. The hypothenar muscles are similar to the thenar muscles in both name and organization.

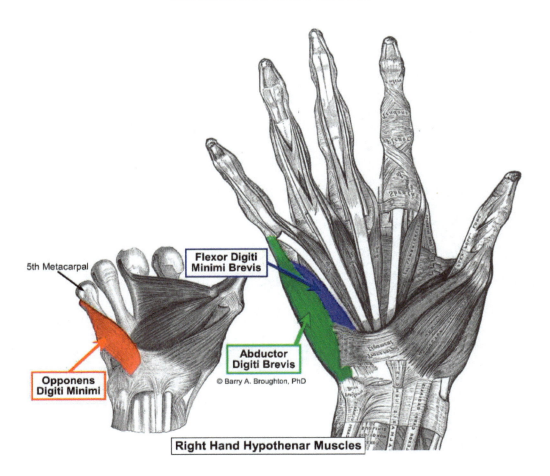

Fig. 5.37 - Hypothenar muscles produces the smaller eminence in the medial palm.

- *Opponens Digiti Minimi:* The opponens digit minimi lies beneath to the other two hypothenar muscles.
    - Attachments: Originates from the hook of hamate and its associated flexor retinaculum. Inserts into the medial margin of the fifth metacarpal.
    - Action: It rotates the metacarpal of the little finger towards the palm, producing opposition towards the thumb.
- *Abductor Digiti Minimi:* The abductor digiti minimi is the most superficial of the hypothenar muscles.
    - Attachments: Originates from the pisiform and the tendon of the flexor carpi ulnaris. It inserts into the base of the proximal phalanx of the little finger.
    - Action: Abducts the little finger.

- *Flexor Digiti Minimi Brevis:* The flexor digiti minimi brevis lies laterally to the abductor digiti minimi.
    - Attachments: Originates from the hook of hamate and the adjacent flexor retinaculum. Inserts into the base of the proximal phalanx of the little finger.
    - Action: Flexes the fifth MCP joint.

- **Interossei**

The interossei muscles are located between the metacarpals and are divided into two groups: the palmar and dorsal interossei.

In addition to their actions of adduction (palmar interossei) and abduction (dorsal interossei) of the fingers, the interossei also assist the lumbricals in flexion at the MCP joints and extension at the interphalangeal (IP) joints.

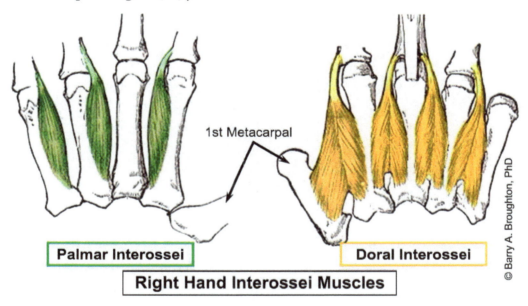

Fig. 5.38 - Interossei muscles of the hand.

- *Palmar Interossei:* The palmar interossei are located anteriorly on the hand.
    - Attachments: Each interossei originates from a medial or lateral surface of a metacarpal and inserts into the extensor hood and proximal phalanx of same finger.
    - Action: Adducts the fingers at the MCP joint.
- *Dorsal Interossei:* The four dorsal interossei muscles lie in the dorsum of the hand.
    - Attachments: Each interossei originates from the lateral and medial surfaces of the metacarpals and inserts into the extensor hood and proximal phalanx of each finger.
    - Action: Abduct the fingers at the MCP joint.

▪ **Lumbricals**

There are four lumbrical muscles in the hand, each associated with a finger. Connecting the extensor tendons to the flexor tendons, the lumbricals are crucial to movement of the fingers.

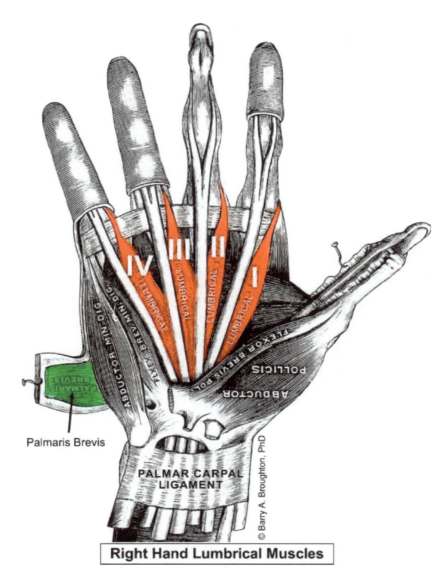

Fig. 5.39 - Lumbrical muscles of the hand.

- *Lumbricals:*
    - Attachments: Each lumbrical originates from a tendon of the flexor digitorum profundus. Each lumbrical passes laterally and dorsally around its associated finger and inserts into the extensor hood.
    - Action: Flexion at the MCP joint and extension at the interphalangeal (IP) joints of each digit.

- **Muscles in the Palm of the Hand**

There are two remaining muscles in the palm of the hand:

- *Adductor Pollicis:* The adductor pollicis is a large triangular muscle containing two heads. The radial artery passes between the two heads forming the deep palmar arch.
    Attachments: One head originates from third metacarpal. The second head originates from the capitate and adjacent areas of second and third metacarpals. They merge and insert into the base of the proximal phalanx of the thumb.
    Action: Adductor of the thumb.

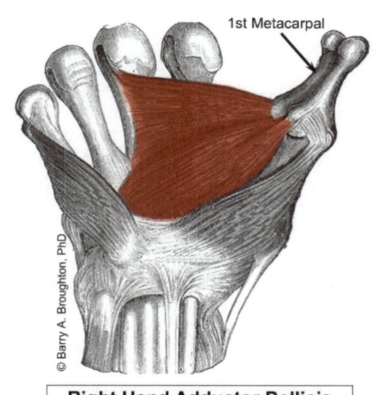

Fig. 5.40 – Adductor pollicis muscle of hand.

- *Palmaris Brevis:* The palmaris brevis is a small, thin, muscle found superficially in the subcutaneous tissue of the hypothenar eminence.
    - Attachments: Originates from the palmar aponeurosis and flexor retinaculum and attaches to the dermis of the skin on the medial margin of the hand.
    - Action: Wrinkles the skin of the hypothenar eminence and deepens the curvature of the hand, improving the grip.

Muscles of the Lower Extremity

The muscles that move the thigh all have their origins on some part of the pelvic girdle, with their insertions into the femur. Anteriorly, the iliopsoas flexes the thigh. The muscles in the medial compartment adduct the thigh. The posterior gluteal muscles (the largest muscle mass) abduct the thigh.

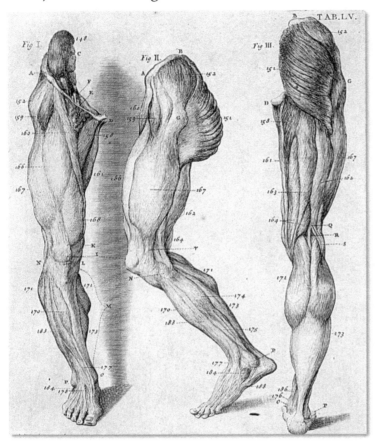

Fig. 5.41 - A 1724 detailed lithograph of muscles of the lower extremity. Titled: Myotomia reformata by W. Cowper Image Credit: Modified/cropped, Fæ, [CC BY 4.0], via Wikimedia Commons

Muscles of the Gluteal Region

The gluteal region, generally referred to as the buttocks, is located on the posterior aspect of the pelvic girdle at the proximal end of the femur. Its boarders include the pelvic girdle anteriorly, the iliac crest superiorly, and the gluteal folds inferiorly.

The muscles of the gluteal region move the lower extremity at the hip joint and are broadly divided into two groups: superficial and deep.

- **Superficial Muscles**

The superficial muscles of the gluteal region consist of the three glutei and the tensor fascia lata, which primarily act to abduct and extend the lower extremity at the hip joint.

- *Gluteus Maximus:* The largest and most superficial of the gluteal muscles, the gluteus maximus produces the mass of the buttocks.
    - Attachments: Originates from the posterolateral surface of sacrum and coccyx, the gluteal (posterior) surface of ilium, thoracolumbar fascia, and sacrotuberous ligament. Fibers run inferolaterally at a 45-degree angle and inserts into the iliotibial tract and the gluteal tuberosity of the femur.
    - Action: Main extensor of the thigh and assists with external/lateral rotation.

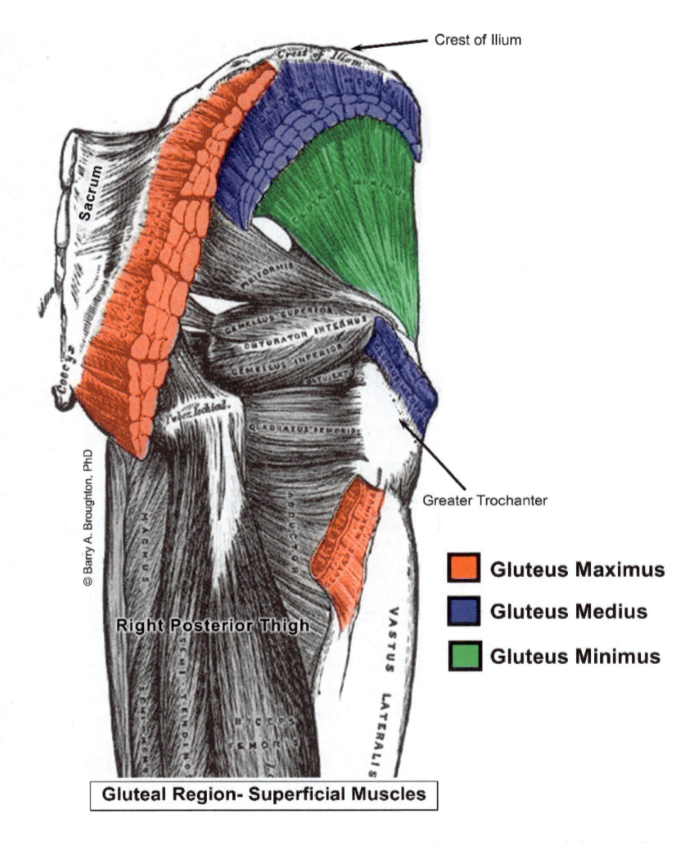

Fig. 5.42 - Superficial muscles of the gluteal region with cut-away of gluteus maximus and gluteus medius.

- *Gluteus Medius:* The gluteus medius is fan-shaped muscle that lies between the other two glutei (gluteus maximus and gluteus minimus).
    - Attachments: Originates from the gluteal (posterior) surface of the ilium and inserts into the lateral surface of the greater trochanter of the femur.
    - Action: Abducts and medially rotates the lower extremity. During locomotion, the gluteus medius stabilizes the pelvis, preventing pelvic drop of the opposite limb. The posterior fibers of the gluteus medius may also produce a small amount of external (lateral) rotation.
- *Gluteus Minimus:* The gluteus minimus is the smallest and deepest of the superficial gluteal muscles. The minimus is similar in shape and function to the gluteus medius.
    - Attachments: Originates from the ilium and converges to form a tendon, inserting into the anterior side of the greater trochanter of the femur.
    - Action: Abducts and internally (medially) rotates the lower extremity. During locomotion it stabilizes the pelvis, preventing pelvic drop of the opposite limb.
- *Tensor Fascia Lata:* Tensor fasciae lata is a small superficial muscle which lies towards the anterior edge of the iliac crest. It functions to tighten the fascia lata, and so abducts and medially rotates the lower extremity.
    - Attachments: Originates from the anterior iliac crest, attaching to the anterior superior iliac spine (ASIS). It inserts into the iliotibial tract, which itself attaches to the lateral condyle of the tibia.
    - Action: The tensor fascia lata assists the gluteus medius and minimus in internal (medial) rotation and abduction of the lower extremity. It also plays a supportive role in the gait cycle.

- **Fascia Lata**

Analogous to a strong elastic stocking, the fascia lata is a fascial plane that surrounds the deep tissues of the thigh. Encapsulating the musculature of the thigh, the fascia lata limits the outward expansion of the contracting muscles, making contraction more efficient.

Attachments: The fascia lata begins proximally around the iliac crest and the inguinal ligament. It receives fibers from gluteus maximus and tensor fascia lata laterally. Distally it inserts into the bony prominences of the tibia. The fascia lata is thickened at its lateral side where it forms the iliotibial band, a structure that runs to the tibia and serves as a site of muscle attachment.

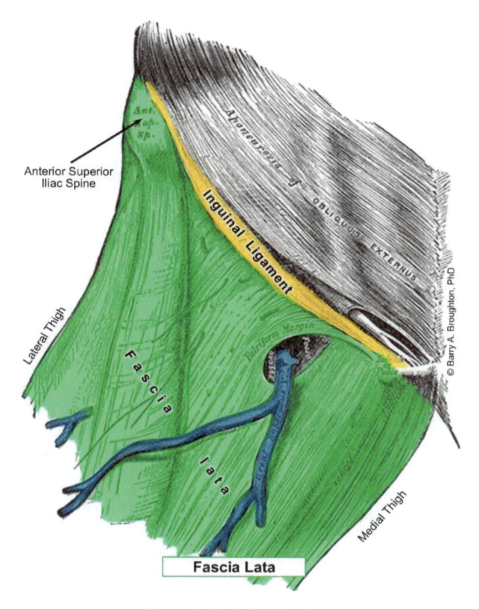

Fig. 5.43 - Right thigh fascia lata.

▪ Iliotibial Band (ITB)

The iliotibial band (or iliotibial tract) is a longitudinal thickening of the fascia lata. It is located in lateral the thigh, extending from the iliac tubercle to the lateral tibial condyle.

> Action: The IT band has three main functions: acts as an extensor, abductor, and external (lateral) rotator of the hip. To a lesser degree, it also provides lateral stabilization to the knee joint.

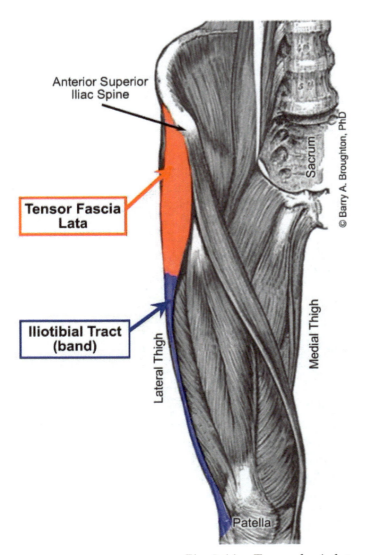

Fig. 5.44 - Tensor fascia lata muscle and iliotibial band.

- **Deep Muscles**

The deep gluteal muscles are a set of five smaller muscles located deep to the gluteus minimus. The primary action of these muscles is to externally rotate the lower extremity. Together they stabilize the hip joint by pulling the femoral head into the acetabulum of the pelvis.

Deep gluteal muscles include: the piriformis, obturator internus, gemellus superior, gemellus inferior, and the quadratus femoris.

- *Piriformis:* The piriformis is the most superior of the deep muscles.
  - Attachments: Originates from the anterior surface of the sacrum. It then travels inferior and laterally through the greater sciatic foramen and inserts into the greater trochanter of the femur.
  - Action: Lateral rotation and abduction.

- *Obturator Internus:* Bilaterally, the obturator internus forms the lateral walls of the pelvic cavity. In some texts, the obturator internus and the gemelli muscles are referred to collectively as the triceps coxae.
    - Attachments: Originates from the pubis and ischium at the obturator foramen. It travels through the lesser sciatic foramen and inserts into the greater trochanter of the femur.
    - Action: Lateral rotation and abduction.

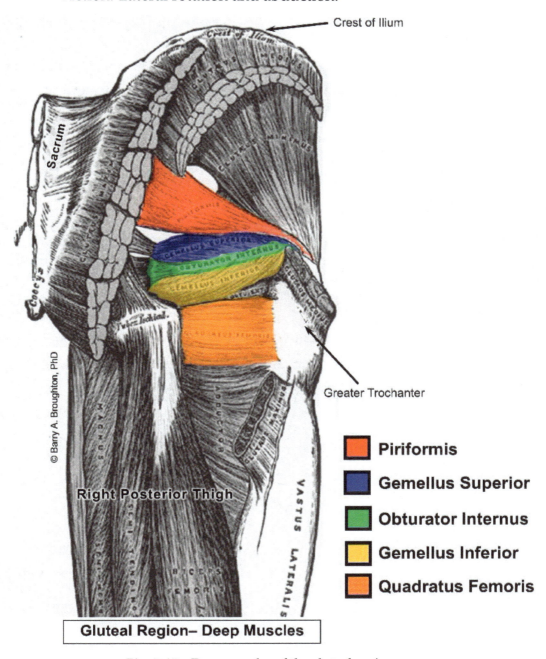

Fig. 5.45 - Deep muscles of the gluteal region.

- *The Gemelli – Superior and Inferior:* The gemelli are two narrow and triangular muscles. They are separated by the obturator internus tendon.
    - Attachments: The superior gemellus muscle originates from the ischial spine, while the inferior originates from the ischial tuberosity. They both insert into the greater trochanter of the femur.
    - Action: Lateral rotation and abduction.
- *Quadratus Femoris:* The quadratus femoris is a flat, square-shaped muscle. Located distal to the gemelli inferior muscle, the quadratus femoris is the most inferior of the deep gluteal muscles.
    - Attachments: It originates from the lateral side of the ischial tuberosity and inserts into the quadrate tuberosity on the intertrochanteric crest of the femur.
    - Action: Lateral rotation.

Muscles of the Thigh

The thigh is located between the hip joint proximally and the knee joint distally. The muscles of the thigh move the lower leg. The thigh muscles are divided into three compartments: the anterior, medial, and posterior compartments.

▪ Anterior Compartment

The muscles in the anterior compartment of the thigh act to extend the leg at the knee joint. There are three major muscles in the anterior thigh – the pectineus, sartorius, and quadriceps femoris. The iliopsoas muscle also passes into the anterior compartment.

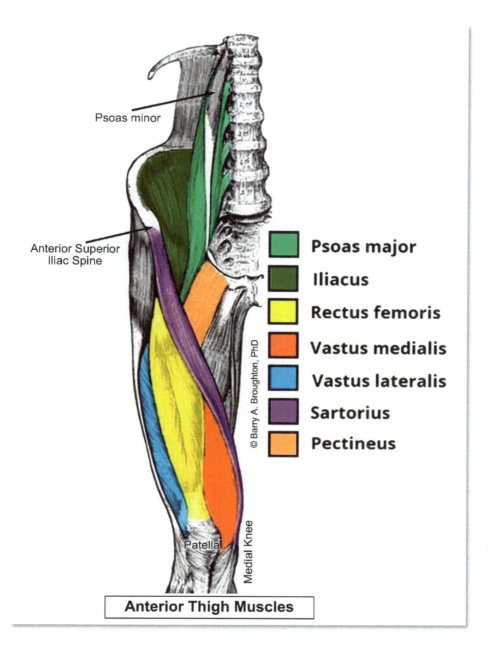

Fig. 5.46 - Muscles of the anterior compartment of the thigh.

- *Iliopsoas:* The iliopsoas muscle is formed by the psoas major and the iliacus muscles. Their origins are in different areas, but merge to form a common tendon, therefore are referred to as single muscle.

  Unlike other muscles of the anterior thigh, the iliopsoas does not extend the leg at the knee joint.
    - Attachments: The psoas major originates from the lumbar vertebrae, while the iliacus originates from the iliac fossa on the anterior surface of the pelvis. They insert together onto the lesser trochanter of the femur.
    - Action: Flexes the thigh at the hip joint.

- *Quadriceps Femoris:* The quadriceps femoris consists of four individual muscles; the rectus femoris and the three vastus muscles. Together, they form the bulk of the thigh, acting as the main extensor of the knee. Collectively the quadriceps is one of the most powerful muscles in the body.

  The four muscles of quadriceps femoris unite distally in the thigh (proximal to the knee joint) forming the quadriceps tendon. The patella (a sesamoid bone) is embedded in the quadriceps tendon acting as a fulcrum for extension of the knee joint. The tendon extends distally and inserts into the tibial tubercle. Because the quadriceps tendon extends beyond the patella and into the tibia, the patella tendon is sometimes referred to as the patella ligament.
  - *Vastus Lateralis:*
    - Proximal attachment: Originates from the greater trochanter and the lateral lip of linea aspera on the posterior femur.
    - Action: Extends the knee joint and stabilizes the patella.
  - *Vastus Intermedius:* Lies beneath the rectus femoris and anterolateral to the femoral shaft.
    - Proximal attachment: Anterior and lateral surfaces of the femoral shaft.
    - Action: Extends the knee joint and stabilizes the patella.
  - *Vastus Medialis:*
    - Proximal attachment: The intertrochanteric line and medial lip of the linea aspera on the posterior femur.
    - Action: Extends the knee joint and stabilizes the patella.
  - *Rectus Femoris:* The only muscle of the quadriceps to cross both the hip and knee joints.
    - Attachments: Originates from the anterior inferior iliac spine and the area just superior to the acetabulum. The rectus femoris extend distally and inserts into the patella via the quadriceps femoris tendon.
    - Action: Flexes the thigh at the hip joint and extends at the knee joint.
- *Sartorius:* The sartorius is the most superficial muscle of the anterior thigh. As the longest muscle in the body, it runs in an inferomedial direction across the anterior thigh.
  - Attachments: Originates from the anterior superior iliac spine, and inserts into the superior, medial surface of the tibia.
  - Action: At the hip joint, it is a flexor, abductor, and lateral rotator. At the knee joint, it is also a flexor.

- *Pectineus:* The pectineus muscle is a flat muscle that forms the base of the femoral triangle.
    - Attachments: It originates from the pectineal line on the anterior surface of the pelvis and inserts into the pectineal line on the posterior femur, just distal to the lesser trochanter.
    - Action: Adduction and flexion at the hip joint.

▪ **Medial Compartment**

The five muscles in the medial compartment of the thigh are collectively known as the hip adductors. The hip adductors include: the adductor magnus, adductor longus, adductor brevis, obturator externus, and the gracilis.

- *Adductor Magnus:* The adductor magnus is the largest muscle in the medial compartment of the thigh. It lies posteriorly to the other adductor muscles. Functionally, the adductor magnus muscle can be divided into two parts: the adductor part, and the hamstring part.
    - Attachments:
    - Adductor part – Originates from the inferior rami of the pubis and the rami of ischium, attaching to the linea aspera of the femur.
    - Hamstring part – Originates from the ischial tuberosity and attaches to the adductor tubercle and medial supracondylar line of the femur.
    - Action: They both adduct the thigh. The adductor component also flexes the thigh, with the hamstring portion extending the thigh.

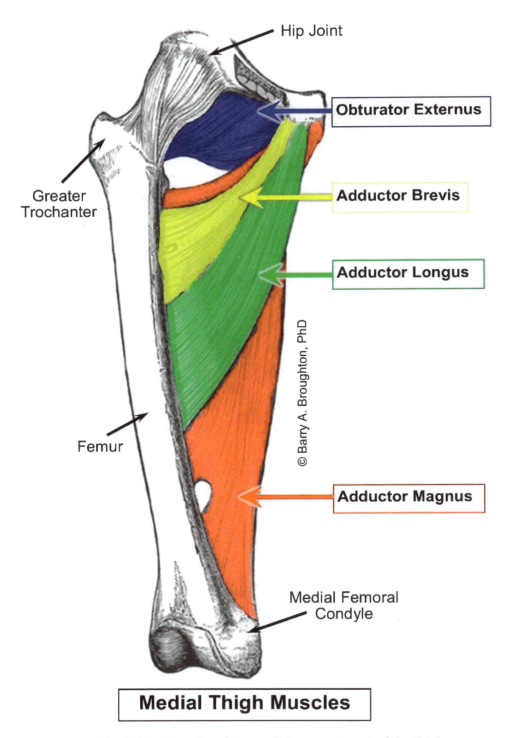

Fig. 5.47 - Muscles of the medial compartment of the thigh.

- *Adductor Longus:* The adductor longus is a large, flat muscle that partially covers the adductor brevis and magnus. The adductor longus forms the medial border of the femoral triangle.
    - Attachments: Originates from the pubis, and expands into a fan shape, attaching broadly to the linea aspera of the femur.
    - Actions: Adduction of the thigh.
- *Adductor Brevis:* The adductor brevis is a short muscle, lying beneath the adductor longus.
    - Attachments: Originates from the body of the pubis and inferior pubic rami and inserts into the linea aspera on the posterior surface of the femur, proximal to the adductor longus.
    - Action: Adduction of the thigh.
- *Obturator Externus:* Located most superiorly of the adductor muscles, the obturator externus is the smallest muscle of the medial thigh.
    - Attachments: It originates from the membrane of the obturator foramen, and adjacent bone of the inferior pubic ramus. It passes under the neck of the femur and inserts into the posterior aspect of the greater trochanter.
    - Action: Adduction and lateral rotation of the thigh.
- *Gracilis:* The gracilis is the most superficial and medial of the muscles in the medial compartment. It crosses both the hip and knee joints.
    - Attachments: It originates from the inferior rami of the pubis and the body of the pubis. It descends almost vertically down the thigh and inserts into the medial surface of the tibia between the tendons of the sartorius (anteriorly) and the semitendinosus (posteriorly).
    - Action: Adduction of the thigh at the hip, and flexion of the leg at the knee.

Clinical Significance and Martial Arts Relevance:

Osteitis Pubis

Osteitis pubis is a condition that affects the symphysis pubis (the joint between the pubic bones). The stress and shearing force of the muscles and tendons attached to it causes inflammation in the joint.

Osteitis pubis commonly occurs as an overuse injury in weight-bearing and kicking sports due to stretching of the pelvis.

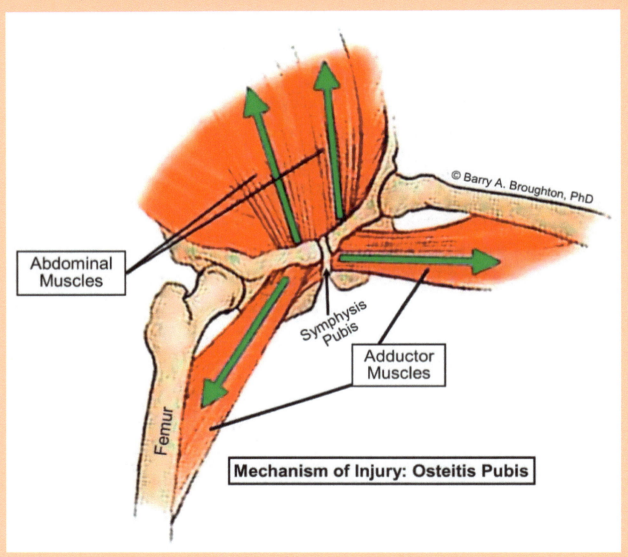

Fig. 5.48 - Osteitis pubis mechanism of injury. Image Credit: Modified by Barry A. Broughton, PhD, Original by Sports Medicine, Mitch Medical Healthcare, 01 May 2021

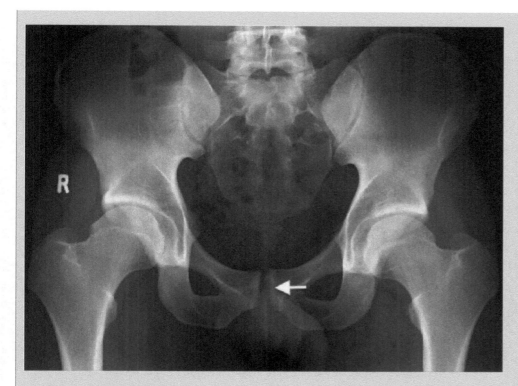

Fig. 5.49 - Pelvic x-ray of 21-year-old male athlete presenting with left groin pain demonstrating cortical changes and new bone formation on the left pubis (white arrow). Image Credit: Creative Commons Attribution (CC BY 4.0)

Injury to the Adductor Muscles - "Pulled Groin"

Strain of the adductor muscles is the underlying cause of what is commonly known as a "pulled groin" or "groin strain". The proximal part of the muscle is most affected, tearing near the bony attachments in the pelvis.

Groin injuries usually occur in sports that require explosive movements, kicking, or extreme stretching.

Myositis ossificans

Myositis ossificans (MO) is a reactive soft tissue bone-forming process that commonly occurs after trauma to the muscle or after sustaining a broken bone. Sixty to seventy-five percent of MO occurs after a significant initial trauma or repeated injury. New bone cells form between the torn muscle fibers at the location of the injury. Within four weeks, radiographic findings reveal a diffuse peripheral calcification at the injury site. By the fifth to sixth month post injury, mature bone is evident on plain radiographs. Young adults (usually 15-35 year old) are most often affected, with a higher prevalence among males.

Symptoms typically present as a painful, tender, enlarging mass (which becomes firm over time), after a blunt force trauma such a kick (or repeated kicks) or blow to the thigh. Approximately 80% of cases are located in large muscles of the extremities such as the quadriceps and gluteal muscles.

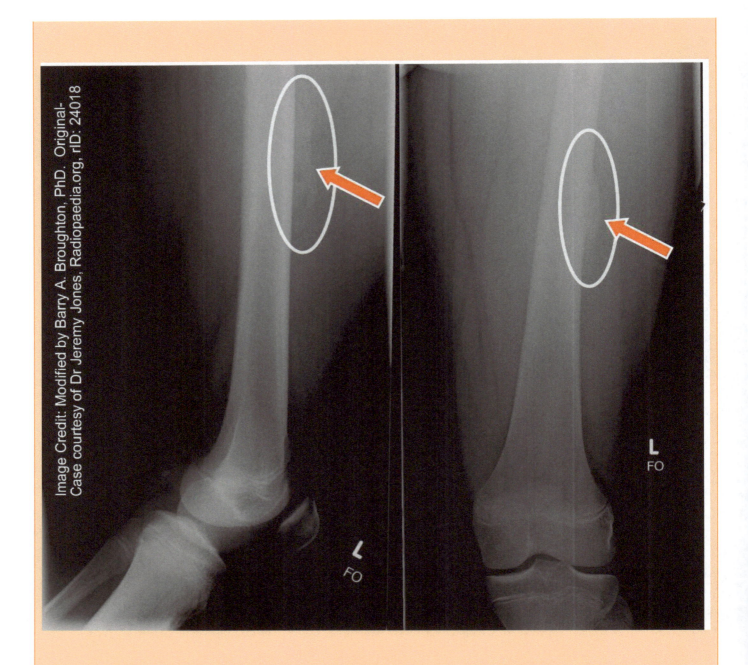

Fig. 5.50 - X-rays of left thigh/femur: Myositis Ossificans left thigh. Left image: Lateral view. Right image: Anteroposterior (AP) view. 15-year-old male with painful mass post blunt trauma to anterolateral thigh. Image Credit: Modified by Barry A. Broughton, PhD. Original: Case courtesy of Dr Jeremy Jones, Radiopaedia.org, rID: 24018

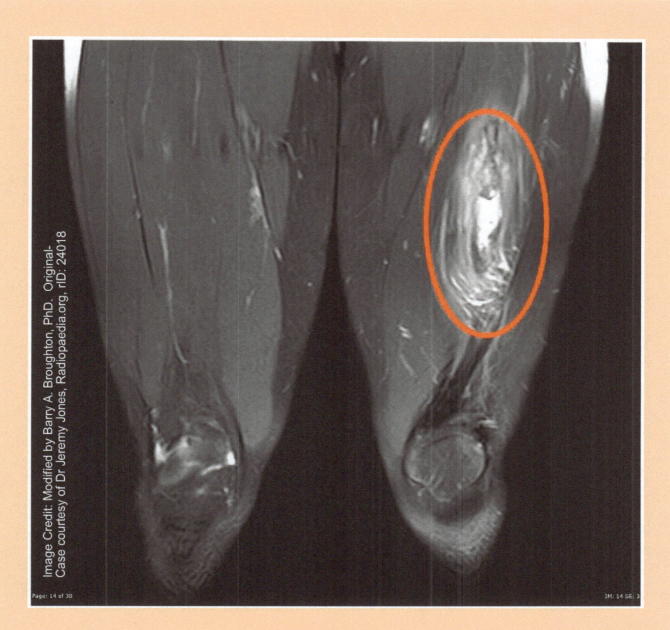

Fig. 5.51 - MRI of Bilateral thighs: Myositis Ossificans left thigh. 15-year-old male with painful mass post blunt trauma to anterolateral thigh. Image Credit: Modified by Barry A. Broughton, PhD. Original: Case courtesy of Dr Jeremy Jones, Radiopaedia.org, rID: 24018

Posterior Compartment

The muscles in the posterior compartment of the thigh form what is known collectively as the hamstring. The biceps femoris, semitendinosus, and semimembranosus, form the tendons that are palpable in the medial and lateral aspects of the posterior knee.

- *Biceps Femoris:* The biceps femoris muscle, like the biceps brachii in the arm, has two heads – a long head and a short head. As the most lateral muscle in the posterior thigh, the common tendon of the two heads can be palpated laterally at the posterior knee.
    - Attachments: The long head originates from the ischial tuberosity of the pelvis. The short head originates from the linea aspera on posterior surface of the femur. The two heads merge to form a tendon that inserts into the head of the fibula.
    - Action: Primary action is flexion of the knee. Secondarily, it extends the thigh at the hip, and externally rotates at the hip and knee.
- *Semitendinosus:* The semitendinosus is a long superficial muscle with a long tendon insertion, giving rise to its name. It lies medial to the biceps femoris in the posterior thigh, covering the majority of the semimembranosus.
    - Attachments: It originates from the ischial tuberosity of the pelvis and inserts into the medial surface of the tibia.
    - Action: Primary action is flexion of the leg at the knee joint, and extension of thigh at the hip. Secondarily it internally rotates the lower extremity.
- *Semimembranosus:* The semimembranosus muscle is the most medial of the hamstring muscles and lies beneath the semitendinosus. It is a flattened broad muscle with a flat tendon at its origin.
    - Attachments: It originates from the ischial tuberosity and inserts into the medial tibial condyle.
    - Actions: Flexion of the leg at the knee joint. Extension of the thigh at the hip. Internal rotation of the lower extremity.

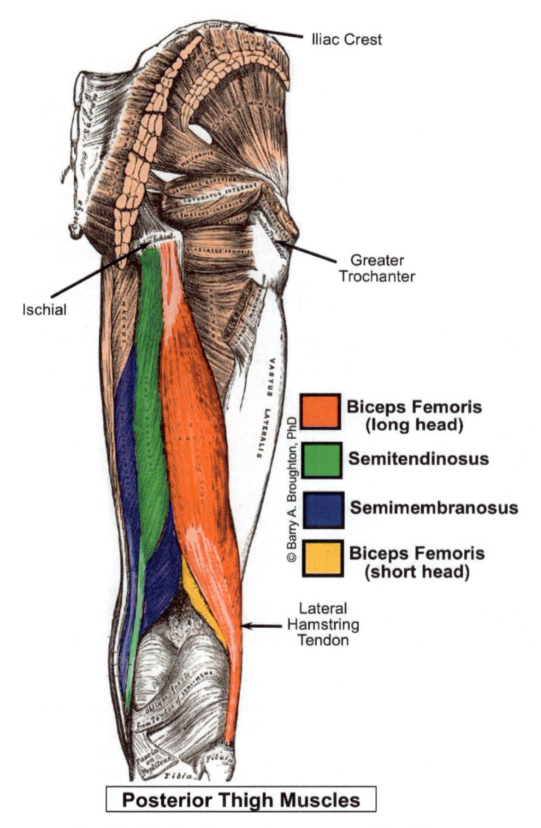

Fig. 5.52 - Muscles of the posterior compartment of the thigh.

Clinical Significance: Hamstring Injury

Hamstring Injury: Muscle Strain

Often seen in athletes involved with kicking or explosive sprinting, a hamstring strain refers to excessive stretching or tearing of the muscle fibers of the one of the hamstring muscles. Injury to the muscle fibers is likely to rupture the surrounding blood vessels producing a hematoma (a collection of blood) within the fascia lata and frequently causes subsequent ecchymosis (black and blue discoloration) to the posterior thigh.

Common treatment of any muscle strain is to utilize the RICE protocol: Rest, Ice, Compression, and Elevation.

Avulsion Fracture of the Ischial Tuberosity

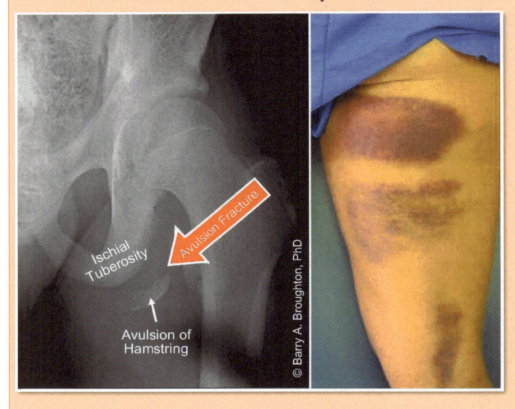

Fig. 5.53 - Left: Radiograph of ischial tuberosity avulsion fracture. Right: Ecchymosis posterior right thigh post hamstring injury.

An avulsion fracture of the ischial tuberosity occurs when the hamstring tendons pulls off a piece of the ischial tuberosity during injury. Such an injury usually occurs during activities that require rapid contraction and relaxation of the muscles, such as with jump kicks, sprinting, hurdling, and football. Avulsion fractures of the ischial tuberosity can be easily misdiagnosed and overlooked as a severe hamstring strain. Therefore, a detailed medical history and radiographic imaging are important for a correct diagnosis and treatment. The degree of displacement of the fracture fragment is a key factor in determining whether the injury needs surgical intervention for internal fixation or if conservative treatment is appropriate.

Muscles of the Leg

The leg is located between the knee joint proximally and the ankle joint distally. Muscles of the leg are responsible for the movements distally of the ankle and foot. The leg muscles are divided into three compartments: the anterior, posterior, and lateral compartments.

The tibialis anterior, which dorsiflexes the foot, is the antagonist to the gastrocnemius and soleus muscles, which plantar flex the foot.

▪ Anterior Compartment

The four muscles of the anterior compartment of the leg includes: the tibialis anterior, extensor digitorum longus, extensor hallucis longus, and the peroneus tertius.

Together, they act to dorsiflex and invert the foot at the ankle joint. The extensor digitorum longus and extensor hallucis longus also extend the toes.

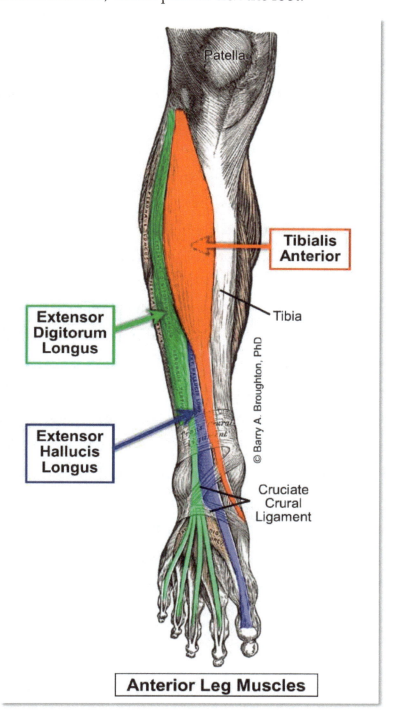

Fig. 5.54 – Muscle of the anterior compartment of the leg.

- *Tibialis Anterior:* The strongest dorsiflexor muscle of the foot, the tibialis anterior muscle is located along the lateral surface of the tibia.
    - Attachments: Originates from the lateral surface of the tibia and inserts into the medial cuneiform and the base of the first metatarsal.
    - Action: Dorsiflexion and inversion of the foot.
- *Extensor Digitorum Longus (EDL):* The extensor digitorum longus lies lateral and deep to the tibialis anterior. The tendons of the EDL can be palpated on the dorsum of the foot.
    - Attachments: Originates from the lateral condyle of the tibia and the medial surface of the fibula. The fibers merge to form a tendon, which travels distally to the dorsum of the foot. Within the cruciate crural ligament (inferior extensor retinaculum), the tendon splits into four smaller tendons, with each inserting into one of the four lateral toes.
    - Action: Extension of the lateral four toes, and dorsiflexion of the foot.
- *Extensor Hallucis Longus (EHL):* The extensor hallucis longus is located deep to the EDL and tibialis anterior.
    - Attachments: Originates from the medial surface of the fibular shaft. The tendon crosses anterior to the ankle joint and inserts at the base of the distal phalanx of the great toe (hallux).
    - Action: Extension of the hallux and dorsiflexion of the foot.
- *Peroneus Tertius:* The peroneus tertius muscle, also known as the fibularis tertius, arises from the most inferior part of the extensor digitorum longus. In some texts the peroneus tertius is considered to be part of the EDL and is not present in all individuals.
    - Attachments: Originates with the extensor digitorum longus from the medial surface of the fibula. The tendon descends with the EDL until they reach the dorsum of the foot. The fibularis tertius tendon then diverges and inserts into fifth metatarsal.
    - Action: Eversion and dorsiflexion of the foot.

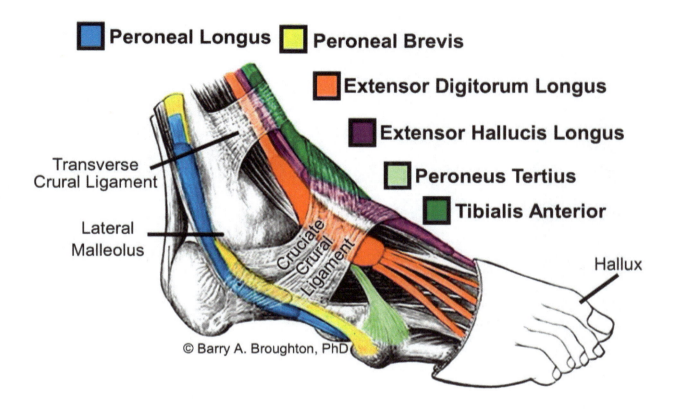

Fig. 5.55 - Lateral view of the leg muscle tendons in the foot.

▪ Lateral Compartment

The two muscles in the lateral compartment of the leg are the peroneal longus and the peroneal brevis (also known as fibularis longus and brevis).

The lateral leg muscles provide for only a few degrees of eversion of the foot (turning the sole of the foot outwards); however, functionally the lateral leg muscles also stabilize the medial margin of the foot during running and prevents excessive inversion.

- *Peroneal Longus:* The peroneal longus is the larger and more superficial muscle within the compartment.
    - Attachments: The peroneal longus originates from the superior and lateral surface of the fibula and the lateral tibial condyle. The fibers merge to form a tendon that descends into the foot, posterior to the lateral malleolus. The tendon then traverses under the foot and inserts into the medial cuneiform and base of first metatarsal.
    - Action: Eversion and plantar flexion of the foot. Supports the lateral and transverse arches of the foot.

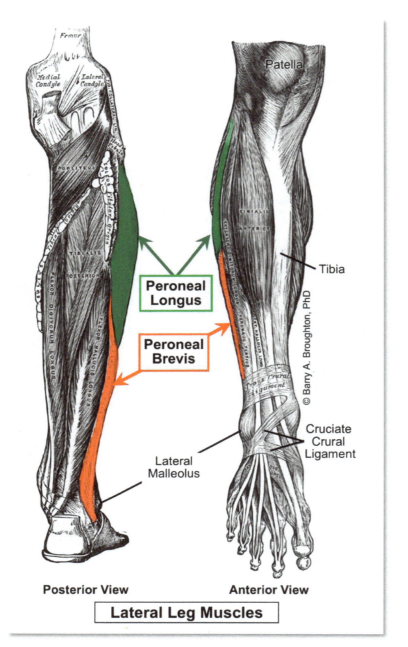

Fig. 5.56 - Lateral muscles of the leg.

- *Peroneal Brevis:* The peroneal brevis muscle is deeper and shorter than the peroneal longus.
    - Attachments: Originates from the inferolateral surface of the fibular shaft. The tendon descends distally along with the peroneal longus posterior to the lateral malleolus and into the foot. The peroneal brevis tendon passes over the calcaneus and the cuboidal bones and inserts into a tubercle on fifth metatarsal.
    - Actions: Eversion of the foot.

Posterior Compartment

The posterior compartment of the leg contains seven muscles, making it the largest of the three compartments. Collectively, the muscles of the posterior compartment plantarflex and invert the foot. Organized into two layers, the superficial and deep compartments are separated by a band of fascia.

Superficial Layer

The superficial muscles of the posterior compartment form the characteristic *"calf"* shape of the leg. The three muscles of the superficial layer insert into the calcaneus of the foot via the Achilles (calcaneal) tendon.

- *Gastrocnemius:* The gastrocnemius is the most superficial muscle in the posterior compartment of the leg. The medial and lateral heads of the gastrocnemius merge to form a single muscle belly.
    - Attachments: The lateral head originates from the lateral femoral condyle, while the medial head's origin is from the medial femoral condyle. The fibers converge and form a single muscle belly. More distally in the leg, the muscle belly combines with the soleus to form the Achilles Tendon, which inserts onto the posterior calcaneus.
    - Action: Plantar flexion of the foot at the ankle joint; and flexion of the leg at the knee.

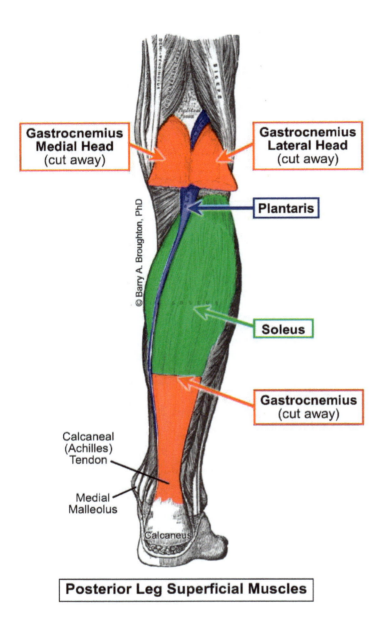

Fig. 5.57 – Superficial muscles of the posterior leg. The body of the gastrocnemius has been cut away to expose the underlying musculature.

- *Plantaris:* The plantaris is a small muscle with a long tendon that descends the posterior leg. The plantaris is absent in 10% of the population.
    - Attachments: Originates from the lateral supracondylar line of the femur. As the muscle descends medially, its long tendon runs down the leg, between the gastrocnemius and soleus muscles. The tendon converges into the Achilles tendon.
    - Actions: Plantar flexion of the foot at the ankle joint, and flexion of the leg at the knee.

- *Soleus:* The soleus is a large flat muscle that lies deep to the gastrocnemius.
  - Attachments: Originates from the soleal line of the tibia and proximal fibular area. The muscle narrows in the lower part of the leg and merges into the Achilles tendon.
  - Action: Plantarflexes the foot at the ankle joint.

To minimize friction during movement, there are two bursae (fluid filled sacs) associated with the Achilles tendon:

  ○ *Subcutaneous calcaneal bursa* – lies between the skin and the Achilles tendon.
  ○ *Retrocalcaneal bursa* – lies between the tendon and the calcaneus.

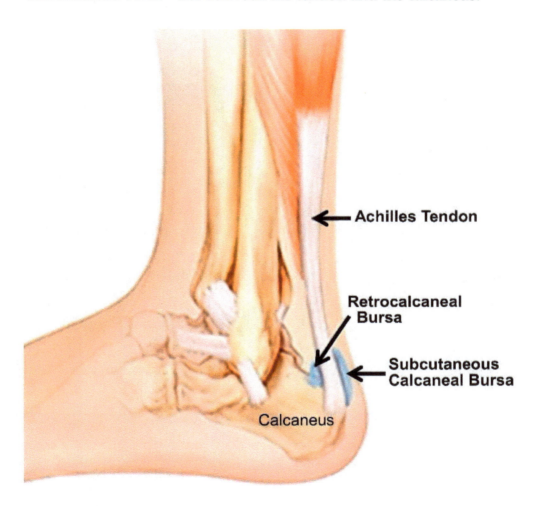

Fig. 5.58 - Bursa associated with the Achilles tendon.

Clinical Significance and Martial Arts Relevance:

Achilles Tendon Rupture

The Achilles tendon is the largest tendon in the body. It functions to control the body as the center of gravity rotates over the foot. Without a functional Achilles Tendon, patients limp and have a markedly dysfunctional gait. A clinical exam is needed to determine if the rupture is partial or complete. The severity of the tear determines conservative treatment vs. surgical repair.

Achilles tendon ruptures usually occur in martial artists (usually males 30 to 40 year old) when they load the Achilles tendon immediately prior to pushing off. This can occur when suddenly changing directions, starting to run (push off), or preparing to jump. A sudden change in direction requires the calf muscle to contract while still lengthening (eccentric loading). This subjects the Achilles tendon to a large loading force, which may cause the tendon to fail.

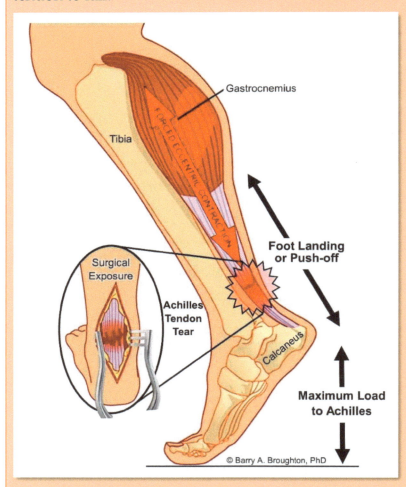

To be clear, the tendon tears because of the large internal forces generated by the eccentric contraction of the calf muscle and applied to the Achilles - and not because of an external force. In such a sense, it may be said that the patient tore the tendon themself. Patients often state that they heard a loud "pop" as if they were "hit (or shot) on the back of the leg" even though no one was near them when the injury occurred.

Fig. 5.59 - Achilles tendon rupture mechanism of injury (Eccentric loading)

Deep Layer

There are four muscles in the deep compartment of the posterior leg. Three of the muscles (tibialis posterior, flexor digitorum longus, and flexor hallucis longus) act on the ankle and foot. The remaining muscle, the popliteus, acts only on the knee joint.

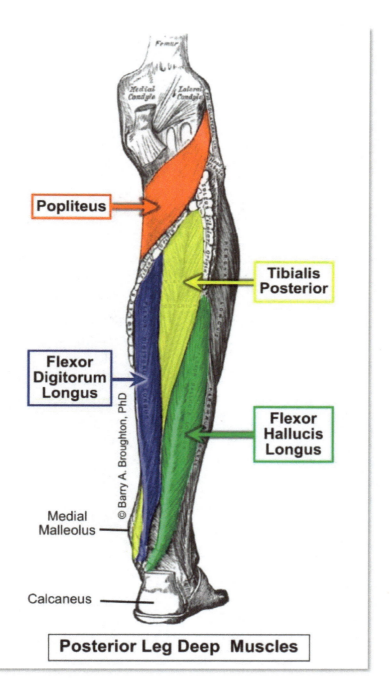

Fig. 5.60 - Deep muscles of the posterior leg.

- *Popliteus:* The popliteus is located more proximally in the leg. It lies posterior in the knee joint, forming the base of the popliteal fossa.
  The popliteus bursa (fluid filled sac) lies between the popliteal tendon and the posterior surface of the knee joint.
    - Attachments: Originates from the lateral condyle of the femur and the posterior horn of the lateral meniscus. It runs inferomedially towards the tibia and inserts into the posterior surface of the proximal tibia just above the origin of the soleus muscle.
    - Action: Externally (laterally) rotates the femur on the tibia. "Unlocks" the knee joint so that flexion can occur. Main stabilizer of the posterior knee.

Clinical Significance and Martial Arts Relevance:

▪ **Baker's Cyst**

A popliteal cyst, also referred to as a Baker's cyst, is swelling in the popliteal fossa of posterior knee. Amongst martial artists and athletes, a Baker's cyst may be the first indicator of intra-articular joint pathology. A Baker's cyst is usually the result of a problem within the knee joint, such as a meniscus tear or arthritis. Both conditions cause the knee to produce excessive synovial fluid, which can lead to a Baker's cyst. The cyst (swelling of the popliteal bursa) is usually treated by addressing the pathology within the knee joint.

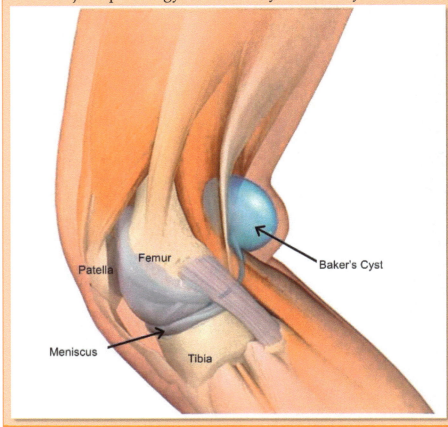

Fig. 5.61 - Popliteal (Baker's) cyst. Image Credit: Modified by Barry A. Broughton, PhD. Original by Mayo Foundation for Medical Education and Research.

- *Tibialis Posterior:* The tibialis posterior lies between the flexor digitorum longus and the flexor hallucis longus.
    - Attachments: Originates from the interosseous membrane between the tibia and fibula, and the posterior surfaces of the two bones. The tendon enters the foot posterior to the medial malleolus and inserts into the plantar surfaces of the medial tarsal bones.
    - Action: Inverts and plantarflexes the foot and maintains the medial arch of the foot.
- *Flexor Digitorum Longus:* The flexor digitorum longus (FDL) is a smaller muscle than the flexor hallucis longus. The FDL is located medially in the posterior leg.
    - Attachments: Originates from the medial surface of the tibia and inserts into the plantar surfaces of the lateral four toes.
    - Action: Flexes the lateral four toes.
- *Flexor Hallucis Longus:* The flexor hallucis longus muscle is located on the lateral side of posterior leg.
    - Attachments: Originates from the posterior surface of the fibula and inserts into the plantar surface of the phalanx of the great toe.
    - Action: Flexes the great toe.

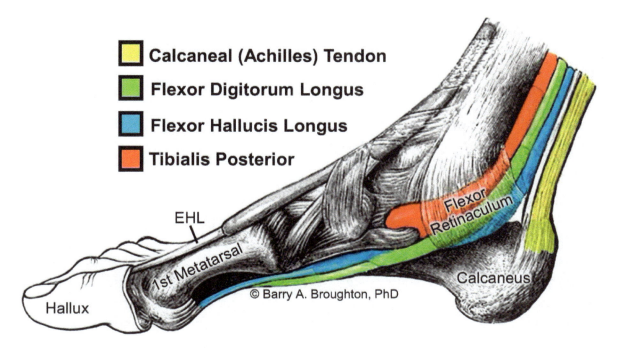

Fig. 5.62 - Medial view of the leg muscle tendons in the foot.

Skeletal Muscles: Their Origins, Insertions, and Actions

The Musculo-Skeletal Connection

The voluntary contraction of skeletal muscles acting upon bones causes movement of the human body. The interaction between the bones and skeletal muscle is ultimately controlled by the nervous system which allows for conscious movements.

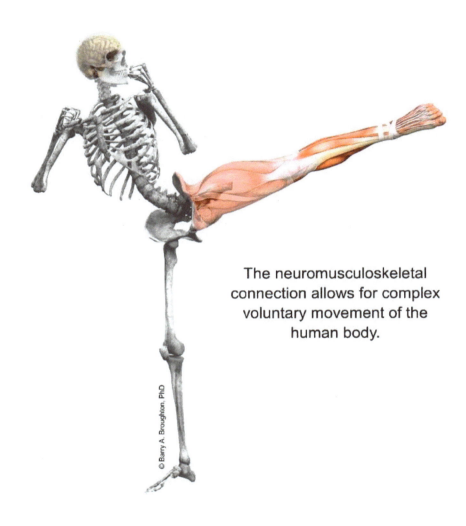

Fig. 5.63 - The neuromusculoskeletal connection.

Muscle contraction occurs when the brain initiates an electrical impulse that passes through a motor neuron in the somatic nervous system (see next chapter). The impulse stimulates the nerve innervating the target muscle signaling its movement. Muscle contraction pulls the tendon that is attached to the more distal bone, causing movement of the distal (movable) bone relative to the stationary proximal bone. The point where the tendon attaches on the proximal bone is called the <u>origin</u>. The point where the tendon attaches to the movable bone is called the <u>insertion</u>.

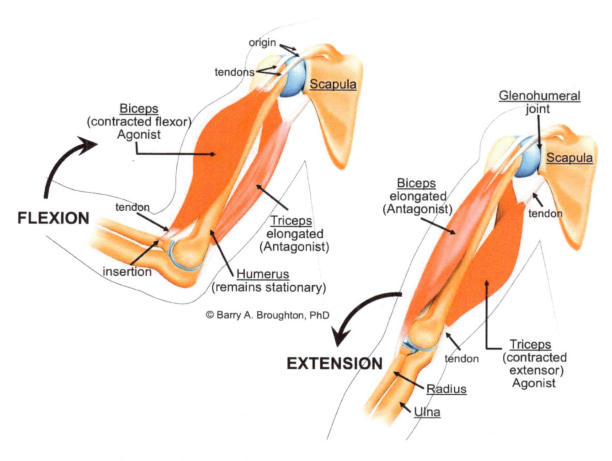

Fig. 5.64 - Agonist and antagonist muscle pairs during a biceps curl.

When initiating complex activities such as kicking, throws, or even walking, there are numerous muscles involved to complete the desired movement effectively and efficiently. Because muscles can only pull (they cannot push) they usually move a joint in tandem with other muscles called antagonistic pairs. To achieve these maneuvers, the involved muscles each adopt the appropriate type of contraction (concentric, eccentric, or isometric) needed to perform their specific role to complete the movement.

There are four distinct roles that a muscle can perform during movement. These roles include:

1. Agonist: Known as the *prime movers*, the agonist is the muscle(s) that provides the major force to complete the movement. While executing a biceps curl with a weighted dumbbell, the agonist biceps muscle contracts to produce flexion at the elbow joint, as seen in Fig. 5.64.
The agonist is not always the muscle that is shortening (concentric contraction). During a dumbbell curl, the bicep is the agonist during flexion as it contracts concentrically; during extension it contracts eccentrically. This is because the biceps is the prime mover in both cases.

2. Antagonist: The antagonist refers to the muscles that oppose the agonist. During elbow flexion where the bicep is the agonist, the triceps muscle is the antagonist. While the agonist contracts causing the movement to occur, the antagonist typically relaxes and elongates so as to not disrupt the agonist, as seen in the image on the previous page.

However, the antagonist muscle does not always relax; another function of antagonist muscles can be to slow down or to stop a movement. If the weight involved in the bicep curl is very heavy; when the weight is being lowered beyond the apex of the curl, the antagonist triceps muscle produces enough tension to control the movement as the weight lowers. This helps to ensure that gravity does not accelerate the movement, causing damage to the elbow joint at the end of the movement.

The triceps becomes the agonist and the bicep the antagonist when the elbow extends against gravity: such as in a push up, a triceps pushdown, or a bench press.

3. Synergist: The synergist muscle stabilizes a joint around which the movement is occurring, in turn helping the agonist muscle to function more effectively. Synergist muscles also help to create the movement. In the bicep curl the synergist muscles are the brachialis and brachioradialis which assist the biceps to create the movement and stabilize the elbow joint. A synergist can also be a fixator that stabilizes the bone that is the attachment for the prime mover's origin.

4. Fixator: The fixator muscle stabilizes the origin of the agonist, as well as the joint that the origin crosses, to help the agonist muscle function more effectively. In the bicep curl this would be the rotator cuff muscles of the shoulder. Most of the fixator muscles are found around the shoulder and hip joints.

Skeletal Muscles Chart: Their Origins, Insertions, and Actions

Refer to the series of charts on the following pages

Skeletal Muscles: Origin, Insertion, and Action

Muscles of Mastication

Muscle	Origin	Insertion	Action
Masseter	Zygomatic Arch	• Mandibular angle • Mandibular ramus	• Elevates mandible
Temporalis	Temporal fossa of the temporal bone	Coronoid process of the mandible	• Elevates mandible • Retracts mandible

Muscles of the Neck

Muscle	Origin	Insertion	Action
Sternocleidomastoid	• Manubrium of sternum • Medial clavicle	Mastoid process of the temporal bone	• Flexes head • Rotates head laterally
Scalenes – anterior, middle, posterior	Transverse processes of the cervical vertebrae	Anterior surface of ribs 1-2	• Elevates ribs 1-2 • Flexes neck • Rotates neck

Muscles of the Thoracic Wall

Muscle	Origin	Insertion	Action
Pectoralis minor	Ribs 3-5	Coracoid process of the scapula	• Depresses scapula • Downwardly rotates scapula
External intercostals	Inferior border of ribs	Superior border of ribs	• Elevates rib cage

Muscles of the Thoracic Wall

Muscle	Origin	Insertion	Action
Internal intercostals	Superior border of ribs	Inferior border of ribs	• Depresses rib cage
Serratus anterior	Ribs 1-8	Vertebral border of the scapula	• Rotates inferior angle of scapula laterally

Muscles of the Abdominal Wall

Muscle	Origin	Insertion	Action
External oblique	Ribs 5-12	• Linea alba • Pubic crest • Pubic tubercle • Iliac crest	• Flexes vertebral column • Compresses abdominal wall
Internal oblique	• Lumbar fascia • Iliac crest • Inguinal ligament	• Linea alba • Pubic crest	• Flexes vertebral column • Compresses abdominal wall
Rectus abdominis	• Pubic crest • Pubic symphysis	• Xiphoid process • Ribs 5-7	• Flexes lumbar region of vertebral column • Rotates lumbar region of vertebral column

Muscles of the Pectoral Girdle

Muscle	Origin	Insertion	Action
Trapezius	• Occipital bone • Spinous processes of C7-T12	• Lateral 1/3 of clavicle • Spine of scapula • Acromion process of scapula	• Elevates scapula • Depresses scapula • Rotates scapula • Adducts scapula

Muscles of the Pectoral Girdle

Muscle	Origin	Insertion	Action
Deltoid	- Lateral 1/3 of clavicle - Spine of scapula - Acromion process of scapula	- Deltoid tuberosity of the humerus	- Abducts arm - Flexes arm at shoulder - Rotates arm medially - Extends arm at shoulder - Rotates arm laterally
Latissimus dorsi	- Spinous processes of T7-T12 - Ribs 9-12 - Iliac crest - Inferior angle of scapula	- Intertubercular groove of the humerus	- Extends arm at shoulder - Adducts arm - Rotates arm medially
Pectoralis major	- Sternal end of the clavicle - Ribs 1-6	- Greater tubercle of humerus	- Flexes arm at shoulder - Rotates arm medially - Adducts arm

Muscles associated with the Scapula

Muscle	Origin	Insertion	Action
Levator scapula(e)	Transverse processes of C1-C4	Vertebral border of the scapula	- Elevates scapula - Downwardly rotates scapula
Rhomboid minor	Spinous processes of C7-T1	Vertebral border of the scapula	- Adducts scapula - Downwardly rotates scapula
Rhomboid major	Spinous processes of T2-T5	Vertebral border of the scapula	- Adducts scapula - Downwardly rotates scapula

Muscles of the Pectoral Girdle

Muscle	Origin	Insertion	Action
Supraspinatus	• Supraspinous fossa of the scapula	• Greater tubercle of the humerus	• Abducts arm
Infraspinatus	• Infraspinous fossa of the scapula	• Greater tubercle of the humerus	• Rotates arm laterally
Teres minor	• Lateral border of the scapula	• Greater tubercle of humerus	• Rotates arm laterally
Teres major	• Inferior angle of the scapula	• Lesser tubercle of the humerus	• Adducts arm • Rotates arm medially • Extends arm at shoulder
Subscapularis	• Subscapular fossa of the scapula	• Lesser tubercle of the humerus	• Rotates arm medially

Muscles of the Anterior compartment of the Arm

Muscle	Origin	Insertion	Action
Biceps brachii **Long head**	Supraglenoid tubercle of the scapula	Radial tuberosity of the radius	• Flexes forearm at elbow • Supinates forearm
Short head	Coracoid process of the scapula		

Muscles of the Anterior compartment of the Arm

Muscle	Origin	Insertion	Action
Brachialis	- Anterior humerus	- Coronoid process of the ulna	- Flexes forearm at elbow
Coracobrachialis	- Coracoid process of the scapula	- Medial humerus	- Flexes arm at shoulder - Adducts arm

Muscles of the Posterior compartment of the Arm

Muscle		Origin	Insertion	Action
Triceps brachii	Long head	Infraglenoid tubercle of the scapula	Olecranon process of the ulna	- Extends forearm at elbow
	Lateral head	Posterior humerus		
	Medial head	Posterior humerus		

Muscles of the Anterior compartment of the Forearm

Muscle	Origin	Insertion	Action
Pronator teres	Medial epicondyle of the humerus	Lateral radius	- Pronates forearm
Flexor carpi radialis	Medial epicondyle of the humerus	2nd and 3rd metacarpals	- Flexes hand at wrist - Abducts hand

Muscles of the Anterior compartment of the Forearm			
Muscle	Origin	Insertion	Action
Palmaris longus	Medial epicondyle of the humerus	Palmar aponeurosis	• Flexes hand at wrist
Flexor carpi ulnaris	• Medial epicondyle of the humerus • Olecranon process of ulna • Shaft of ulna	• Pisiform • Hamate • 5th metacarpal	• Flexes hand at wrist • Adducts hand
Flexor digitorum superficialis	• Medial epicondyle of the humerus • Coronoid process of ulna • Shaft of radius	Middle phalanges of 2nd to 5th digit	• Flexes hand at wrist • Flexes proximal interphalangeal joints
Flexor digitorum profundus	• Ulna • Interosseous membrane	Distal phalanges of 2nd to 5th digit	• Flexes distal interphalangeal joints
Flexor pollicis longus	• Anterior radius • Interosseous membrane	Distal phalanx of pollex	• Flexes 1st interphalangeal joints

Muscles of the Anterior compartment of the Forearm

Muscle	Origin	Insertion	Action
Pronator quadratus	Distal and anterior ulnar shaft	Distal and anterior radius	• Pronates forearm

Muscles of the Posterior compartment of the Forearm

Muscle	Origin	Insertion	Action
Brachioradialis	• Lateral supracondylar ridge of the humerus	• Styloid process of the radius	• Flexes forearm at elbow • Stabilizes elbow during flexion and extension
Extensor carpi radialis longus	• Lateral supracondylar ridge of the humerus	2nd metacarpal	• Extends hand at wrist • Abducts hand
Extensor carpi radialis brevis	• Lateral epicondyle of the humerus	3rd metacarpal	• Extends hand at wrist • Abducts hand
Extensor digitorum	• Lateral epicondyle of the humerus	Distal phalanges of 2nd to 5th digit	• Extends distal interphalangeal joints • Extends hand at wrist

Muscles of the Posterior compartment of the Forearm

Muscle	Origin	Insertion	Action
Extensor carpi ulnaris	• Lateral epicondyle of the humerus • Posterior ulna	5th metacarpal	• Extends hand at wrist • Adducts hand
Supinator	• Lateral epicondyle of the humerus • Proximal ulna	Proximal end of radius	• Supinates forearm
Abductor pollicis longus	• Posterior radius • Posterior ulna • Interosseus membrane	• Trapezium • 1st metacarpal	• Abducts pollex
Extensor pollicis brevis	• Posterior radius • Posterior ulna • Interosseus membrane	Proximal phalanx of pollex	• Extends 1st metacarpal-phalangeal joint
Extensor pollicis longus	• Posterior radius • Posterior ulna • Interosseus membrane	Distal phalanx of pollex	• Extends 1st interphalangeal joint

Muscles of the Posterior compartment of the Forearm

Muscle	Origin	Insertion	Action
Extensor indicis	• Posterior ulna • Interosseus membrane	Distal phalanx of 2nd digit	• Extends 2nd distal interphalangeal joint
Extensor digiti minimi	• Lateral epicondyle of humerus	Distal phalanx of 5th digit	• Extends 5th distal interphalangeal joint

Intrinsic Muscles of the Hand

Muscle	Origin	Insertion	Action
Abductor pollicis brevis	• Scaphoid • Trapezium • Flexor retinaculum	Proximal phalanx of pollex	• Abducts pollex
Opponens pollicis	• Trapezium • Flexor retinaculum	1st metacarpal	• Opposes pollex
Flexor pollicis brevis	• Trapezium • Flexor retinaculum	Proximal phalanx of pollex	• Flexes 1st metacarpal-phalangeal joint
Adductor pollicis	• Capitate • 2nd - 4th metacarpals	Proximal phalanx of pollex	• Adducts pollex • Opposes pollex

Muscles associated with the Anterior compartment of the Thigh			
Muscle	Origin	Insertion	Action
Iliopsoas (Major and Minor)	• Iliac fossa • Ala of the sacrum • Transverse processes of T12-L5	Lesser trochanter of the femur	• Flexes thigh at hip • Flexes vertebral column
Sartorius	• Anterior superior iliac spine	Medial tibia	• Flexes thigh at hip • Rotates thigh laterally • Flexes leg at knee
Quadriceps femoris		All four:	
Rectus femoris	• Anterior inferior iliac spine	Patella and tibial tuberosity via tendon of quadriceps femoris and patellar ligament	• Extends leg at knee • Flexes thigh at hip
Vastus lateralis	• Greater trochanter of the femur • Intertrochanteric line • Linea aspera of femur		• Extends leg at knee • Stabilizes knee
Vastus medialis	• Linea aspera of femur • Intertrochanteric line		• Extends leg at knee • Stabilizes patella
Vastus intermedius	• Shaft of the femur		• Extends leg at knee
Pectineus	• Superior ramus of pubis	Linea aspera of femur	• Adducts thigh • Flexes thigh at hip • Rotates thigh medially

Muscles associated with the Anterior compartment of the Thigh

Muscle	Origin	Insertion	Action
Tensor fascia latae	• Anterior superior iliac spine • Iliac crest	Iliotibial tract	• Flexes thigh at hip • Abducts thigh • Rotates thigh medially

Muscles associated with the Medial compartment of the Thigh

Muscle	Origin	Insertion	Action
Gracilis	• Inferior ramus of pubis • Body of the pubis	Medial surface of tibia	• Adducts thigh • Flexes leg at knee • Rotates leg medially
Adductor longus	• Pubis – near pubic symphysis	Linea aspera of femur	• Adducts thigh • Flexes thigh at hip • Rotates thigh medially
Adductor brevis	• Inferior ramus of pubis • Body of the pubis	Linea aspera of femur	• Adducts thigh • Rotates thigh medially
Adductor magnus	• Inferior ramus of pubis • Ischial ramus • Ischial tuberosity	Linea aspera of femur	• Adducts thigh • Rotates thigh laterally • Flexes thigh at hip

Muscles associated with the Gluteal region and Posterior compartment of the Thigh

Muscle	Origin	Insertion	Action
Gluteus maximus	• Posterior ilium • Sacrum • Coccyx	• Iliotibial tract • Gluteal tuberosity of femur	• Extends thigh at hip • Rotates thigh laterally • Abducts thigh

Muscles associated with the Gluteal region and Posterior compartment of the Thigh			
Muscle	Origin	Insertion	Action
Gluteus medius	• Lateral surface of ilium	Greater trochanter of femur	• Abducts thigh • Rotates thigh medially
Gluteus minimis	• Lateral surface of ilium	Greater trochanter of femur	• Abducts thigh • Rotates thigh medially
Biceps femoris Long head Short head	• Ischial tuberosity • Linea aspera	• Head of fibula • Lateral condyle of tibia	• Extends thigh at hip • Flexes leg at knee • Rotates leg laterally
Semitendinosus	• Ischial tuberosity	Medial tibia	• Extends thigh at hip • Flexes leg at knee • Rotates leg medially
Semimembranosus	• Ischial tuberosity	Medial condyle of tibia	• Extends thigh at hip • Flexes leg at knee • Rotates leg medially
Piriformis	• Lateral surface of sacrum	Greater trochanter of femur	• Rotates thigh laterally when hip is extended
Quadratus femoris	• Ischial tuberosity	Intertrochanteric crest of the femur	• Rotates thigh laterally • Stabilizes hip

Muscles associated with the Anterior compartment of the Leg

Muscle	Origin	Insertion	Action
Tibialis anterior	• Lateral condyle of tibia • Interosseous membrane	• Medial cuneiform • 1st metatarsal	• Dorsiflexes foot at ankle • Inverts foot
Extensor hallucis longus	• Anterior fibula • Interosseous membrane	Distal phalanx of hallux	• Dorsiflexes foot at ankle • Extends 1st interphalangeal joint
Extensor digitorum longus	• Lateral condyle of tibia • Proximal fibula • Interosseous membrane	Middle and distal phalanges of 2nd-5th digits	• Extends 2nd-5th distal interphalangeal joints
Fibularis (peroneus) tertius	• Anterior fibula • Interosseous membrane	5th metatarsal	• Dorsiflexes foot at ankle • Everts foot

Muscles associated with the Lateral compartment of the Leg

Muscle	Origin	Insertion	Action
Fibularis (peroneus) longus	• Head of fibula	• Medial cuneiform • 1st metatarsal	• Plantar flexes foot at ankle • Everts foot
Fibularis (peroneus) brevis	• Distal fibula	5th metatarsal	• Plantar flexes foot at ankle • Everts foot

Muscles associated with the Posterior compartment of the Leg			
Muscle	Origin	Insertion	Action
Gastrocnemius	• Lateral condyle of femur • Medial condyle of femur	Calcaneus	• Plantar flexes foot at ankle
Soleus	• Proximal tibia • Proximal fibula • Interosseous membrane	Calcaneus	• Plantar flexes foot at ankle
Flexor digitorum longus	• Posterior tibia	Distal phalanges of 2nd-5th digits	• Plantar flexes foot at ankle • Inverts foot • Flexes 2nd-5th distal interphalangeal joints
Flexor hallucis longus	• Middle shaft of fibula • Interosseous membrane	Distal phalanx of hallux	• Plantar flexes foot at ankle • Inverts foot • Flexes all joints of hallux
Tibialis posterior	• Proximal tibia • Proximal fibula • Interosseous membrane	• Navicular bone • 2nd-4th metatarsals	• Plantar flexes foot at ankle • Inverts foot

Intrinsic Muscles of the Back

Muscle	Origin	Insertion	Action
Erector spinae (group)			
Iliocostalis	• Iliac crest • Ribs 3-12	• Inferior border of ribs • Transverse processes of C4-C6	• Extends vertebral column • Laterally flexes vertebral column
Longissimus	• Transverse processes of C4-L5	Mastoid process of temporal bone	• Extends vertebral column • Laterally flexes vertebral column
Spinalis	• Spinous processes of T7-L3	Spinous processes of C4-T6	• Extends vertebral column
Splenius capitis	• Spinous processes of C6-T7	• Mastoid process of temporal bone • Occipital bone	• Extends or hyperextends vertebral column
Semispinalis capitis	• Transverse processes of C7-T12	Occipital bone	• Extends vertebral column

Chart Credit: Laurie Boriskie, Muscle Origin Insertion Actions, Created 6/15/09, 1278 KB, 15 pgs., colorado.edu

Chapter 6

Introduction to the Nervous System

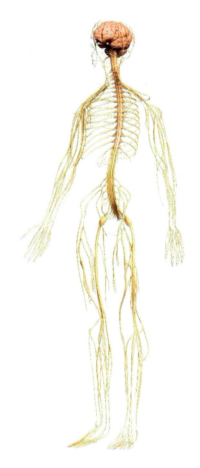

Fig. 6.1 - Introduction to the Nervous System.

The nervous system functions as the body's command center, coordinating all its activities, movements, and bodily functions. Responsible for all mental activity including thought, learning, and memory, the nervous system relays messages via electrical impulses throughout the body. Through its receptors, with the aid of the endocrine system, the nervous system prepares and regulates the body to respond and adapt to its environment, both external and internal.

Like other systems in the body, the nervous system is composed of organs, primarily the brain, spinal cord, nerves, and ganglia. In turn, these structures consist of various tissues, including nerve cells, blood, and connective tissue. Together they carry out the complex activities of the nervous system that can be grouped together as three general overlapping functions:

- Sensory
- Integrative
- Motor

The human body contains millions of *sensory* receptors that detect changes, called stimuli, which occur in the environment (both internally and externally). They monitor such things as light, sound, and temperature from the external environment. Internally, the receptors detect variations in pressure, carbon dioxide concentration, the levels of various electrolytes, and the acid-base balance of the body. The information gathered is referred to as sensory input.

Sensory input is converted into electrical signals, called nerve impulses, which are then transmitted to the brain. Within the brain, the process of *integration* combines nerve impulses, sensory perceptions, and higher cognitive functions such as memories, emotion, and learning to produce a response.

Based on the sensory input and integration, the nervous system responds by sending signals to specific glands, causing them to produce secretions, or to muscles causing them to contract. Muscles and glands are called effectors because they cause an effect in response to the instructions given by the nervous system. This is the motor output or *motor* function.

How does the human body create electricity?

The human body needs an energy source to move, punch, kick, throw, and think. The bioelectricity within the human body is simply the flow of electrical charges. The energy created by chemicals is due to the reactions of the atoms and molecules present in the body.

The most common form of electricity that most people are familiar with is via plugging the cord of an electrical appliance into a wall socket. The electrical current runs from the power plant throughout the electric grid, to the copper wires of a house, waiting to be tapped into at the wall socket or light switch. That is *not* the kind of electricity that is produced in the human body. In the neurological system, nerves carry the electrical current. The electrical charges in the human body are present on *charged* atoms. A charged atom is called an ion, which can have either a positive or negative charge.

When food is ingested, the large molecules get broken down during the digestive process creating smaller similar molecules (See the *Introduction to the Digestive System* chapter). Those smaller molecules are used in the cells via cellular respiration. All the elements taken into the human body, such as oxygen, sodium, potassium, and calcium have a specific electrical charge; meaning they have a specific number of electrons, protons, and neutrons. Those specific charges, whether positive or negative, reacts to the charges of adjacent molecules. This reaction is what creates the energy needed to produce bioelectricity.

Nerve Tissue

Although the nervous system is highly complex, there are only two primary types of cells in nerve tissue. The neuron is the actual structural unit of the nervous system that conducts and transmits impulses. The neuroglia, or glial cells, are nonconductive cells that provide a support system for the neurons. They are a special type of connective tissue for the nervous system.

▪ Neurons

Neurons are highly specialized cells that carry out the functions of the nervous system by conducting nerve impulses. If a neuron is destroyed, it cannot be replaced or regenerated.

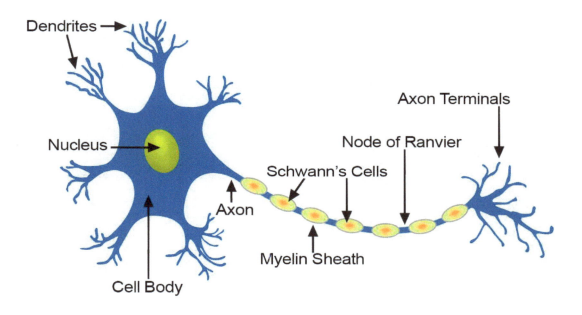

Fig. 6.2 - Structure of a typical neuron.

Each neuron has three basic parts: the cell body, one or more dendrites, and a single axon.

- *Cell Body:* The cell body of a neuron has a nucleus with at least one nucleolus. Except for centrioles, it contains many of the typical cytoplasmic organelles.

Dendrites and axons are cytoplasmic extensions, or processes, that project from the cell body.

- Dendrites: Also referred to as fibers, dendrites are usually short and branching, which increases their surface area to receive signals from other neurons. The number of dendrites on a neuron varies. Dendrites are called afferent processes because they transmit impulses to the neuron cell body.

- *Axon:* There is only one axon that projects from each neuron cell body. Because it carries impulses away from the cell body, it is called an efferent process. An axon may have infrequent branches called axon collaterals. Axons and axon collaterals terminate in many short branches called telodendria. The distal ends of the telodendria are slightly enlarged to form synaptic bulbs. Many axons are surrounded by a segmented, fatty, white substance called myelin that forms the myelin sheath. Myelinated fibers make up the white matter in the central nervous system (CNS), while cell bodies and unmyelinated fibers form the gray matter. The unmyelinated gaps between the myelin segments are called the nodes of Ranvier.

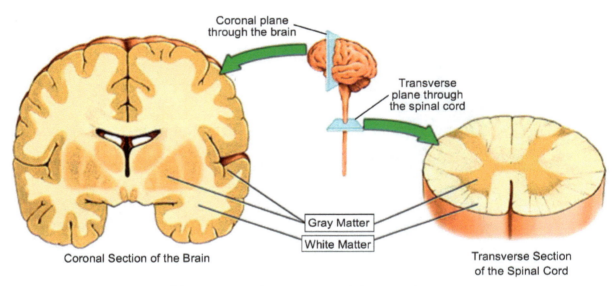

Fig. 6.3 - *White matter and gray matter of the central nervous system.*

In the *peripheral nervous system*, the myelin is produced by Schwann cells. The cytoplasm, nucleus, and outer cell membrane of the Schwann cell form the neurilemma, a tight covering around the myelin and around the axon itself at the nodes of Ranvier. The neurilemma plays an important role in the regeneration of nerve fibers. In the *central nervous system*, oligodendrocytes produce myelin, but there is no neurilemma, which is why fibers within the CNS do not regenerate.

Functionally, *neurons* are classified as afferent, efferent, or interneurons (association neurons) based on the direction in which they transmit impulses relative to the central nervous system.

- *Afferent* (or sensory) neurons carry impulses from the peripheral sense receptors to the central nervous system. They usually have long dendrites and relatively short axons.
- *Efferent* (or motor) neurons transmit impulses from the central nervous system to effector organs such as muscles and glands. Efferent neurons usually have short dendrites and long axons.
- *Interneurons* (association neurons) are located entirely within the CNS in which they form the connecting link between the afferent and efferent neurons. They have short dendrites and may have either a short or long axon.

▪ Neuroglia

Neuroglia cells do not conduct nerve impulses. They provide physical and metabolic support to the neuron. Neuroglia also insulate and protect the neurons. They are far more numerous than neurons and, unlike neurons, are capable of mitosis (dividing into two identical cells).

Organization of the Nervous System

The nervous system is divided into two divisions, the central nervous system (CNS) and the peripheral nervous system (PNS). The PNS is further subdivided into subsequent smaller divisions. Although terminology may seem to indicate otherwise, there is only one nervous system in the human body. All of the smaller systems belong to the single, highly integrated Nervous System. Each subdivision has functional as well as structural characteristics that distinguishes it from the others.

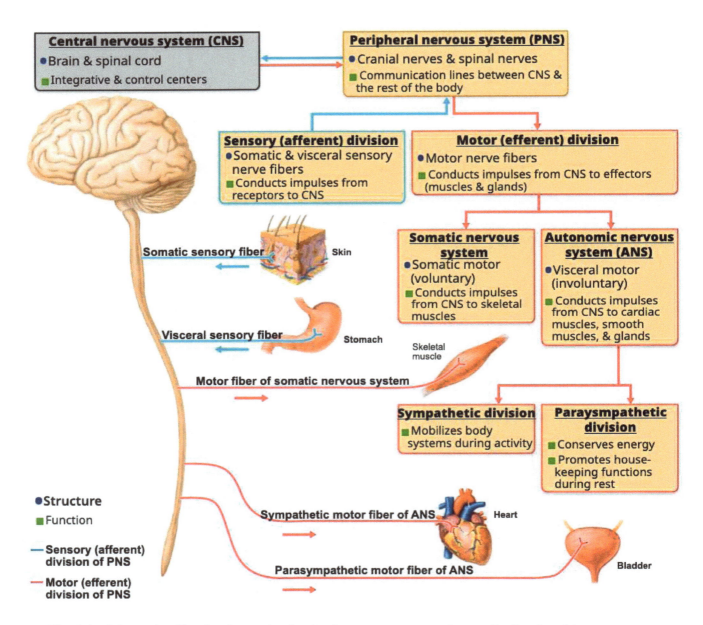

Fig. 6.4 - Schematic of levels of organization in the nervous system. Image Credit: clpccd.instructure.com

Central Nervous System Overview

The organs of the central nervous system include the brain and spinal cord. Because of their vulnerability, and vital importance, both structures are encased in bone for protection. The brain is in the cranial vault, while the spinal cord is surrounded by the vertebral canal of the vertebral column. Although considered to be two separate organs, the spinal cord extends from the brain at the medulla oblongata.

Peripheral Nervous System Overview

The organs of the peripheral nervous system include the nerves and ganglia. Much like muscles are bundles of muscle fibers, nerves are bundles of nerve fibers. Cranial nerves and spinal nerves extend from the central nervous system to the peripheral organs such as muscles and glands. Ganglia are collections of nerve cell bodies outside the CNS.

The peripheral nervous system is subdivided into an *afferent (sensory) division* and an *efferent (motor) division*. The afferent, or sensory, division transmits impulses from *peripheral organs* to the CNS. The e<u>ffe</u>rent, or motor, division transmits impulses from the CNS to the *peripheral organs* to cause an action (or e<u>ffe</u>ct).

The efferent (motor) division is further subdivided into the *somatic nervous system* and the *autonomic nervous system*.

> The somatic nervous system, also called the somatic efferent (or somatomotor) nervous system, supplies motor impulses to the skeletal muscles. Because these nerves allow for conscious control of the skeletal muscles, it is also called the voluntary nervous system.

> The autonomic nervous system (ANS), also called the visceral efferent nervous system, provides motor impulses to cardiac muscle, smooth muscle, and to glandular epithelium. Because the ANS regulates automatic, or involuntary functions, it is also called the involuntary nervous system. The ANS is further subdivided again into *sympathetic* and *parasympathetic divisions*.

The Central Nervous System

The organs of the CNS are located within the dorsal cavity of the body. The brain is surrounded by the bones of the cranium, while the spinal cord is protected by the vertebrae. In addition to bone, the central nervous system is also surrounded by connective tissue membranes, called meninges, and by cerebrospinal fluid.

• Meninges

There are three layers of meninges that cover the brain and spinal cord. These membranes protect and anchor the brain while providing a support system for nerves, blood vessels, lymphatics, and the cerebrospinal fluid that surrounds the central nervous system.

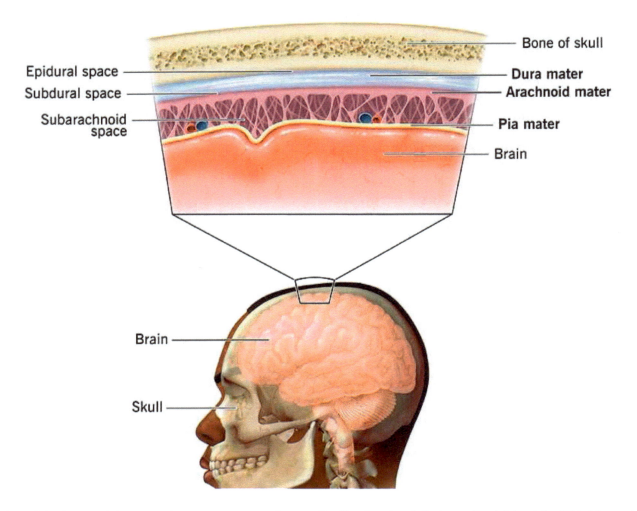

Fig. 6.5 - Meninges of the central nervous system. Image Credit: clevelandclinic.org/health/articles/22266-meninges

The *dura mater* is the outermost layer closest to the skull. It is composed of two layers of tough white fibrous connective tissue. One side of the dura mater attaches to the skull, while the other side attaches to the middle meningeal layer. The dura mater contains the dural venous sinuses; a drainage system that allows blood to leave the brain, and cerebrospinal fluid to re-enter the circulation.

The *arachnoid mater* is the middle layer of meninges and does not contain blood vessels or nerves. Resembling a spiderweb in appearance, the arachnoid mater is a thin layer with numerous threadlike strands that attach it to the innermost layer. The space between the arachnoid and innermost layer, the *subarachnoid space*, contains blood vessels and is filled with cerebrospinal fluid to cushion the brain.

The *pia mater* is the innermost layer of meninges. This delicate, thin membrane is tightly bound to the surface of the brain and spinal cord. The pia mater helps to contain cerebrospinal fluid and maintain the stiffness of the spinal cord. Blood vessels pass through the pia mater to profuse the brain tissue.

Clinical Significance and Martial Arts Relevance:

- **Extradural and Subdural Hematomas**

A hematoma is a collection of blood which forms as a result of bleeding into an organ or cavity. Intracranial hematomas are serious conditions that can cause compression on the underlying brain.

The most common cause of extradural and subdural hematomas are head injuries caused by blunt force trauma. A martial arts throw (or fall) causing the head to strike the floor (or mat), or a significant kick to the head are both sufficient enough traumas to cause an intracranial hematoma. Because the cranial vault is essentially a closed space, a hematoma can cause a rapid increase in intracranial pressure. Intracranial hematomas may be associated with a brief episode in loss of consciousness; however, it does not always occur. If left untreated, it may result in death.

There are two types of hematomas involving the dura mater:
- *Extradural Hematomas* are most often a result of arterial blood that collects between the skull and periosteal layer of the dura mater. The vessel commonly injured is the middle meningeal artery that is torn as a result of brain trauma.

- *Subdural Hematomas* are the most common type of intracranial hematoma among athletes. A significant head injury results in arterial or venous blood collecting between the dura mater and the arachnoid mater below. There are three types of subdural hematomas:
    - *Acute*: Generally caused by a severe head injury. Signs and symptoms usually appear immediately. Acute subdural hematomas are the most dangerous type of intracranial hematomas.
    - *Subacute*: Signs and symptoms take time to develop, sometimes days or weeks after your injury.
    - *Chronic*: The result of less severe head injuries, this type of hematoma can cause slow bleeding, and symptoms can take weeks and even months to appear.
    - All three types require medical attention as soon as signs and symptoms appear so that permanent brain damage can be prevented

Classical symptoms of an epidural hematoma include a brief loss of consciousness post injury, followed by a "lucid interval", then development of progressive headaches, weakness, numbness, increasing drowsiness, and a dilated pupil in the eye. The progression of symptoms is a sign of hematoma expansion, and worsening pressure and compression of the brain. Acute subdural hematomas may have similar symptoms, but without the "lucid interval". Urgent medical attention is required for both conditions.

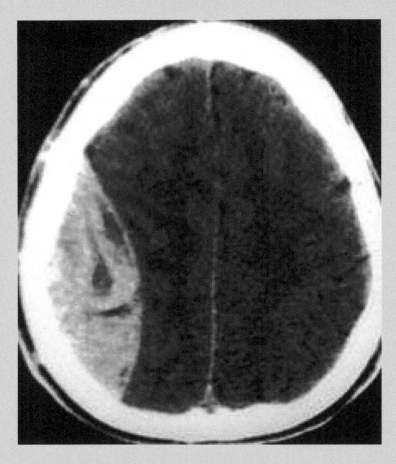

Fig. 6.6 – CT scan of a massive extradural hematoma.

Brain

The brain is divided into four regions: the cerebrum, diencephalons, cerebellum, and the brain stem.

- *Cerebrum:* The cerebrum is the largest and most obvious portion of the brain. It is divided by a deep longitudinal fissure separating it into two cerebral hemispheres. The two hemispheres are separate entities but are connected beneath the cerebral cortex by a thick bundle of nerve fibers, called the corpus callosum. The corpus collosum provides a pathway for communication between the two hemispheres.

  Each cerebral hemisphere is divided into five lobes, four of which have the same name as the bone over them: the *frontal lobe, parietal lobe, occipital lobe,* and the *temporal lobe*. The fifth lobe, the insula (or Island of Reil) lies deep within the lateral sulcus.

  The *frontal lobe* is primarily responsible for reasoning and thought. The *parietal lobe* is primarily responsible for integrating sensory information. The *temporal lobe* is primarily responsible for processing auditory information from the ears. The *occipital lobe* is responsible for processing visual information from the eyes. The insula controls autonomic functions through the regulation of the sympathetic and parasympathetic nervous systems.

- *Diencephalon:* The diencephalons is centrally located in the brain between the cerebrum and the midbrain. The diencephalon contains the *thalamus*, the *hypothalamus*, and *epithalamus*.

  The *thalamus* consists of two oval masses of gray matter that serve as relay stations for sensory impulses (except for the sense of smell) going to the cerebral cortex.

  The *hypothalamus* is a small region below the thalamus. It maintains homeostasis by controlling autonomic nervous system functions such as blood vessel constriction and dilation, body temperature, water balance, appetite, and sleep. The hypothalamus also plays a role in the expression of emotions such as pleasure, affection, pain, fear, and anger.

  The *epithalamus* is small gland in the most dorsal portion of the diencephalons and functions as a biological clock. The epithalamus is involved with the onset of puberty and rhythmic cycles in the body.

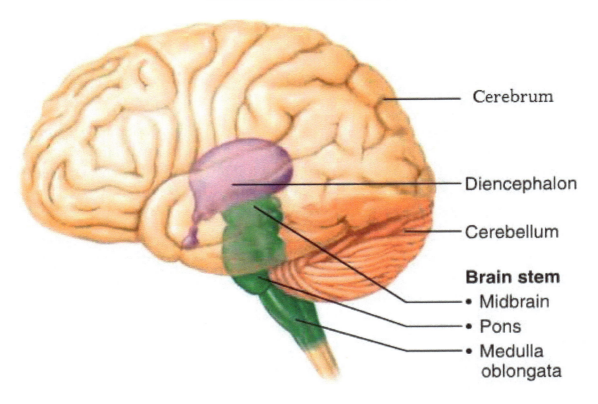

Fig. 6.7 - Regions of the human brain.

- *Cerebellum:* The cerebellum, the second largest portion of the brain, is located posteriorly below the occipital lobes of the cerebrum. Three paired bundles of myelinated nerve fibers, called cerebellar peduncles, form the communication pathways between the cerebellum and other parts of the central nervous system. The cerebellum is responsible for muscle coordination, balance, posture, and muscle tone.

- *Brain Stem:* The brain stem is the region between the diencephalons and the spinal cord. It contains three parts: the *midbrain*, *pons*, and the *medulla oblongata*.

The *midbrain* is the most superior portion of the brain stem and is responsible for certain eye and auditory reflexes.

The *pons* is the bulging middle portion of the brain stem below the midbrain. It primarily consists of nerve fibers that form conduction tracts between the higher brain centers and the spinal cord. The pons is responsible for certain reflex actions such as chewing, tasting, and saliva production.

- The *medulla oblongata* (or medulla) extends inferiorly from the pons. It is continuous with the spinal cord and is responsible for regulating blood pressure, cardiac and blood vessel function, swallowing, digestion, coughing, and sneezing. It's also known as the center for respiration.

  All the ascending (sensory) and descending (motor) nerve fibers connecting the brain and spinal cord pass through the medulla oblongata.

Ventricles and Cerebrospinal Fluid: A series of four interconnected, fluid-filled cavities are located within the brain. The cavities, called ventricles, are structures that produce cerebrospinal fluid, and transport it throughout the cranial cavity and spinal canal. Cerebrospinal fluid (CSF) is a clear, colorless liquid that helps cushion the brain and spinal cord from injury and provides nutrients to the CNS.

Clinical Significance and Martial Arts Relevance:

- **Concussion**

A concussion is a traumatic brain injury that disrupts the normal function of the brain. In combat sports this is often associated with direct strikes (kicks or punches) to the head, or from the head hitting the floor via a throw or fall. A concussion is an obvious result of getting knocked out; however, loss of consciousness does not need to occur for a concussion to be present.

Although concussions are most often caused by a direct blow to the head, an indirect blow to other areas of the body that subsequently jars the head can also cause a significant enough force that would impact the brain. An abrupt acceleration and/or deceleration creates an impact and shearing force on the brain. The forces that impact the head can be linear or rotational, and most often consists of a combination of both.

In head injuries, a "coup" injury refers to the brain lesion that occurs directly under the area of impact. In contrast, a "contrecoup" injury occurs on the opposite side of the brain from where the head was struck. These injuries can occur separately as only a coup injury, or only as a contrecoup injury; however, if the blow is significant enough, they can occur together as a "coup-contrecoup" injury.

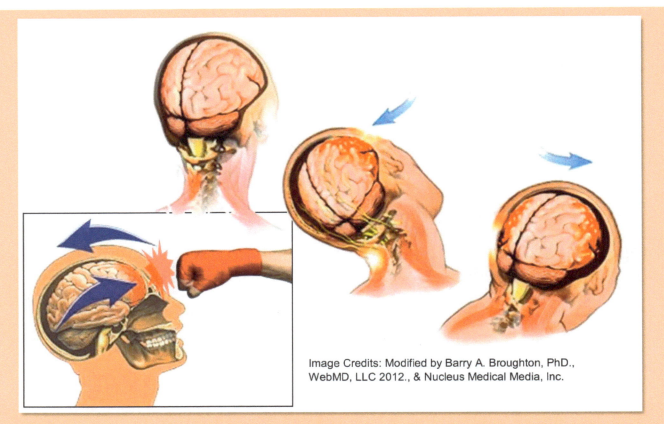

Fig. 6.8 - Concussion and traumatic brain injury mechanism of injury: Impact forces causing primary and secondary (coup-contrecoup) brain injury.

    Brain tissue has a similar consistency as gelatin or soft tofu. The two heavy hemispheres rest upon the brainstem where it is connected inferiorly. Surrounded by cerebral fluid, the brain essentially floats within the skull as a means to protect the vulnerable brain tissue. When the head is moved in a forceful violent fashion, the brain moves around inside the skull. Because of its suspension within the cranial vault, there is little constraint from keeping the brain from moving within that closed space. When an impact force strikes the head, it pushes the brain against the interior wall of the cranium. The skull in turn, pushes it back. In doing so, the heavy hemispheres put a significant amount of pressure on the brainstem, which can be twisted and pulled as the rest of the brain moves out of place during the forceful blow. The accelerations, decelerations, and collisions involved in the secondary injury phase can be equally damaging to the brain and nervous system.

    Mild concussions and brain injuries can cause temporary effects such as changes of mental status, headache, difficulty concentrating, or loss of consciousness. Nausea, vomiting, noise and light sensitivity, and slurred or slow speech may also be present. More severe brain injuries can create long-term effects that impact thinking, memory, coordination, balance, vision, speech, hearing, and emotional instability. Severe concussions may result in extended durations of unconsciousness, coma, and even death.

Activities of daily living such as exercise, driving, and working are all impacted by the disability created by concussions. Any head injury that causes even the slightest change in mental acuity needs a thorough medical evaluation. A qualified healthcare provider will give the approval to return to normal activities once symptoms have subsided. It is vitally important to allow enough time for the brain tissue to heal. It is equally important to avoid another significant blow to the head. Multiple concussions significantly increase the risk of long-term sequalae.

The Dangers of Repeat Concussions in Combat Sports

Martial artists and athletes who participate in combat sports are at a higher risk for repeat concussions. Repeat concussions have a higher risk of complications such a cerebral edema, permanent brain injury, and death. Repeated concussions can also result in early dementia-like symptoms that can occur many years after the injuries.

Repeated concussions (even mild) are linked to chronic traumatic encephalopathy (CTE), a degenerative disease of the brain. CTE causes permanent changes in the brain that leads to memory loss, impaired judgement, depression, aggression, and dementia. Unfortunately, CTE can only be diagnosed after death.

Self-inflicted Concussion via Headbutting

Contrary to what is seen in many action movies, intentional straight-on *forehead-to-forehead* headbutting is not advisable. The human cranium is different than that of a bighorn sheep in that it cannot absorb the forceful blow of two craniums colliding together. In humans, headbutting can cause a concussion to both parties. The person initiating the headbutt starts by throwing their head back, and then immediately forward into another head that is stationary. The initiator can cause a self-inflicted coupe-contrecoup injury as their brain bounces back and forth in their skull with more force.

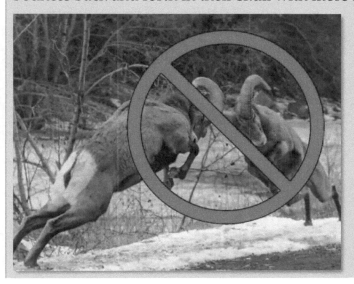

Research has shown that the powerful neck muscles and cranial sutures in headbutting animals redistribute the energy from the blows. Additionally, the horns of rams are made of semi-elastic spongy keratin which helps to absorb the energy of the shock; something that the human skull is lacking.

Fig. 6.9 - Avoid intentional forehead-to-forehead headbutting as a self-defense technique.

Concussion Policies

Many athletic and sporting organizations now recognize the dangers of concussions and repeat concussions. In addition to taking steps to prevent concussions, many organizations have developed concussion policies detailing what should be done after an injury, as well as who decides when the injured athlete can return to sport. The most responsible organizations now leave the decision up to the team medical staff rather than up to the coaches who do not usually have the medical training required to make such decisions.

Spinal Cord

The spinal cord extends from the medulla oblongata of the brain stem, through the foramen magnum at the base of the skull to the level of the first lumbar vertebra. The spinal cord, like the brain, is surrounded by bone, meninges, and cerebrospinal fluid.

The spinal cord is divided into 31 segments with each segment having a pair of spinal nerves. At the distal end of the spinal cord, a bundle of spinal nerves extends to form the cauda equina (resembling horse's tail).

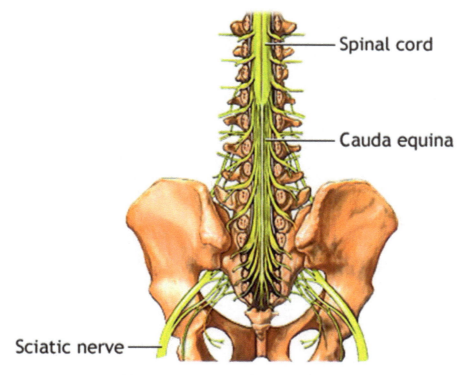

Fig. 6.10 - Spinal cord and cauda equina.

The two main functions of the spinal cord include:

- The spinal cord serves as a conduction pathway for impulses going to and from the brain. Sensory impulses travel to the brain on ascending tracts in the cord, while motor impulses travel on descending tracts.
- The spinal cord also serves as a reflex center. The reflex arc is the functional unit of the nervous system. Reflexes are responses to stimuli that do not require conscious thought and, consequently, they occur more quickly than reactions that require thought processes. A classic example is the *withdrawal reflex*: the reflex action withdraws the affected part before being aware of the pain, such as when touching a hot stove. Many reflexes are mediated in the spinal cord without going to the higher brain centers.

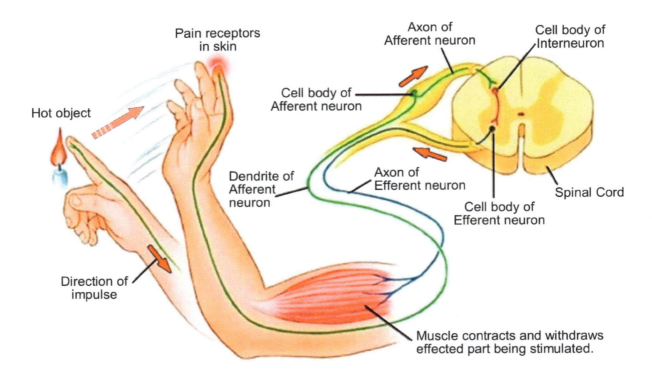

Fig. 6.11 - Withdrawal reflex involves the sensory (afferent) neuron, the interneuron in the spinal cord, and the motor (efferent) neuron.

The Peripheral Nervous System

The peripheral nervous system is the communication network between the central nervous system and the remaining parts of the body. It consists of the nerves that branch out from the brain and spinal cord. The peripheral nervous system is further subdivided into the autonomic nervous system and the somatic nervous system.

The *autonomic* nervous system (ANS) regulates and controls unconscious bodily functions. It consists of nerves that connect the CNS to the visceral organs responsible for breathing, heartbeat and blood pressure, and digestive processes.

The *somatic* (motor) nervous system consists of nerves that go to the skin and muscles involved in conscious (voluntary) activities.

Structure of a Nerve

A nerve contains bundles of nerve fibers (either axons or dendrites) surrounded by a connective tissue sheath called the epineurium. Each bundle of nerve fibers is called a fasciculus and is surrounded by a layer of connective tissue called the perineurium. Within the fasciculus, each individual nerve fiber, with its myelin and neurilemma, is surrounded by connective tissue called the endoneurium.

Sensory nerves contain only afferent fibers, long dendrites of sensory neurons. Motor nerves have only efferent fibers, long axons of motor neurons. Mixed nerves contain both types of fibers. A nerve may also have blood vessels enclosed in its connective tissue wrappings.

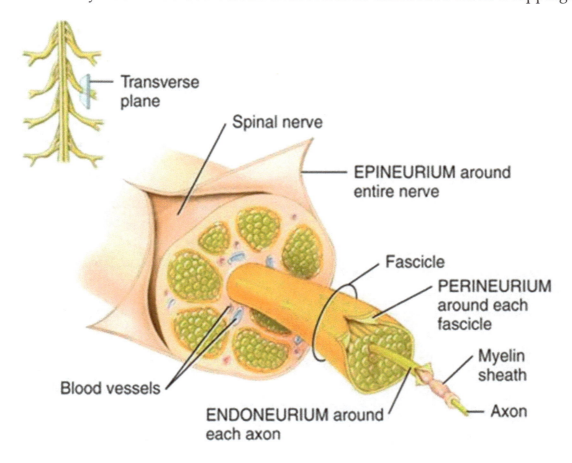

Fig. 6.12 - Transverse section showing the coverings of a spinal nerve.

- **Cranial Nerves**

There are twelve pairs of cranial nerves that emerge from the inferior surface of the brain. All of the cranial nerves, except for the vagus nerve, pass through foramina of the skull to innervate structures in the head, neck, and facial region.

The cranial nerves are designated by Roman numerals according to the order in which they appear on the inferior surface of the brain. They also have specific names based on their function, course, or structure. Most of the cranial nerves have both sensory and motor components; however, three of the nerves associated with the special senses of smell, vision, hearing, and equilibrium have only sensory fibers. Five of the cranial nerves are primarily motor in function but do have some sensory fibers for proprioception. The remaining four cranial nerves consist of significant amounts of both sensory and motor fibers.

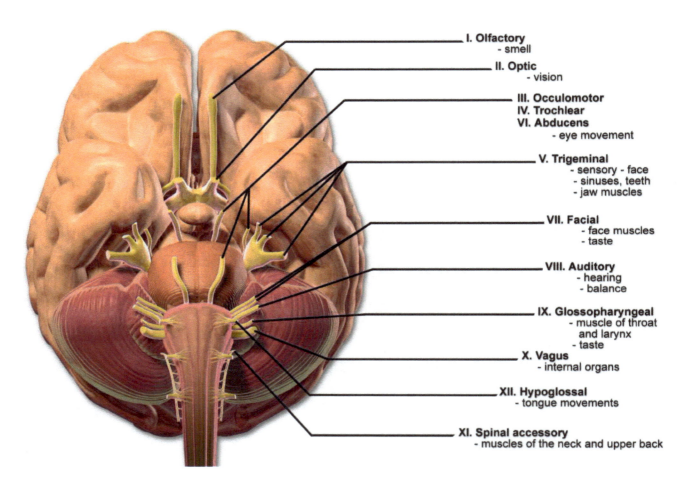

Fig. 6.13 - The 12 cranial nerves and their function. Image Credit: BruceBlaus "Medical gallery of Blausen 2014". WikiJournal of Medicine 1 (2). [CC BY 3.0].

Cranial Nerve	Function	Origin
I – Olfactory Nerve	Special Sensory	Cerebrum
II – Optic Nerve	Special Sensory	Cerebrum
III – Oculomotor Nerve	Motor	Midbrain
IV – Trochlear Nerve	Motor	Midbrain
V – Trigeminal Nerve	Sensory and motor	Pons
VI – Abducens Nerve	Motor	Pons
VII – Facial Nerve	Sensory, special sensory and motor	Pons
VIII – Vestibulocochlear Nerve	Special sensory	Pons
IX – Glossopharyngeal Nerve	Sensory, special sensory, autonomic, and motor	Medulla
X – Vagus Nerve	Sensory, motor, autonomic	Medulla
XI – Accessory Nerve	Motor	Medulla
XII – Hypoglossal Nerve	Motor	Medulla

Fig. 6.14 - Cranial nerves function and origin.

▪ Spinal Nerves

There are 31 pairs of spinal nerves that emerge laterally from the spinal cord. Each pair of nerves corresponds to a segment of the spinal cord and are named accordingly. This means there are 8 cervical nerves, 12 thoracic nerves, 5 lumbar nerves, 5 sacral nerves, and 1 coccygeal nerve.

Each spinal nerve is connected to the spinal cord by a dorsal (posterior) root and a ventral (anterior) root. The cell bodies of the sensory neurons are in the dorsal root ganglion, but the motor neuron cell bodies are in the gray matter. The two roots merge to form the spinal nerve just prior to the nerve exiting the vertebral column. Because all spinal nerves carry motor, sensory, and autonomic nerve impulses between the body and the spinal cord, they are all considered mixed nerves.

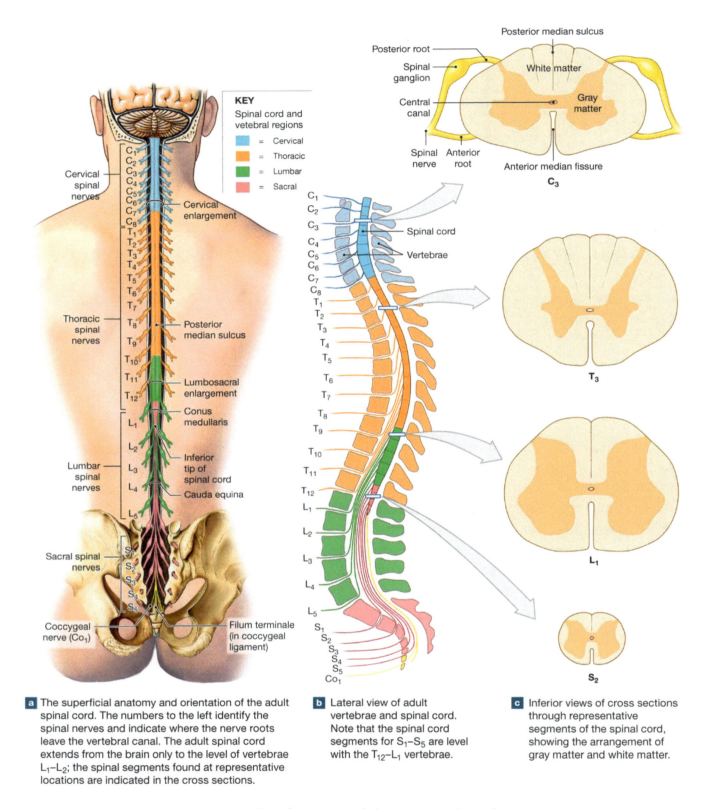

Fig. 6.15 - Spinals nerves and their associated vertebrae.

Dermatomes and Myotomes

A *dermatome* is a specific area on the skin that is innervated by branches of a single spinal sensory nerve root. The sensory nerves transmit signals from the area of sensation to the spinal cord.

Myotome refers to the group of muscles that are innervated by a specific spinal nerve root.

Dermatomes have overlapping regions innervated by one single spinal nerve; however, most *myotome* are innervated by more than one spinal nerve.

Dermatomes are responsible for the coordination of senses whereas myotomes are responsible for the coordination of voluntary muscular movement.

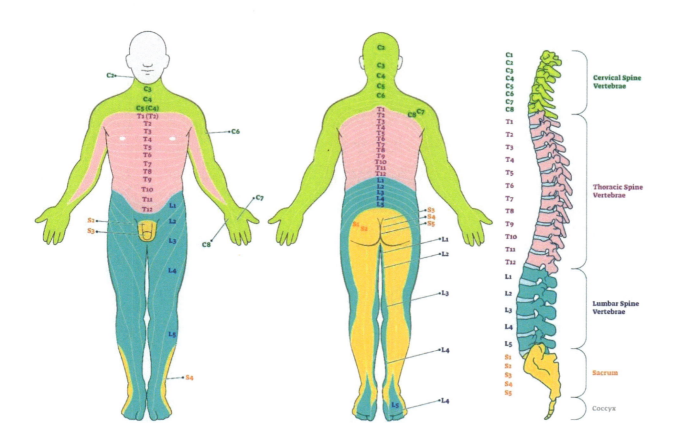

Fig. 6.16 - Dermatomes of the of the human body.

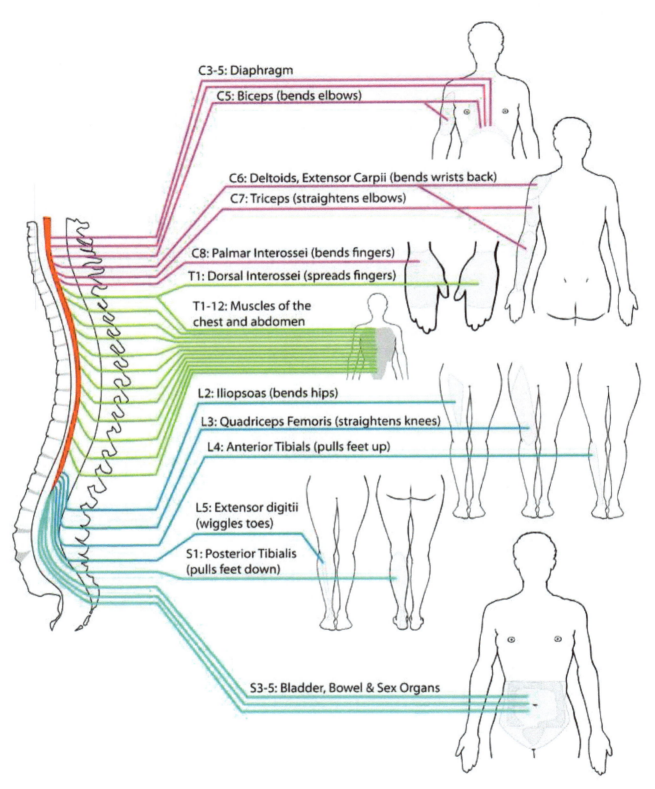

Fig. 6.17 - *Myotomes of the human body.*

Nerve Root	Muscle	Muscle Action	Peripheral Nerve
C4	Levator Scapulae	Neck side bending	Dorsal Scapular n.
C5	Deltoid Biceps	Shoulder abduction Elbow flexion	Axillary n. Musculocutaneous n.
C6	Biceps Extensor Carpi Radialis Longus	Supination Wrist extension	Musculocutaneous n. Radial n.
C7	Triceps Flexor Carpi Ulnaris	Elbow extension Wrist flexion	Radial n. Ulnar n.
C8	Extensor Pollicis Longus Flexor Digitorum	Thumb extension Grip	Radial n. Median n.
T1	Intrinsics	Finger abduction and adduction	Deep Ulnar n.
L2	Psoas	Hip flexion	Anterior Rami L2-4
L3	Quadriceps Adductor Longus and Magnus	Knee extension Hip adduction	Femoral n. Obturator n.
L4	Anterior Tibialis	Ankle dorsiflexion	Deep Peroneal n.
L5	Glut Medius Peroneals Extensor Hallicus Longus	Hip abduction Ankle eversion Great toe extension	Superior Gluteal n. Deep Peroneal n. Superficial Peroneal n.
S1	Gastrocnemius Hamstrings	Ankle plantarflexion Knee flex	Tibial n. Sciatic n.
S2	Glut maximus	Hip extension	Inferior Gluteal n.

Fig. 6.18 - Common nerve roots, peripheral nerves, innervated muscles, and their actions.

Autonomic Nervous System

The autonomic nervous system sends motor impulses to the visceral organs, which means it is a visceral efferent system. It functions automatically and continuously to innervate smooth muscle, cardiac muscle, and glands without conscious effort. It regulates the heart rate, breathing rate, blood pressure, body temperature, and other visceral activities that work together to maintain homeostasis.

The autonomic nervous system is subdivided into the *sympathetic* and the *parasympathetic* division. Many visceral organs are innervated by fibers from both divisions: one stimulates while the other inhibits. This antagonistic functional relationship serves as a balance to help maintain homeostasis. The sympathetic nervous system governs the "fight or flight" response, while the parasympathetic system controls the "rest and digest" response.

The sympathetic nervous system (SNS) is vital to survival. Fibers from the SNS innervate tissues in almost every organ system and provides physiological regulation over diverse bodily processes including pupil diameter, gut motility, and urinary output. The main objective of the SNS is to prepare the body for physical activity. It revs up the body when confronted with imminent danger to either defend or to escape the threat.

The parasympathetic nervous system is the counterbalance to the sympathetic response to danger, whether real or imagined. Once the threat is resolved, the parasympathetic system brings all the organ systems of the body back to normal. The parasympathetic nervous system promotes digestion and other "housekeeping" functions when the body is at rest.

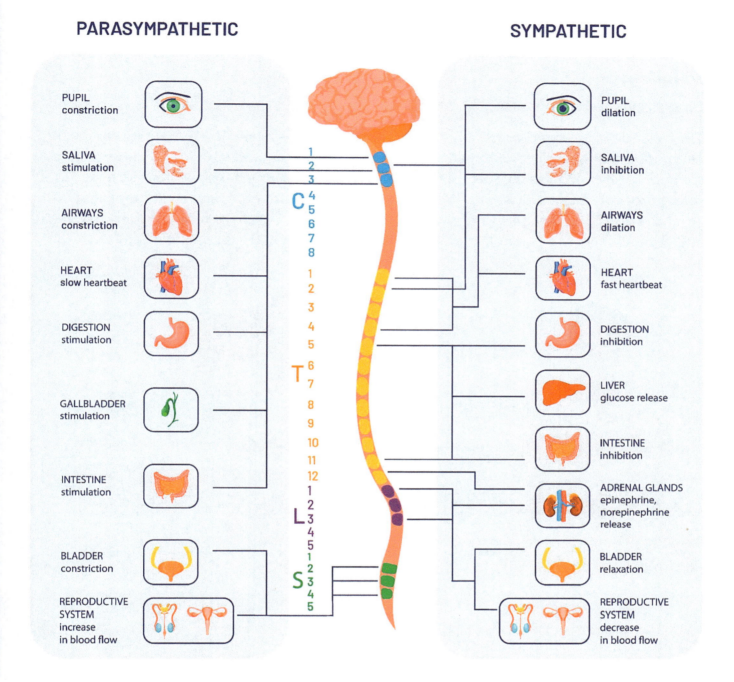

Fig. 6.19 - Comparison of sympathetic and parasympathetic nervous system functions

Clinical Significance and Martial Arts Relevance:

Solar Plexus

Innervation of the Abdomen

The celiac (solar) plexus is part of the sympathetic nervous system. It is a complex bundle of nerves found in the upper abdomen posterior to the pancreas, and anterior of the aorta. It is commonly referred to as the solar plexus because of its radiating network of nerve fibers. The solar plexus innervates the stomach, liver, gallbladder, intestines, pancreas, kidneys, and adrenal glands. It transmits visceral sensory impulses such as pain or reflexes from the foregut and midgut, increases glandular secretion, and promotes peristalsis and digestion.

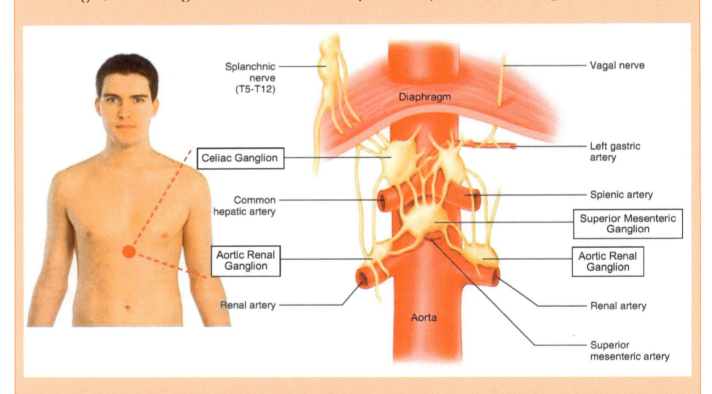

Fig. 6.20 - *Approximate location of the celiac (solar) plexus, posterior to the pancreas and anterior to the aorta. The celiac plexus consists of celiac, superior mesenteric, and renal ganglia found surrounding the roots of the celiac trunk, superior mesenteric, and renal arteries.*

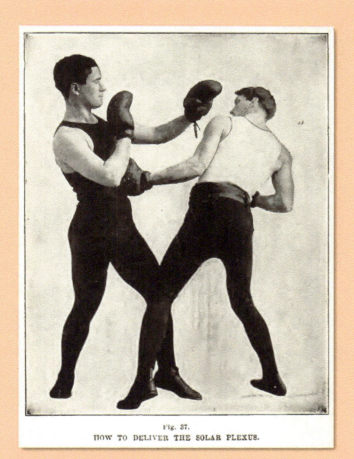

In the context of sparring or injury, a strike to the mid abdomen around the solar plexus (not solar "plex") region may cause the diaphragm to spasm, resulting in difficulty breathing — a sensation frequently referred to as "getting the wind knocked out of you". As the diaphragm spasms, it makes it difficult to inhale and "catch your breath". It may also affect the celiac plexus itself, which can cause great pain and interfere with the functioning of the viscera.

Fig. 6.21 - Punch to the solar plexus. Image Credit: Boxing: A Guide to the Manly Art of Self Defense. New York, American Sports Publishing Co., 1917. Pg. 108.

The Somatic Nervous System

The somatic nervous system (or voluntary nervous system) is responsible for carrying motor and sensory information both to and from the central nervous system. This system is made up of nerves that connect to the skin, sensory organs, and all skeletal muscles. In addition to processing sensory information that arrives via external stimuli (including hearing, touch, and sight), the somatic system is also responsible for nearly all voluntary muscle movements. The structures that allow this communication to happen between the nerves throughout the body and the CNS are known as the afferent sensory neurons and the efferent motor neurons.

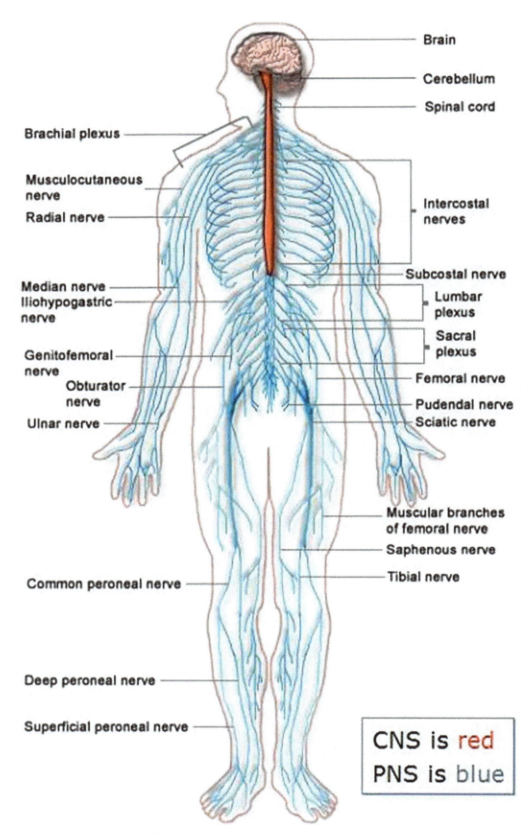

Fig. 6.22 - Major peripheral nerves of the human body.

Brachial Plexus

The Brachial Plexus is formed by the anterior primary rami of the 5th, 6th, 7th and 8th cervical roots and part of the 1st thoracic root. The nerves which arise from above the clavicle (supraclavicular branches) supply the Supraspinatus and Infraspinatus via the Suprascapular nerve which also supply the shoulder joint and acromio clavicular joint. The Subclavius muscle is supplied by its own nerve and the Serratus Anterior is supplied by the Long Thoracic nerve from C5, 6 & 7.

The nerves which arise from below the clavicle (Infraclavicular branches) are the Musculocutaneous nerve, Ulnar nerve, Median nerve, Radial nerve, Circumflex (axillary) nerve, Subscapular nerve and nerve to the Latissimus Dorsi muscle.

1 Terminal Branches
2 Axilla
3 Lateral Posterior Medial Cords
4 Divisions First Rib
5 Superior Middle Inferior
6 Trunks Scalene Muscles
7 Anterior Primary Rami
8 Roots

Definitions

ROOTS – The cervical spinal nerves after they have given off their branches to the prevertebral muscles constitute the roots of the plexus.

TRUNKS – Formed by union of the roots, the upper trunk C5 and C6, central C7 and lower trunk C8 & T1

DIVISIONS – Each of the three trunks divides into an anterior and posterior division behind the clavicle

CORDS – The upper two divisions unite to form the Lateral cord. The anterior division of the lower trunk runs on as the Medial cord and all three posterior divisions unite to form the Posterior Cord

Musculocutaneous N.

Originating from the lateral cord of the Brachial Plexus, it contains fibres from the 5th, 6th and 7th cervical roots.

Supplies:
- Coracobrachialis muscle
- Also provides branches to Biceps and Brachialis muscles.
- Becomes Lateral Cutaneous nerve of forearm after it appears on outside of Biceps near the elbow joint.
- Just below the elbow it inserts into the deep fascia of Biceps tendon and continues as the Lateral Cutaneous nerve of the forearm.

Long Thoracic Nerve

Arises usually by three roots from the 5th, 6th and 7th cervical roots. The 5th and 6th roots supply the Scalenus Medius. The main muscle it supplies is the Serratus Anterior.

Ulnar Nerve

Arises from the medial cord of Brachial Plexus. The source of its fibres are from the 7th and 8th cervical and 1st thoracic roots. It runs down the medial side of the arm and forearm, behind the medial epicondyles of the humerus and continues into the hand.

Two muscular branches just below the elbow supply:
- Flexor Carpi Ulnaris
- Flexor Digitorum Profundus (also supplied by Median nerve)

As it enters the hand the deep terminal branch supplies at its source the three short muscles of the little finger.

As it crosses the hand it supplies:
- Adductor Pollicis
- Flexor Pollicis Brevis

It terminates by supplying the 3rd and 4th lumbricals and all the interosscii both palmar and dorsal. Superficial branch supplies palmaris brevis and the sensory fibres of the little finger and adjacent side of ring finger.

Median Nerve

Originates from the medial cord and contains fibres from the 5th to the 8th cervical roots and the 1st thoracic root.

Supplies fibres to:
- Pronator Teres
- Flexor Carpi Radialis
- Palmaris Longus
- Flexor Digitorum Superficialis

Via a branch on the front of the interosseous membrane in the forearm it supplies:
- Lateral side of Flexor Digitorum Profundus (also supplied from Ulnar nerve)
- Flexor Pollicis Longus
- Pronator Quadratus

Once in the hand the nerve divides to supply the muscles of the thenar eminence:
- Abductor Pollicis Brevis
- Flexor Pollicis Brevis
- Opponens Pollicis
- 1st and 2nd Lumbricals

Nerves of the Anterior Upper Extremity

Cervical Plexus

It is formed by the anterior primary rami of the first four cervical nerves and is situated in front of the Levator Scapulae and Scalenus Medius muscles and behind the Sterno-mastoid muscle. It supplies the skin of the back and side of the scalp, side and front of the neck. It supplies the deep and superficial muscles of the neck and has an important branch via C3, 4 & 5 which form the Phrenic nerve that passes through the thorax to the diaphram.

Upper & Lower Subscapular Nerve

These two nerves arise from C5-C6 as shown in the Brachial Plexus. Upper Subscapular nerve supplies the Subscapularis muscle. Lower Subscapular nerve supplies the Teres Major.

Accessory Nerve

The accessory nerve is formed by the fusion of the 11th cranial and spinal (cervical) roots. The pathway of this nerve in the neck runs down and through the sternocleidomastoid muscle then into the front of the trapezius muscle.

Supplies:
- Sternocleidomastoid (C2-C3)
- Upper, mid and lower Trapezius muscle together with branches from C3-C4

Suprascapular Nerve

This is a large nerve arising from upper part of Brachial Plexus (C5-C6).

Supplies via branches:
- Supraspinatus
- Infraspinatus

Via filaments:
- Shoulder joint and Acromio-clavicular joint
- Scapula

Dorsal Scapular Nerve

Arises from C5

Supplies:
- Scalenus medius
- Levator scapulae
- Rhomboids – minor and major

Axillary Nerve

Arises from the posterior aspect of the Brachial Plexus, its fibres coming from C5-C6.

Radial Nerve

Arises from the posterior cord of the brachial plexus and passes behind the clavicle and down round the posterior surface of the Humerus below Teres Minor. It continues between the origins of the lateral and medial heads of the Triceps muscle. It travels down the lateral side of the upper arm, then moves to the front of the lateral epicondyle of the humerus between the Brachio-radialis and Brachialis muscles, (where it gives off the Posterior Interosseous nerve) continues down the side of the forearm, passing to the back of the wrist and divides into the digital branches of the hand. *

Supraclavicular Branches

(above the clavicle) supply:
- Supraspinatus, Infraspinatus, Shoulder and Acromio-clavicular joints.
- Subclavius and Serratus Anterior muscles.

Infraclavicular Branches

Arising below the clavicle are the Musculocutaneous nerve, Ulnar, Median and Radial nerves, Circumflex and Subscapular nerves as well as the nerve to the Latissimus Dorsi muscle.

Posterior Interosseous Nerve

Supplies:
- Extensor Carpi Radialis Brevis
- Supinator
- Extensor Carpi Ulnaris
- Extensor Digiti Minimi
- Extensor Digitorum
- Extensor Pollicis Longus
- Abductor Pollicis Longus
- Extensor Pollicis Brevis
- Extensor Indicis

* Radial Nerve Cont'd.

Supplies:
- Three heads of Triceps muscle
- Anconeus
- Brachioradialis
- Extensor Carpi Radialis Longus

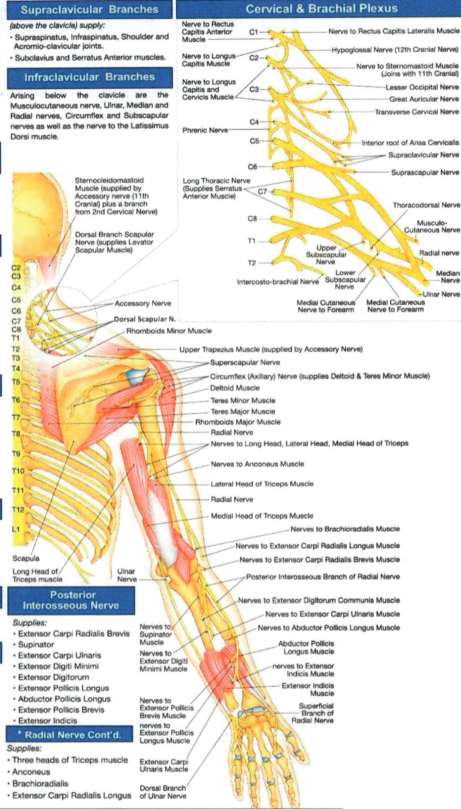

Nerves of the Posterior Upper Extremity

COMPREHENSIVE ANATOMY FOR MARTIAL ARTS

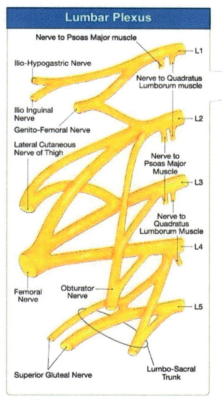

Lumbar Plexus

Femoral Nerve

Arises from the anterior branches of the L1, 2, 3 &. 4 roots. It goes through fibres of Psoas Major and continues down between it and the Iliacus muscle. The Femoral nerve is like the fingers of a hand.

Supplies the major anterior thigh muscles:
- Rectus Femoris
- Vastus Lateralis, Medialis and Intermedius
- Pectineus
- Sartorius

It also supplies the Cutaneous Branches to the anterior skin of the thigh. Lateral Cutaneous nerve of the thigh arises from the anterior branches of the L2-3 roots and passes into the lateral side of the thigh under or through the inguinal ligament.

Common Peroneal Nerve

Arises from L4 and 5 and S1 and S2. It runs down the outside of the back of the thigh in the Sciatic nerve, then across the popliteal fossa to the head of the fibula before wrapping round the neck of the fibula.

Supplies all the major extensor muscles of the foot and ankle situated on the front of the lower leg through its deep peroneal branch.

The superficial peroneal branch supplies Peroneus Longus and Brevis whose tendons pass behind the Lateral Malleolus of the ankle and evert the foot and ankle.

Nerves of the Anterior Lower Extremity

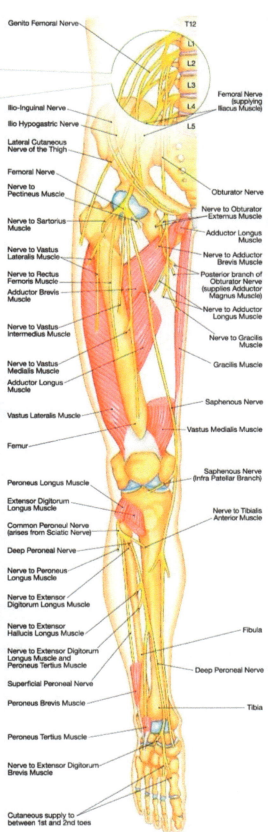

Genitofemoral Nerve

Arises from L1 and L2. It often divides close to its origin into two branches. The genital and femoral branches supply the pelvis and genital organs.

Ilioinguinal Nerve

Arises with the Iliohypogastric nerve from L1. Together these two nerves emerge from the Psoas major and pass across the Quadratus Lumborum.

They supply:
- Transversus Abdominis
- Obliquus Internus Abdominis

Obturator Nerve

Arises from the Lumbar plexus, L2, 3 & 4. It runs through and around the inside of the pelvis and down through the Obturator foramen.

Anterior branch supplies:
- Adductor Longus
- Adductor Brevis
- Gracilis
- Sensation on the medial side of the thigh
- Capsule of the hip joint

Posterior branch supplies:
- Obturator
- Part of Adductor Magnus
- Capsule of the knee joint

Saphenous Nerve

It is the largest sensory branch of the Femoral nerve. It runs down the leg beside the femoral artery, then goes across the adductor muscles to the medial side of the knee before going down to the medial border of the tibia. At the knee is gives off the Infra Patellar branch. It also has a large sensory element supplying the medial side of the lower leg and foot.

Deep Peroneal Nerve

Arises at the bifurcation of the Common Peroneal nerve between the fibula and proximal fibres of the Peroneus Longus muscle.

Supplies:
- Tibialis Anterior
- Extensor Hallucis Longus
- Extensor Digitorum Longus
- Peroneus Tertius

Lateral terminal branch supplies:
- Extensor Digitorum Brevis

Medial terminal branch supplies:
- Muscles of the great and second toes

Superior Gluteal Nerve

Arises from Dorsal branches of L4, 5 & S1. It is divided into a superior and an inferior branch.

Superior branch supplies:
- Gluteus Medius

Inferior branch supplies:
- Gluteus Minimus
- Tensor Fascia Latae

Inferior Gluteal Nerve

Arises from dorsal branches of L5, S1 and S2.

Supplies:
- Piriformis
- Gluteus Maximus

Posterior Femoral Cutaneous Nerve

Arises from S1, 2 and 3.

Supplies sensation to the skin over the anal region, the buttocks, back of the thigh and upper part of the calf.

Pudendal Nerve

Arises from roots of S2, 3 and 4. Supplies the muscles and body of the genitalia and anus as well as the skin of the perineum.

Sciatic Nerve

This is the largest nerve in the body. At its starting point it is 2cm wide. It arises from L4 & 5 and S1, 2 & 3. Two nerves make up the Sciatic nerve:

Common Peroneal and Tibial nerves. The main sciatic trunk, the tibial division, supplies the hamstrings:
- Semitendinosus
- Semimembranosus
- Biceps Femoris (long head), and
- part of Adductor Magnus (in conjunction with the Obturator nerve)

In the lower leg it supplies:
- Gastrocnemius
- Soleus
- Plantaris
- Popliteus
- Tibialis Posterior
- Flexor Hallucis Longus
- Flexor Digitorum Longus

Tibial Nerve

divides into:
1. The Medial Plantar Nerve
which supplies:
- Abductor Hallucis
- Flexor Digitorum Brevis
- 1st Lumbrical muscle

2. The Lateral Plantar Nerve
which supplies:
- Abductor Digiti Minimi
- Adductor Hallucis
- Flexor Digiti Minimi Brevis
- Interosseous muscles of the foot.

Common Peroneal

Supplies:
- Short head of Biceps Femoris
- Anterior Peroneal Muscle

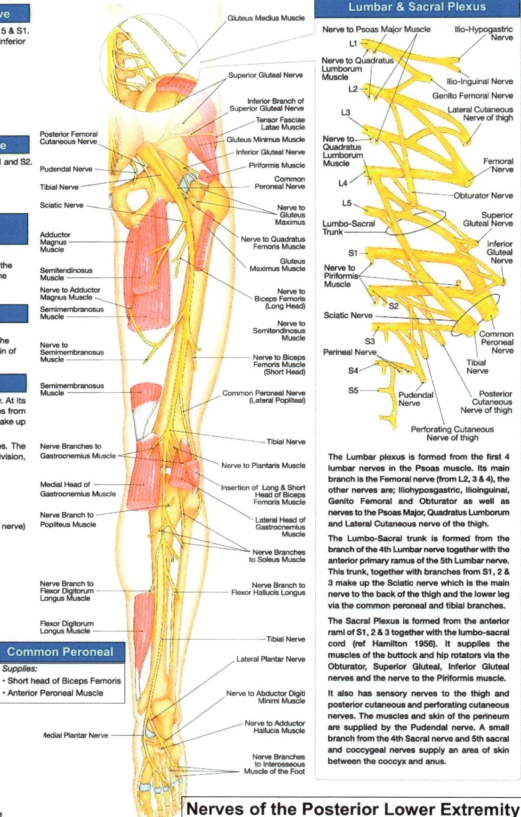

Lumbar & Sacral Plexus

The Lumbar plexus is formed from the first 4 lumbar nerves in the Psoas muscle. Its main branch is the Femoral nerve (from L2, 3 & 4), the other nerves are; Iliohyposgastric, Ilioinguinal, Genito Femoral and Obturator as well as nerves to the Psoas Major, Quadratus Lumborum and Lateral Cutaneous nerve of the thigh.

The Lumbo-Sacral trunk is formed from the branch of the 4th Lumbar nerve together with the anterior primary ramus of the 5th Lumbar nerve. This trunk, together with branches from S1, 2 & 3 make up the Sciatic nerve which is the main nerve to the back of the thigh and the lower leg via the common peroneal and tibial branches.

The Sacral Plexus is formed from the anterior rami of S1, 2 & 3 together with the lumbo-sacral cord (ref Hamilton 1956). It supplies the muscles of the buttock and hip rotators via the Obturator, Superior Gluteal, Inferior Gluteal nerves and the nerve to the Piriformis muscle.

It also has sensory nerves to the thigh and posterior cutaneous and perforating cutaneous nerves. The muscles and skin of the perineum are supplied by the Pudendal nerve. A small branch from the 4th Sacral nerve and 5th sacral and coccygeal nerves supply an area of skin between the coccyx and anus.

Nerves of the Posterior Lower Extremity

Chapter 7

Special Sensory Organs

The human body has two major types of senses: special senses and general senses. In the study of anatomy, and within the medical profession, the special senses are considered the senses that have specialized organs devoted to them, i.e., vision (eyes), hearing and balance (ears), smell (nose), and taste (tongue). General senses are all associated with touch and lack special sensory organs. All senses depend on sensory receptor cells to detect sensory stimuli, and in turn transform them into nerve impulses.

Special sensory organs are a prime example of how multiple anatomy systems (nervous, muscular, skeletal, circulatory) must work together to achieve a specific function.

The special sensory organs most relevant for martial artists and combat sport athletes include the ears and eyes.

The Ears

The human ear can be divided into main three parts: the external (outer) ear, middle ear, and inner (internal) ear.

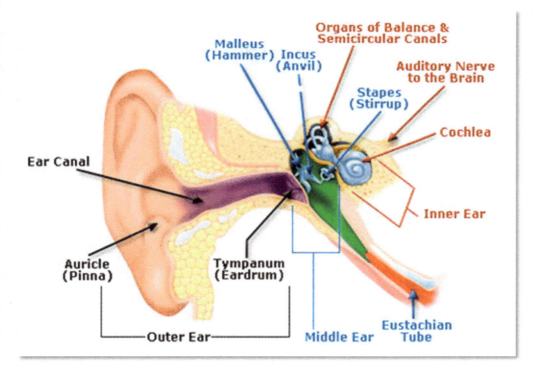

Fig. 7.1 - Anatomy of the human ear. Image Credit: Public domain, Wikimedia Commons.

External Ear

The external ear can be divided both structurally and functionally into two parts: the visible auricle (or pinna), and the external acoustic meatus, which ends at the tympanic membrane.

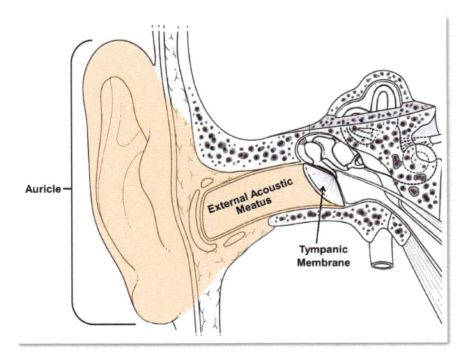

Fig. 7.2 – Structures of the external ear.

- **Auricle**

The *auricle* are paired structures found on either side of the head that function to capture and direct sound waves towards the *external acoustic meatus* (ear canal).

The auricles are mostly cartilaginous in their structure, with the *lobule* being the only part not supported by cartilage. The cartilaginous portion of the auricle that forms an outer curvature is known as the *helix*. The innermost curvature that runs parallel with the helix is called the *antihelix*. The antihelix is divided into two *cura*; the *inferoanterior* (lying below and in front) *crus*, and the *superoposterior* (lying above and behind) *crus*.

The *concha* is the hollow depression in the middle of the auricle. It acts to direct sound into the external acoustic meatus. Immediately anterior to the beginning of the external acoustic meatus is an elevation of cartilaginous tissue known as the *tragus*. Opposite the tragus is the *antitragus*.

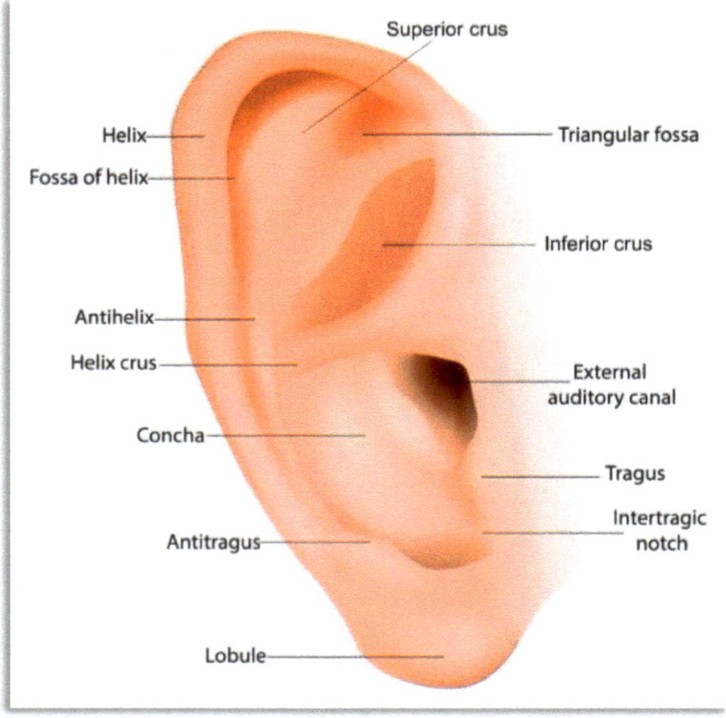

Fig. 7.3 – Anterior surface of the auricle of the external ear.

Clinical Significance and Martial Arts Relevance:

Auricular Hematoma and Cauliflower Ear

An auricular hematoma refers to a collection of blood between the cartilage of the ear and the overlying perichondrium. It usually occurs as a result of trauma, commonly seen in contact and combat sports.

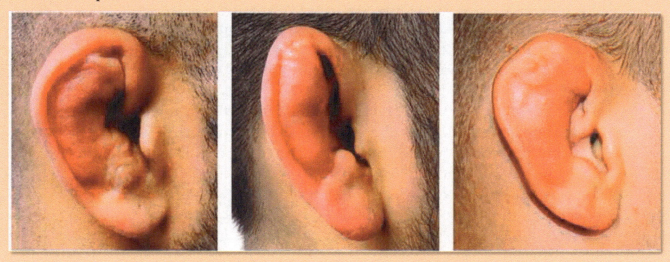

Fig. 7.4 - An untreated auricular hematoma can lead to cauliflower ear. Above, three patients with permanent and solid cauliflower ears as a result of failure to evacuate the hematoma. Image Credit: Christoffer Ingvaldsen, MD, PhD

The resulting hematoma can disrupt the blood supply to the cartilage and requires prompt drainage. Untreated auricular hematomas can result in avascular necrosis of the cartilage, resulting in a "cauliflower ear" deformity. The collection of blood separates the tissue planes in the auricle of the ear, which fills with blood, loses tissue, eventually scars, solidifies, and causes the signature unusual shape and swelling.

Draining the swollen area by surgical incision and drainage, or aspiration, followed by a compression bolster dressing is the most common treatment for auricular hematoma to help prevent cauliflower ear.

Because of the decreased blood supply and the fact that people often return too quickly to training in a dirty environment (like a gym or locker room) with an unhealed wound; even with the appropriate treatment, there is still a significant risk of infection.

Unfortunately, there is a current trend among some martial artists and grapplers who consider cauliflower ear as a badge of honor. Wrestlers have been reported to rub each other's ears trying to give each other cauliflower ear. There is a video on social media platforms of grapplers smashing each other's ears with bottles attempting to cause auricular hematoma.

Too often ill-informed coaches and instructors have cavalier attitudes about the potential sequalae associated with these injuries among young athletes.

Cauliflower ear can affect the training of affected athletes and their training partners. It can break open and bleed while training and be at a higher risk for infection. It can also make things like sleeping comfortably or even wearing headphones a challenge in more severe cases.

While the treatment can be straightforward, the consequences are not something to be taken lightly. A study by the Asian Journal of Sports Medicine in 2015 showed athletes with cauliflower ear are more likely to have ear infections; because it "may increase the probability of collection of pathogenic microorganisms in the ear canal and thereby increase the rate of infection in such ears."

Worse, the same study confirmed previous research that demonstrated an increased likelihood of hearing loss associated with cauliflower ear. Reconstructive surgery is an option in severe cases, but the procedure can be difficult and involves reshaping the damaged ear tissue, replacing it with artificial cartilage, or part of the ribs.

Cauliflower ear does not need to be an inevitable result of long-term training in combat sports. Prevention strategies includes education and awareness. Fortunately, wearing low-profile ear protection/headgear is becoming more popular in the grappling related arts. Protecting the ear when defending against strikes to the side of the head can diminish direct blows to the auricle. Being aware and cautious when clinching, tying up, and escaping chokes can also reduce the potential for injury.

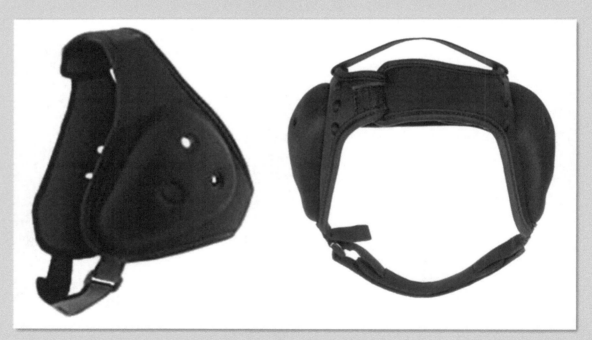

Fig. 7.5 - Low profile soft grappling headgear can prevent the occurrence of auricle hematoma.

- **External Acoustic Meatus**

The external acoustic meatus (ear canal) is an S-shaped tube that extends from the deep part of the concha to the tympanic membrane. The walls of the external one-third of the canal is formed by cartilage, whereas the inner two-thirds are formed by the temporal bone.

- **Tympanic Membrane**

The tympanic membrane (eardrum) forms the distal end of the external acoustic meatus. The eardrum is a connective tissue structure, covered with skin on the outside and a mucous membrane on the inside. It is connected to the surrounding temporal bone by a fibrocartilaginous ring.

The thin tympanic membrane is translucent, which allows the structures within the middle ear to be observed during otoscopic examination. The handle of malleus bone attaches to the inner surface tympanic membrane at a point called the *umbo* of the tympanic membrane.

The *handle of malleus* continues superiorly from the umbo. At its highest point, a small projection called the *lateral process* of the malleus can be seen. The parts of the tympanic membrane moving away from the lateral process are called the anterior and posterior malleolar folds.

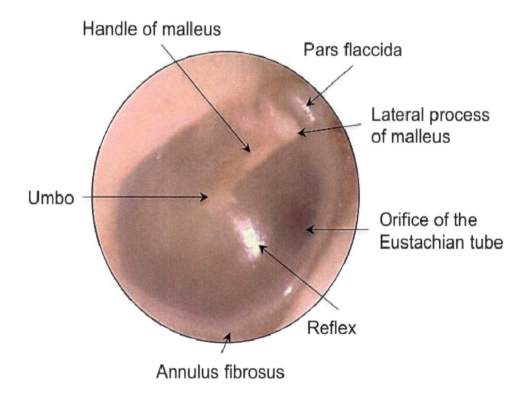

Fig. 7.6 – The surface anatomy of a normal tympanic membrane.
Image Credit: Semantic Scholar Corpus ID: 32512477

Clinical Significance and Martial Arts Relevance:

Perforation of the Tympanic Membrane

The tympanic membrane (TM) is a relatively thin connective tissue structure that is susceptible to perforation, usually by trauma or infection.

An infection of the middle ear (otitis media) can cause fluid and pus to build up behind the tympanic membrane. This causes an increase in pressure within the middle ear and can eventually cause the eardrum to rupture. In most cases the tympanic membrane heals itself, but in larger perforations surgical grafting may be required.

Rupture or perforation of the eardrum can also be caused by an abrupt forceful blow or slap to the external ear. A traumatic eardrum rupture can cause a significant amount of pain. However, in and of itself, a ruptured TM does *not* cause a loss of balance or the inability to walk as is often taught in martial arts. Patients are treated daily around the world who have sustained isolated traumatic ruptured eardrums and none of them need to "learn how to walk again". Additionally, eardrums do *not* "*shatter*". When martial arts instructors make such claims, they are automatically discredited by those who are more informed. As with any sharp blow to the head, there can be a momentary sense of being disoriented; but it is not due to a disruption in the integrity of the TM itself. The vestibule and the semicircular canals in the inner ear control balance, not the tympanic membrane. See *The Inner Ear* section for more details.

Middle Ear

The middle ear lies within the temporal bone. It extends from the tympanic membrane to the lateral wall of the inner ear. The primary function of the middle ear is to transmit vibrations from the tympanic membrane to the inner ear via the auditory ossicles (bones).

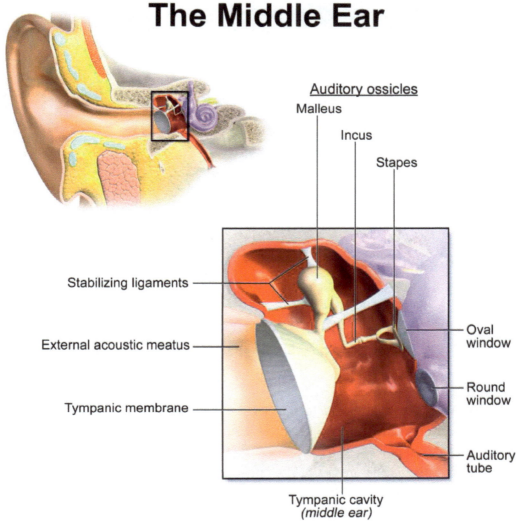

Fig. 7.7 – Structures of the middle ear. Image Credit: Medical gallery of Blausen Medical 2014. WikiJournal of Medicine 1 (2). [CC BY 3.0] via Wikimedia Commons

The middle ear can be divided into two areas: the tympanic cavity and the epitympanic recess.

The **tympanic cavity** is located medial to the tympanic membrane. It contains three small bones known as the auditory ossicles: the *malleus*, the *incus*, and the *stapes*. Together the ossicles transmit sound vibrations through the middle ear.

The **epitympanic recess** is the space superior to the tympanic cavity, which lies next to the mastoid air cells. The malleus and incus extend partially superiorly into the epitympanic recess.

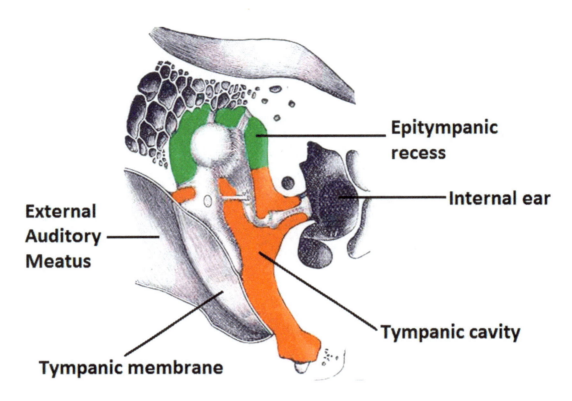

Fig. 7.8 – The two primary areas of the middle ear include the tympanic cavity and the epitympanic recess. Image Credit:

▪ **Auditory Ossicles**

The bones of the middle ear are the auditory ossicles: the *malleus* (hammer), *incus* (anvil), and the *stapes* (stirrup). Connected in a chain-like fashion, they link the tympanic membrane to the oval window of the internal ear.

Sound vibrations cause a movement of the tympanic membrane, which then in turn creates movement (oscillation) in the auditory ossicles. This movement transmits the sound waves from the tympanic membrane of the external ear to the oval window of the internal ear.

The malleus is the largest and most lateral of the ossicles and attaches to the tympanic membrane, via the handle of malleus. The head of the malleus lies in the epitympanic recess where it articulates with the incus.

The incus consists of a body and two limbs. The body of the incus articulates with the malleus. The short limb attaches to the posterior wall of the middle ear, while the long limb of the incus articulates with the stapes.

The stapes is the smallest bone in the human body. It connects the incus to the oval window of the inner ear. It is stirrup-shaped with a head, two limbs, and a base. The head articulates with the incus, and the base connects with the oval window.

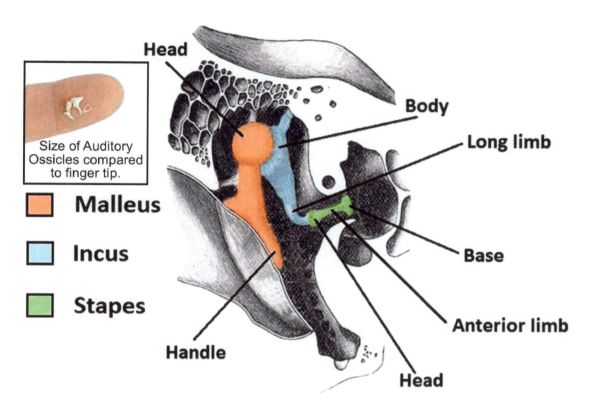

Fig. 7.9 – Bones of the middle ear.

- **Mastoid Air Cells**

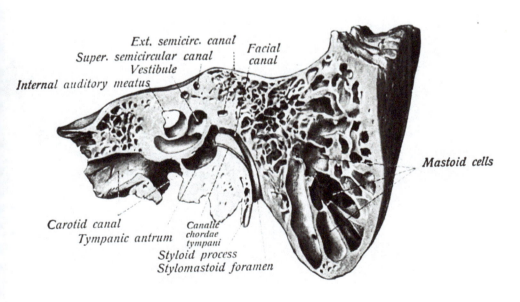

Fig. 7.10 – Coronal section showing the mastoid air cells in detail.

The mastoid air cells are located posterior to epitympanic recess. They are a collection of air-filled spaces in the mastoid process of the temporal bone. The mastoid cells protect the structures of the ear and regulate pressure within the middle ear. The air cells are contained within a cavity called the mastoid antrum.

Muscles of the Middle Ear

The *tensor tympani* and *stapedius* are two muscles which provide a protective function within the middle ear. Known as the acoustic reflex, the muscles contract in response to loud noise, inhibiting the vibrations of the malleus, incus, and stapes; thereby reducing the transmission of sound to the inner ear.

The tensor tympani muscle originates from the eustachian tube and attaches to the handle of malleus, pulling it medially as it contracts. The stapedius muscle inserts into the stapes and is innervated by the facial nerve. The tensor tympani muscle is innervated by the tensor tympani nerve, a branch of the mandibular nerve.

Eustachian Tube

The eustachian tube (auditory tube) is a cartilaginous and bony tube that connects the middle ear to the nasopharynx. It functions to equalize the pressure within the middle ear to that of the external auditory meatus.

The eustachian tube extends from the anterior wall of the middle ear in an anterior, medioinferior direction, opening into the lateral wall of the nasopharynx.

The Inner Ear

The inner ear (internal ear) is the innermost part of the ear and contains the vestibulocochlear organs. The structures of the inner ear convert *mechanical* signals from the middle ear into *electrical* signals, which transmits information to the auditory pathway in the brain. They also assist in maintaining balance, detecting motion and body position.

The inner ear is located within the *petrous* part of the temporal bone. It is situated between the middle ear (laterally) and the internal acoustic meatus (medially). The inner ear contains two main components: the bony labyrinth and membranous labyrinth.

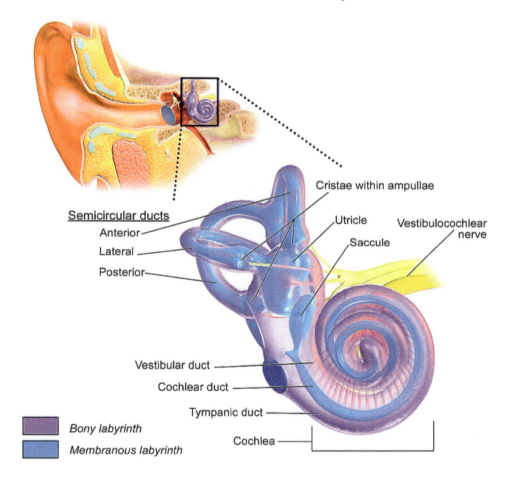

Fig. 7.11 – Structures of the Inner ear. Image Credit: Medical gallery of Blausen Medical 2014. WikiJournal of Medicine 1 (2). [CC BY 3.0] via Wikimedia Commons.

The **bony labyrinth** consists of a series of bony cavities which includes: the cochlea, vestibule, and three semicircular canals. All three structures contain a fluid called perilymph and are lined internally with periosteum.

The **membranous labyrinth** lies within the bony labyrinth and consists of the cochlear duct, semicircular ducts, the saccule, and the utricle. The membranous labyrinth is filled with fluid called endolymph.

There are two openings between the middle ear and the inner ear that are both covered by membranes. The *oval window* lies between the middle ear and the vestibule, while the *round window* separates the middle ear from the scala tympani (part of the cochlear duct).

▪ Bony Labyrinth

The bony labyrinth is a series of bony cavities that consists of three parts: the cochlea, vestibule, and the three semicircular canals.

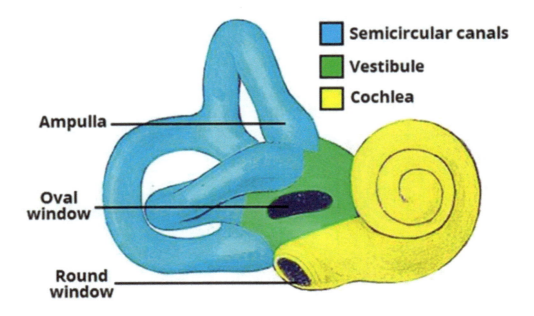

Fig. 7.12 – The three parts of the bony labyrinth include the cochlea, vestibule, and semicircular canals

- *Vestibule:* The vestibule is the central part of the bony labyrinth. It is separated from the middle ear by the oval window and communicates anteriorly with the cochlea and posteriorly with the semicircular canals.

    Two parts of the membranous labyrinth; the *saccule* and *utricle*, are located within the vestibule.

- *Cochlea:* The cochlea houses the cochlea duct of the membranous labyrinth. It twists upon itself around a central portion of bone called the *modiolus*, producing a cone shape which points in an anterolateral direction. Branches from the cochlear portion of the vestibulocochlear (VIII) nerve are found at the base of the modiolus.

The spiral lamina is a bony shelf that projects from the modiolus to the interior of the canal. It projects about half-way toward the outer wall of the canal, and partially divides its cavity into two passages (or scalae). The presence of the cochlear duct creates two perilymph-filled chambers superiorly and inferiorly:

- The *scala vestibuli* is located superiorly to the cochlear duct and is continuous with the vestibule.
- The *scala tympani* is located inferiorly to the cochlear duct and terminates at the round window.

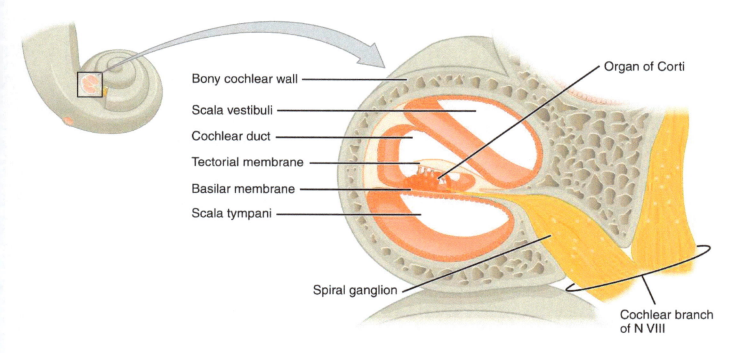

Fig. 7.13 - Anatomy of the cochlea. Image Credit: OpenStax, [CC BY 4.0] via Wikimedia Commons.

- *Semicircular Canals:* There are three semicircular canals which include: the anterior, lateral, and posterior canal. They contain the *semicircular ducts* which, along with the utricle and saccule, are responsible for balance.

    The canals are situated superoposterior to the vestibule, at right angles to each other. The enlargement at one end is known as the *ampulla*.

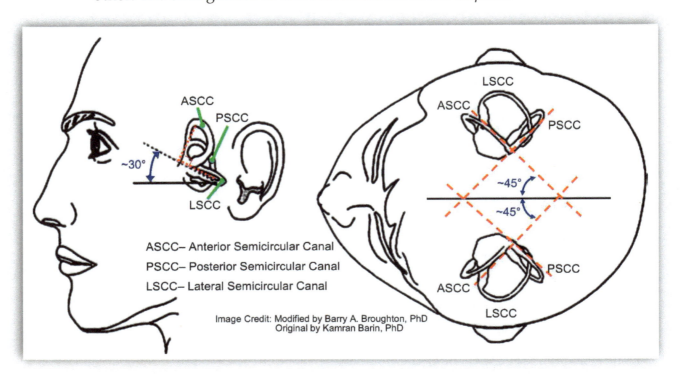

Fig. 7.14 - Orientation of semicircular canals. The lateral semicircular canals lie in the same horizontal plane. The right anterior canal lies parallel to the left posterior canal, and the left anterior canal lies parallel to the right posterior canal. Image Credit: Modified by Barry A. Broughton, PhD. Original by Kamran Barin, Ph.D.

Membranous Labyrinth

The membranous labyrinth is a continuous system of ducts, filled with *endolymph*, which lies within the bony labyrinth. Surrounded by perilymph, the membranous labyrinth is composed of the cochlear duct, the three semicircular ducts, saccule, and the utricle.

The cochlear duct is situated within the cochlea and functions as an organ of hearing. Known as the *vestibular apparatus*: the semicircular ducts, saccule, and utricle are the organs of balance.

- *Cochlear Duct:* The cochlear duct is located within the bony scaffolding of the cochlea and is held in place by the spiral lamina. The presence of the duct creates two canals (the scala vestibuli and scala tympani) above and below it. The cochlear duct has a triangular shape formed by the:

- *Lateral wall* – Formed by thickened periosteum known as the spiral ligament.
- *Roof* – Formed by Reissner's membrane which separates the cochlear duct from the scala vestibuli.
- *Floor* – Formed by the basilar membrane which separates the cochlear duct from the scala tympani.

The basilar membrane houses the epithelial cells of hearing – the *Organ of Corti*.

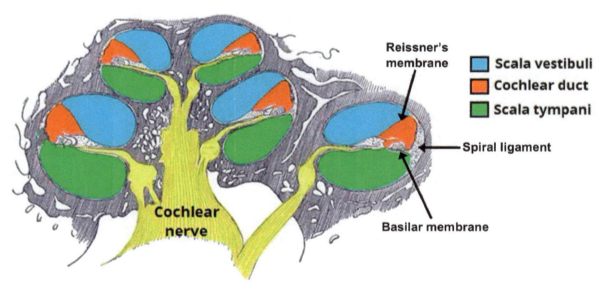

Fig. 7.15 – Structure of the cochlea, and borders of the cochlear duct. Image Credit: Public domain.

- *Saccule and Utricle:* The saccule and utricle are two membranous sacs located within the vestibule. As organs of balance, they detect movement or acceleration of the head in the vertical and horizontal planes, respectively.
  The utricle is the larger of the two membranous sacs, receiving the three semicircular ducts. The saccule is globular in shape and receives the cochlear duct. Endolymph drains from the utricle and saccule into the *endolymphatic duct*. The endolymphatic duct travels through the *vestibular aqueduct* to the posterior aspect of the petrous part of the temporal bone. The duct then expands to a sac where endolymph can be secreted and absorbed.
- *Semicircular Ducts:* The semicircular ducts are located within the semicircular canals. The flow of *endolymph* within the ducts changes speed and/or direction upon movement of the head. Sensory receptors within the ampullae of the semicircular canals detect the change in position, then sends signals to the brain, which allows for the processing of balance.

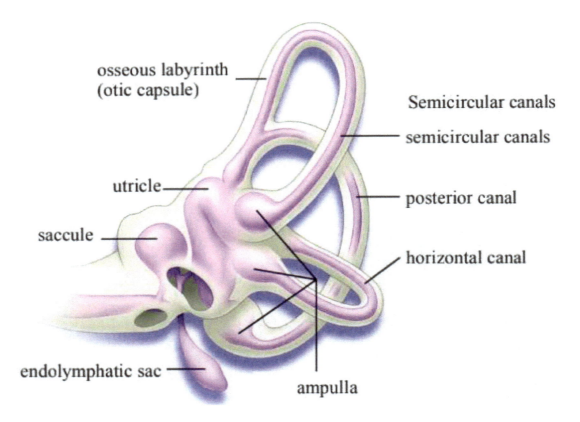

Fig. 7.16 – The components of the membranous labyrinth. Image Credit: Christine Kenney, [CC by 3.0] JAMC, 30 Sept. 2003, 169 (7).

Innervation of the Ear

Entering the ear via the internal acoustic meatus, the inner ear is innervated by the vestibulocochlear nerve (CN VIII). It then divides into the *vestibular nerve*, which is responsible for balance, and the *cochlear nerve* which is responsible for hearing.

- The *vestibular nerve* enlarges to form the vestibular ganglion. It then splits into superior and inferior parts to supply the utricle, saccule, and three semicircular ducts.
- The *cochlear nerve* enters at the base of the modiolus, and its branches pass through the lamina to supply the receptors of the Organ of Corti.

Overview of the Mechanism of Hearing

Sound waves are essentially vibrations that are carried through the air. The process in which the brain interprets those vibrations to sound can be divided into three phases: 1) collecting the vibrations, 2) converting those vibrations into mechanical energy, and 3) relaying each as an electrical impulse to be interpreted as sound by the brain.

The following is the route of sound waves through the ear and subsequent activation of the cochlear hair cells.

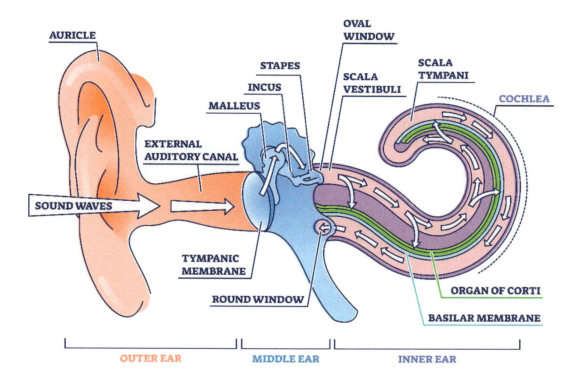

Fig. 7.17 - Diagram of the mechanism of hearing as sound waves travel through the external, middle, and inner ear. The cochlea is drawn as though it were uncoiled to make the events of sound transmission occurring there easier to follow.

Sound waves are funneled into the ear via the auricle and through the external auditory canal to the tympanic membrane (eardrum) where the vibrations are then converted into mechanical energy. To excite the hair cells in the organ of Corti in the inner ear, sound wave vibrations must pass through air, membranes, bone, and fluid.

The tympanic membrane is attached to the first of the three small bones known as the ossicular chain. The three bones (the malleus, incus, and stapes) propel each other sequentially, ultimately striking the oval window.

The bottom layer of the cochlea is carpeted by a layer of microscopic hair cells, each stimulated by specific frequencies, or pitches, of sound waves/vibrations.

> *Low frequency sound waves*: Low frequency sound waves that are below the level of hearing travel entirely around the cochlear duct without exciting hair cells.
>
> *High frequency sound waves*: Higher frequency sounds result in pressure waves that penetrate through the cochlear duct and the basilar membrane to reach the scala tympani; this causes the basilar membrane to vibrate maximally in certain areas in response to certain frequencies of sound, stimulating specific hair cells and sensory neurons.

Once stimulated by the movement of the perilymph fluid, the hair cells relay that information to the brain via the auditory nerve to be interpreted in the brain as sound.

Clinical Significance and Martial Arts Relevance:

Mechanisms of Equilibrium

The equilibrium receptors within the inner ear, collectively referred to as the vestibular apparatus, can be divided into two functional arms, one arm responsible for monitoring static equilibrium and the other involved with dynamic equilibrium.

Static Equilibrium

Within the membrane sacs of the vestibule are receptors called maculae that are essential to our sense of static equilibrium.

The *maculae* report on changes in the position of the head in space with respect to the pull of gravity when the body is not moving. Each macula is a patch of receptor (hair) cells with their "hairs" embedded in the *otolithic hair membrane,* a jelly-like mass studded with *otoliths* (tiny stones made of calcium salts). As the head moves, the otoliths roll in response to changes in the pull of gravity; this movement creates a pull on the gel, which in turn slides like a greased plate over the hair cells, bending their hairs.

This event activates the hair cells, which send impulses along the *vestibular nerve* (a division of cranial nerve VIII) to the cerebellum of the brain, informing it of the position of the head in space.

PLEASE REFER to the diagram on the following page.

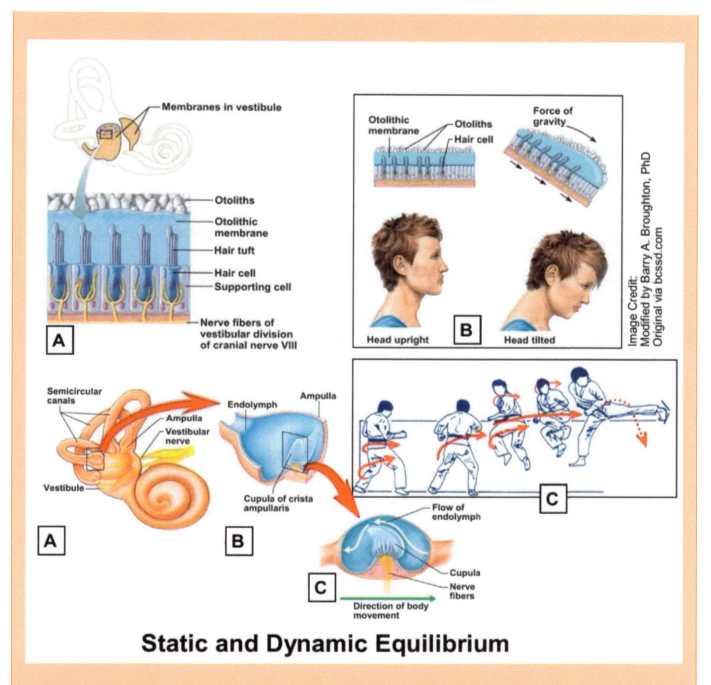

Fig. 7.18 - Static and dynamic equilibrium. Image Credit: Modified by Barry A. Broughton, PhD; Original by bcssd.com

Dynamic Equilibrium

The dynamic equilibrium receptors, found in the semicircular canals, respond to angular or rotatory movements of the head rather than to straight-line movements.

The *semicircular canals* are oriented in the three planes of space; thus, regardless of which plane one moves in, there will be receptors to detect the movement. Within the ampulla, a swollen region at the base of each membranous semicircular canal is a receptor region called *crista ampullaris*, which consists of a tuft of hair cells covered with a gelatinous cap called the *cupula*. When the head moves in an arc-like or angular direction, the endolymph in the canal lags behind. As the cupula drags against the stationary endolymph, the cupula bends with the body's motion.

This motion stimulates the hair cells, and impulses are transmitted up the vestibular nerve to the cerebellum.

The Eyes

The human eyes are bilateral spherical organs which house the structures responsible for the special sense of vision. Of all the sensory receptors in the body, approximately 70% are in the eyes.

Anatomy of the Eye

For purposes of this text, anatomical structures of the eye are divided into two categories: the *external and accessory structures*, and the *internal structures*.

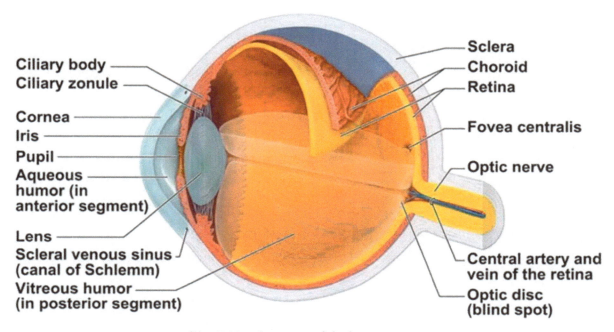

Fig. 7.19 - Anatomy of the human eye.

▪ External and Accessory Structures

The accessory structures of the eye include the eyelids, conjunctiva, lacrimal apparatus, and extrinsic eye muscles.

> **Eyelids:** The eyelids are thin, mobile folds that cover the eyeball anteriorly and meet at the medial and lateral corners of the eye, known as the *medial* and *lateral canthus*. They provide protection from injury or excessive light and maintain lubrication by distributing tears over the surface of the eyeball. Projecting from the border of each eyelid are the eyelashes.
> The *tarsal glands* are modified sebaceous glands that are located along the rim of the eyelid. These glands produce an oily secretion that lubricates the eye. The *ciliary glands* are modified sweat glands that lie between the eyelashes.
> **Conjunctiva:** The conjunctiva is a delicate membrane that lines the eyelids and covers part of the outer surface of the eyeball. It ends at the edge of the cornea by fusing with the corneal epithelium.

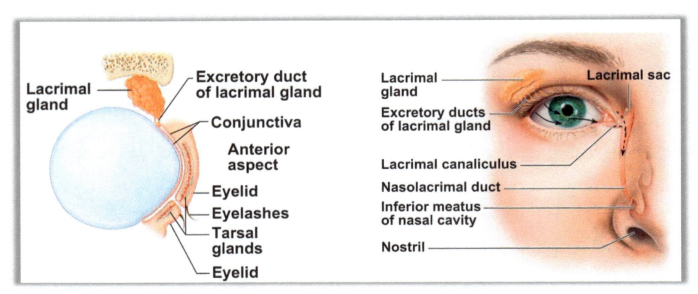

Fig. 7.20 - External anatomy and accessory structures of the human eye.

Lacrimal apparatus. The lacrimal apparatus consists of the lacrimal gland and numerous ducts that drain the lacrimal secretions into the nasal cavity.

- *Lacrimal glands:* The lacrimal glands are located above the lateral edge of each eye. They continually release tears onto the anterior surface of the eyeball through several small ducts.
- *Lacrimal canaliculi:* The tears flush across the eyeball into the lacrimal canaliculi medially, then into the *lacrimal sac,* and finally into the *nasolacrimal duct,* which empties into the nasal cavity.
- *Lysozyme:* Lacrimal secretion also contains antibodies and lysozyme, an enzyme that destroys bacteria. In addition to moistening and lubricating the eye, the lacrimal secretions also cleanse and protect the surface of the eye.

Extrinsic eye muscle. There are six extrinsic (external) eye muscles that are attached to the outer surface of the eye. These muscles produce gross eye movements and make it possible for the eyes to follow a moving object. The extrinsic muscles of the eye include: the *lateral rectus, medial rectus, superior rectus, inferior rectus, inferior oblique,* and the *superior oblique* muscles.

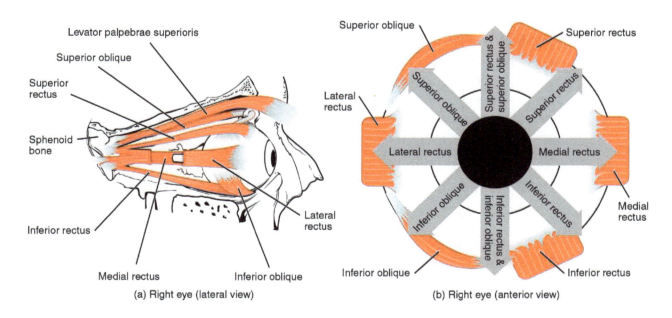

Fig. 7.21 - Extrinsic muscles of the eye and associated movements. Image Credit: OpenStax, [CC BY 4.0] via Wikimedia Commons.

▪ Internal Structures: The Eyeball

The eyeball itself is a hollow sphere. Its wall is composed of three distinct layers and is filled with fluids (called humors) that maintain the shape of the eye.

Layers of the Eyeball

The eyeball is formed by three layers: the fibrous, vascular, and inner layers. Each of these layers has a specialized structure and function.

> **Fibrous layer.** The outermost layer, called the fibrous layer, consists of the protective sclera and the transparent cornea.
> - *Sclera:* The sclera comprises approximately 85% of the fibrous layer. It is the thick, glistening, white connective tissue seen anteriorly as the "white of the eye". It provides attachments for the extraocular (extrinsic) muscles.
> - *Cornea:* The cornea is the transparent central anterior portion of the fibrous layer. Light entering the eye is refracted by the cornea.

Vascular layer. The vascular layer of the eyeball lies beneath the fibrous layer. It has three distinguishable regions: the choroid, the ciliary body, and the iris.

- *Choroid:* Most posterior is the choroid, a blood-rich nutritive tunic that provides nourishment to the outer layers of the retina. The choroid contains a dark pigment that prevents light from scattering inside the eye.

- *Ciliary body:* The ciliary body is comprised of two parts, the ciliary muscle and ciliary processes. The ciliary muscle consists of a collection of smooth muscles fibers that are attached to the lens of the eye by the ciliary processes. The ciliary body controls the shape of the lens and contributes to the formation of aqueous humor.

- *Iris:* The pigmented iris is a circular structure with an aperture (the pupil) in the center, through which light passes. The diameter of the pupil is altered by smooth muscle fibers within the iris which are innervated by the autonomic nervous system. The iris is situated between the lens and the cornea.

Inner layer. The innermost sensory layer of the eye is formed by the light detecting component called the retina. The inner layer is subdivided into two layers: the pigmented layer and the neural layer.

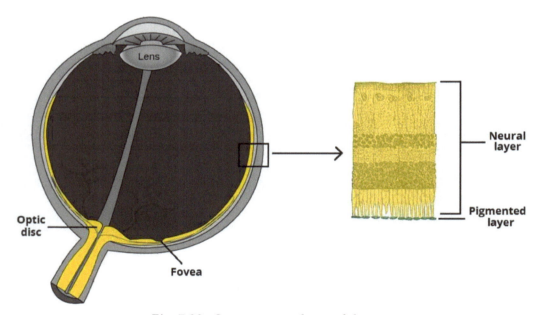

Fig. 7.22 - Inner sensory layer of the eye.

- *Pigmented layer:* The outer pigmented layer of the retina is composed of as single layer of pigmented cells that (like those of the choroid) absorb light and prevent light from scattering inside the eye. The pigmented layer continues around the whole inner surface of the eye.

- *Neural layer:* The transparent inner neural layer of the retina contains millions of receptor cells called *rods* and *cones*. These light detecting photoreceptors are located laterally and posteriorly in the eye.

Electrical signals pass from the photoreceptors via a *two-neuron chain (bipolar cells* and then *ganglion cells)* before leaving the retina as nerve impulses via the *optic nerve*. The nerve impulses are transmitted to the optic cortex of the brain and results in vision.

The photoreceptor cells are distributed over the entire retina, with the exception of where the optic nerve leaves the eyeball; this site is called the *optic disc* (or blind spot). Lateral to each blind spot is the *fovea centralis*, a tiny pit that contains only cones.

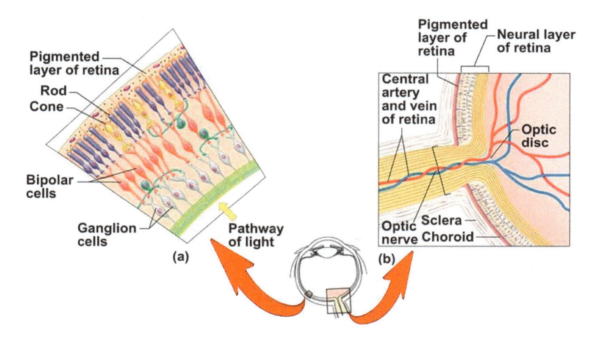

Fig. 7.23 - Photoreceptors of the eye.
Image A: Rods, cones, and the two-neuron chain. *Image B:* Optic nerve and optic disc.

Structures of the Eyeball

- Aqueous humor: Aqueous humor is a plasma-like fluid that helps maintain intraocular pressure (or the pressure inside the eye). The aqueous humor is produced constantly, and drains via the *trabecular meshwork*, an area of tissue at the base of the cornea, near the anterior chamber.

- Vitreous humor: Vitreous humor is a transparent gel that fills the posterior segment of the eye. It helps prevent the eyeball from collapsing inward by reinforcing it internally.

- **Canal of Schlemm:** Aqueous humor is reabsorbed into the venous blood through the scleral venous sinus, or Canal of Schlemm, located at the junction of the sclera and cornea.

- **Lens:** The lens is a flexible biconvex, crystal-like structure. Light entering the eye is focused on the retina by the lens.

- **Chambers:** The inside of the eye is divided into three chambers or sections. The lens divides the eye in to two sections: the *anterior (aqueous) section*, and the *posterior (vitreous) section*. The anterior section is further divided in to the anterior and posterior chambers.

- *Anterior chamber:* The anterior chamber is the part of the eye located between the cornea and the iris.
- *Posterior chamber:* The posterior chamber is located between the iris and lens.

The chambers in front of the lens are filled with aqueous humor, a clear watery-like fluid that nourishes the eye. If the drainage of aqueous humor is obstructed, it can cause increased pressure within the eye, a condition known as glaucoma. Glaucoma damages the optic nerve and can lead to permanent vision loss or blindness.

- Posterior (vitreous) Section: The vitreous chamber is located between the lens and the back of the eye. It is filled with a gel-like substance called either vitreous humor or the vitreous body.

Clinical Significance and Martial Arts Relevance:

Hyphema

Hyphema is the presence of blood within the aqueous fluid of the anterior chamber. The most common cause of hyphema is blunt eye trauma related to sporting activities. Hyphema is a medical emergency that should not be treated without the evaluation of an eye doctor.

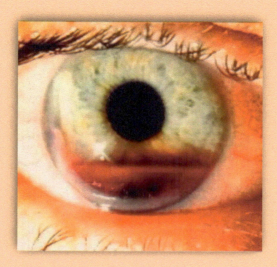

Fig. 7.24 - Hyphema: blood in the anterior chamber of the eye is a medical emergency.

Eye Reflexes

Both the external (extrinsic) and internal (intrinsic) eye muscles are necessary for proper eye function.

Photo-pupillary reflex: When the eyes are suddenly exposed to bright light, the pupils immediately constrict; this is the photo-pupillary reflex. This protective reflex prevents excessively bright light from damaging the delicate photoreceptors.

Accommodation pupillary reflex: The pupils also constrict reflexively when viewing close objects; this accommodation pupillary reflex provides for more acute vision.

Chapter 8

Introduction to the Respiratory System

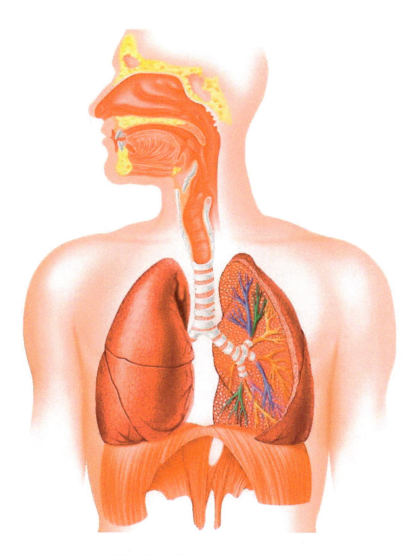

Fig. 8.1 - The respiratory system.

The respiratory system contains the specialized organs and tissue that aids in the entire process of respiration. The cells of the human body need a continuous supply of oxygen for the metabolic processes that are necessary to maintain life. The respiratory and the circulatory systems work together to provide oxygen, and to remove the waste products of metabolism. It also helps to regulate the pH level of the blood.

Respiration is the series of events that results in the exchange of oxygen and carbon dioxide between the atmosphere and the cells. Nerve impulses stimulate the ventilation process (breathing), which moves air through numerous anatomical structures into and out of the lungs. Within the lungs there is an exchange of gases between the lungs and the blood. This process is referred to as *external respiration*. Blood within the circulatory system transports the gases to and from the tissue cells. The exchange of gases between the blood and tissue cells is referred to as *internal respiration*. The cells then utilize the oxygen for their specific activities through the process of cellular metabolism (cellular respiration). These activities together constitute the process of respiration.

Mechanics of Ventilation

Ventilation (breathing) is the process of moving air through the conducting passages between the atmosphere and the lungs. Air moves through the respiratory passages because of pressure gradients that are produced by the downward contraction of the diaphragm, and thoracic and intercostal muscles.

Pulmonary ventilation

Pulmonary ventilation is the process of air flowing into the lungs during inhalation (inspiration), and out of the lungs during exhalation (expiration). Air flows because of the difference in pressure between the atmosphere and the gases inside the lungs.

Note: Air in the earth's atmosphere is composed of about 78% nitrogen, 21% oxygen, .93% argon, .04% carbon dioxide, and a small number of other gases and water vapor. Humans use only about 4% of the oxygen they inhale.

Air, like other gases, flows from an area of higher pressure to an area of lower pressure. The mechanical movements of the chest wall and the recoil of elastic tissues create the changes in pressure that result in ventilation. Pulmonary ventilation involves three different pressures:

- *Atmospheric pressure* - the pressure of the air outside the body.

- *Intraalveolar (intrapulmonary) pressure* - the pressure inside the alveoli of the lungs.

- *Intrapleural pressure* - the pressure within the pleural cavity.

Inhalation

Inhalation (inspiration) is the process of drawing air into the lungs. Inhaling is the active phase of ventilation as it is the result of muscle contraction. During normal inhalation, the diaphragm contracts and the thoracic wall expands as in external intercostal muscles elevate the ribs, increasing in volume within the thoracic cavity. This decreases the intraalveolar pressure so that air is drawn into the lungs.

During rigorous activities, or in the case of significant trauma, other accessory muscles also assist with active respiration. The accessory muscles for inhalation include: the scalene, the sternocleidomastoid, the pectoralis major, the trapezius, and serratus anterior.

Exhalation

Exhalation (expiration) is the process of forcing air out of the lungs during the respiratory cycle. During exhalation, relaxation of the diaphragm and the elastic recoil of tissue decreases the intrathoracic volume and increases the intraalveolar pressure.

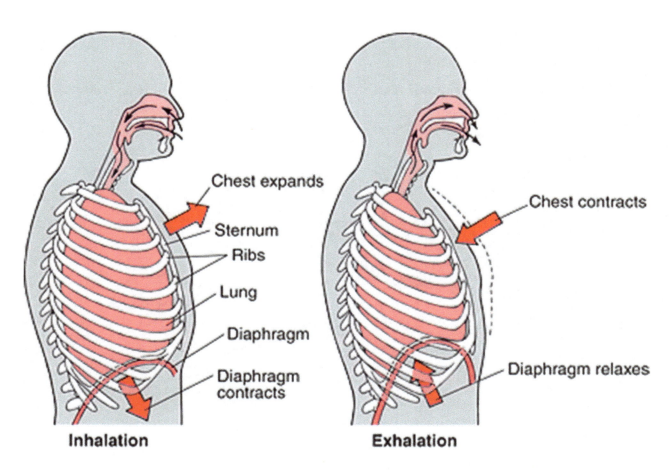

Fig. 8.2 - *Mechanics of ventilation.*

Respiratory Volumes and Capacities

Under normal conditions, the average adult takes 12 to 15 breaths a minute. A breath is one complete respiratory cycle that consists of one inhalation and one exhalation.

Factors such as age, sex, body build, and physical conditioning all influence lung volume and capacities. Lungs usually reach their maximum in capacity in early adulthood and then decline with age.

Clinical Significance and Martial Arts Relevance:

Compression of the Chest

Restricting chest wall excursion by maintaining compression on the chest of an assailant (or opponent), makes it difficult for the defender to inhale and complete a full respiratory cycle. In this instance, the defender is unable to draw in enough oxygen, and blow off enough carbon dioxide, which can make them feel as though they are being suffocated.

The opportunity to employ such a strategy is most often applied in grappling related arts. Techniques such as leg scissors (or using legs to Figure-4) to the chest/abdomen, and scarf holds (kesa gatame) are sufficient enough to fatigue the muscles of respiration and disrupt mechanical ventilation.

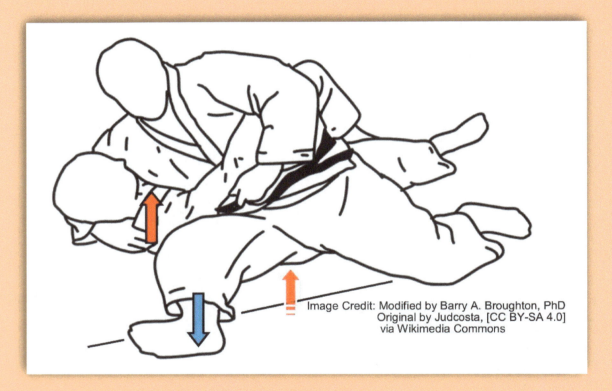

Fig. 8.3 - Scarf Hold (kesa gatame) applying compression to the chest. Image Credit: Modified by Barry A. Broughton, PhD; Original by Judcosta, [CC BY-SA 4.0], via Wikimedia Commons

Because of its efficacy and known potential for harm, many law enforcement agencies no longer allow officers to kneel or put weight on the chest or posterior thorax of a detainee.

Respiratory Passages

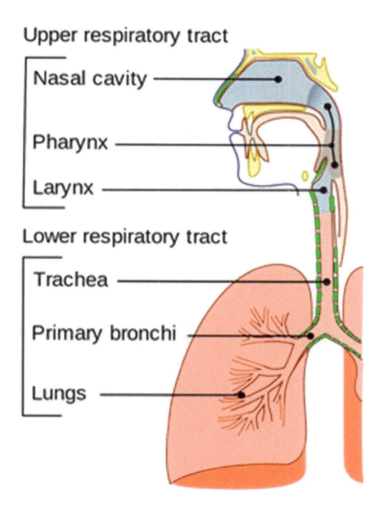

Fig. 8.4 - Upper and lower respiratory tracts.

The respiratory passages are divided into the *upper* and *lower respiratory tracts*. The upper respiratory tract includes the *nose, pharynx*, and *larynx*. The lower respiratory tract includes the *trachea, bronchial tree,* and the *lungs*. Both the upper and lower tracts are lined with mucous membranes. In some regions, the membrane has hairs that help filter the air, while other regions may have cilia to propel mucus.

Nose, Nasal Cavities, & Paranasal Sinuses

Nose and Nasal Cavities

The framework of the nose consists of both bone and cartilage. Two small nasal bones and extensions of the maxillae form the bony bridge of the nose. The remaining cartilaginous framework is the flexible portion of the nose. Connective tissue and skin cover the framework of the nose.

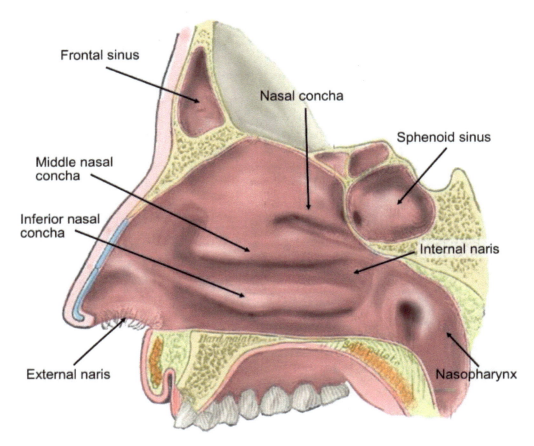

Fig. 8.5 - Nose and nasal cavities. Image Credit: Modified by Barry A. Broughton, PhD; Original by Cypressvine, [CC BY-SA 4.0] via Wikimedia Commons.

Air enters the nasal cavity from the outside through two openings: the nostrils or external nares. The openings from the nasal cavity into the pharynx are the internal nares. Nose hairs at the entrance to the nose trap large, inhaled particles.

Clinical Significance and Martial Arts Relevance:

Nasal Fracture

Because of the prominence of the external nasal skeleton, nasal fractures are common occurrence in martial arts and combat sports. Nasal fractures are the most common facial fracture. Fractures of the nasal bones usually occur as a result of blunt force trauma to the nose. A common sequela of nasal fractures is permanent deformity, due to disruption of the bone and cartilaginous architecture.

Contrary to the popular urban myth, and antiquated self-defense teachings, there are no nasal bones that are able to puncture through the skull and penetrate the brain causing death. Consider the amount of full-contact contact sports that occur daily without anyone dying specifically from a nasal bone being pushed up into the brain.

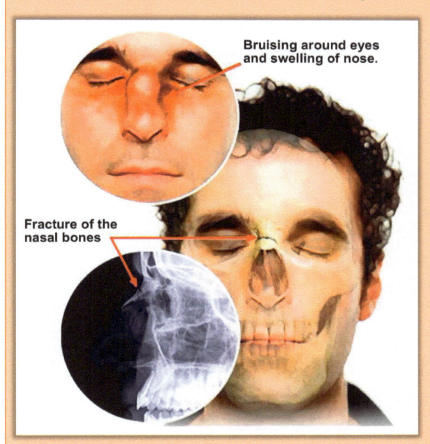

Fig. 8.6 - Nasal bone fracture. Image Credit: Modified by Barry A. Broughton, PhD; Original by MedicineNet, Inc, 2011

Epistaxis

Epistaxis is the medical term for a nosebleed. Because of the rich vascular network of arteries (Kiesselbach's plexus) providing blood supply to the nasal tissue, nose bleeds are a common occurrence in sports. Epistasis is most likely to occur in the anterior third of the nasal cavity known as the Kiesselbach area.

The most common cause of epistaxis is local blunt trauma to the nose and facial area.

Paranasal Sinuses

The paranasal sinuses are air-filled cavities in the maxillae, frontal, ethmoid, and sphenoid bones. These sinuses, named as the same bones in which they are located, surround the nasal cavity and open into it. They produce mucus, and influence voice quality by acting as resonating chambers. The sinuses also function to reduce the weight of the skull.

Pharynx

The pharynx, or throat, is the passageway that extends from the base of the skull inferiorly to the level of the sixth cervical vertebra. The pharynx serves both the respiratory and digestive systems by receiving air from the nasal cavity, as well as air, food, and water from the oral cavity. Inferiorly the pharynx opens into the larynx and the esophagus. It is divided into three regions according to location: the *naso*pharynx, *oro*pharynx, and the *laryngo*pharynx (hypopharynx)

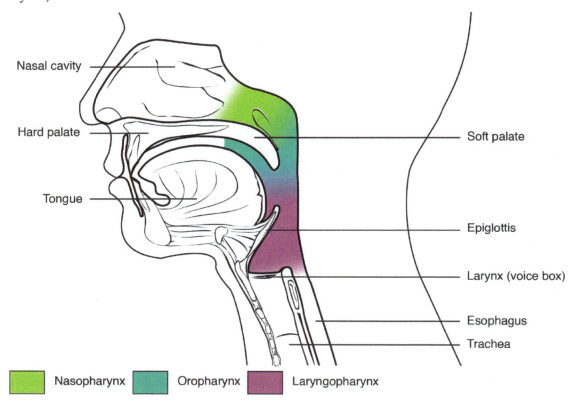

Fig. 8.7 - The pharynx is divided into the nasopharynx, oropharynx, and the laryngopharynx. Image Credit: OpenStax College, [CC BY 3.0], via Wikimedia Commons

- The *nasopharynx* is the portion of the pharynx that is posterior to the nasal cavity and extends inferiorly to the uvula.

- The *oropharynx* is the portion of the pharynx that is posterior to the oral cavity.

- The *laryngopharynx* is the most inferior portion of the pharynx that extends from the hyoid bone down to the lower margin of the larynx.

The upper part of the pharynx (throat) lets only air pass through, while the lower portion permits air, foods, and fluids to pass.

The pharyngeal, palatine, tubal, and lingual tonsils (called Waldeyer's Ring) are located in the pharynx. The ring acts as a first line of defense against microbes that enters the body through the nasal and oral routes.

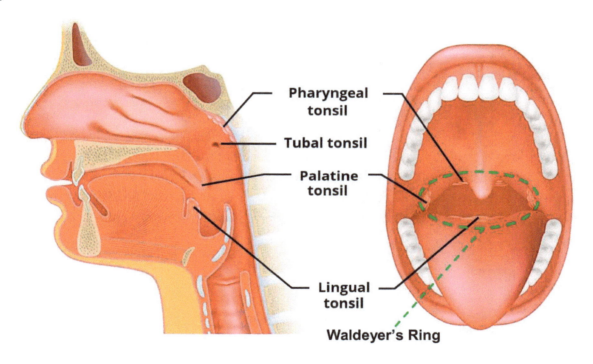

Fig. 8.8 - Waldeyer's Ring includes the pharyngeal, palatine, tubal, and lingual tonsils.

Larynx & Trachea

Larynx

The larynx (glottis), or voice box, is the passageway for air between the pharynx superiorly and the trachea inferiorly. It extends from the fourth to the sixth vertebral levels. The larynx is often divided into three sections: supraglottis, glottis, and subglottis. It is formed by nine cartilages that are connected to each other by muscles and ligaments.

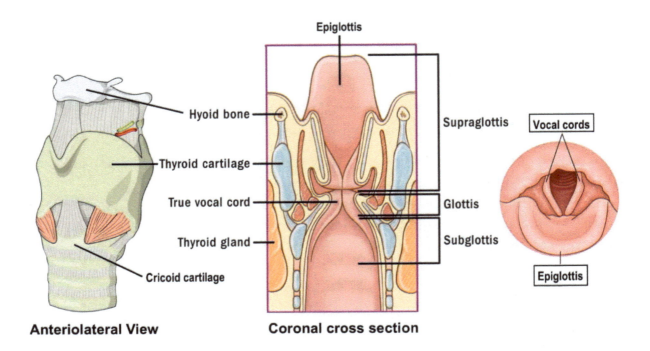

Fig. 8.9 - The Larynx and vocal cords.

The larynx plays a crucial role in human speech. During vocalization, the vocal cords close together and vibrate as air is expelled from the lungs and passes between them.

The epiglottis is a flap of cartilage that acts like a trap door to keep food and other particles from entering the larynx and trachea. The thyroid cartilage is commonly called the Adam's apple.

Trachea

The trachea (windpipe) is a long cartilaginous tube that is the main airway to the lungs. Superiorly it connects to the larynx. Inferiorly, it divides into the right and left bronchi, channeling air to the right or left lung.

The hyaline cartilage rings in the tracheal wall provides support and prevents the trachea from collapsing. The posterior soft tissue elastic fibers of the trachea allow for expansion of the esophagus, which is positioned immediately posterior to the trachea.

The mucous membrane that lines the trachea is ciliated epithelium, similar to that in the nasal cavity and nasopharynx. Goblet cells produce mucus that traps airborne particles and microorganisms. The cilia (microscopic hair-like structures) propel the mucus upward, where it is either swallowed or expelled.

Clinical Significance and Martial Arts Relevance:

Airway Chokes

Arguably, the most used choke in combat sports is some variation of a rear choke or rear naked choke. Although most rear naked choke variations are indeed "blood chokes"; *not all rear choke* variations are "blood chokes". In medicine, a *choke* is the interruption, or prevention, of *respiration* by *obstruction or compression of the airway*.

Note: Please see the discussions on Vascular Neck Restraints and Strangulations in the *Introduction to the Circulatory System* chapter, and in *Section Four- Physiology of Specific Techniques*.

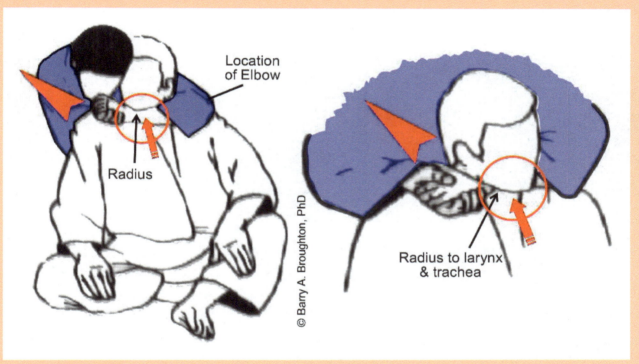

Fig. 8.10 - Rear choke attacking the airway.

There are a host of chokes that directly attack the larynx and trachea (windpipe) that can disrupt the opponent's ability to breathe. In grappling related martial arts, these are often referred to as "airway chokes" or "air chokes". Because of the potential for severe injury, or even death associated with "airway chokes", they are often illegal in combat sport competition; and therefore, are often neglected and frequently are not taught.

Airway chokes, either intentionally or inadvertently, directly attack the soft tissue, cartilaginous, and bony structures of the airway. Numerous anatomical structures within the neck can be severely injured during the application of airway chokes.

By applying direct pressure over the laryngotracheal region, airway chokes can directly injure the hyoid bone, thyroid cartilage, cricoid cartilage, trachea, and surrounding membranes. Injury to any of these structures can be severe and require immediate medical intervention.

Research by Travis, et. al., evaluated static and dynamic impact trauma of the human larynx. Their findings revealed that fracture of the cricoid and thyroid cartilages occurred at 20.8 kg (45.85 lbs.) and 15.8 kg (34.8 lbs.) of force, respectively. Structural collapse of the larynx occurs at 55 kg (121.25 lbs.) of force. Occlusion of the trachea requires 33 pounds of force, and just 35 pounds to fracture the tracheal cartilage. All relatively easily achieved when it has been reported that trained practitioners can apply chokes in excess of 100 pounds of force.

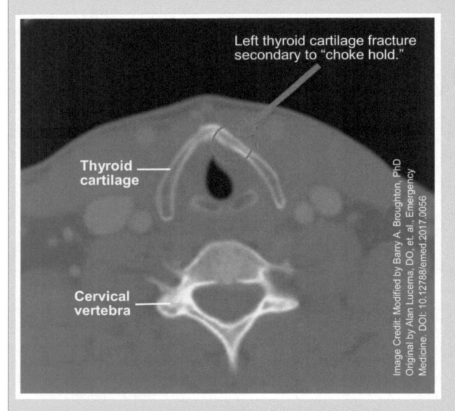

Fig. 8.11 - Computed tomography image showing a minimally displaced fracture of the left thyroid cartilage with soft-tissue swelling and minimal narrowing of the subglottic trachea. Case History: A 38-year-old man presented with a complaint of throat pain after his 15-year-old son applied a "choke hold" while wrestling. He reported that he felt a "crack" in his anterior neck, and soon afterwards felt throat pain with swallowing, along with discomfort with breathing.

Image Credit: Modified by Barry A. Broughton, PhD Original by Alan Lucerna, DO, et. al., Emergency Medicine. DOI: 10.12788/emed.2017.0056

When employing any variation of airway chokes, in addition to the local trauma that occurs from the direct pressure, underlying medical conditions can also be exacerbated. Airway chokes applied to those with comorbidities such as asthma can have deleterious effect.

Bronchi, Bronchial Tree, & Lungs

Bronchi and Bronchial Tree

Within the mediastinum the trachea divides into the right and left primary bronchi, the tubes that carry air from the trachea to the lungs. The bronchi branch into subsequently smaller and smaller passageways until they terminate in tiny air sacs called alveoli.

The cartilage and mucous membrane of the primary bronchi are similar to that in the trachea. As the branching continues throughout the bronchial tree, the amount of hyaline cartilage in the walls decreases until it is absent in the smallest bronchioles. As the cartilage decreases, the amount of smooth muscle increases.

The alveolar ducts and alveoli consist primarily of simple squamous epithelium, which allow for the rapid diffusion of oxygen and carbon dioxide across the membrane. The exchange of gases between the air in the lungs, and the blood in the capillaries, occurs within the walls of the alveolar ducts and alveoli.

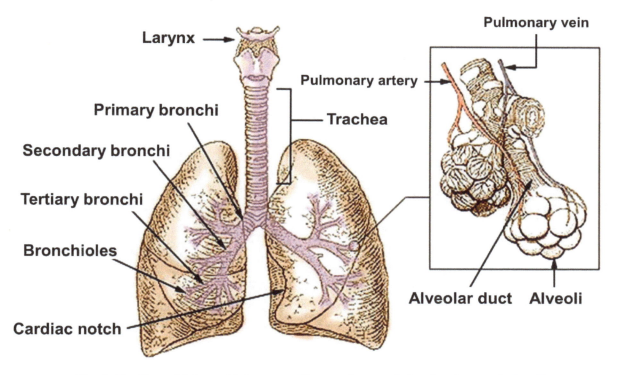

Fig. 8.12 - Bronchi, bronchial tree, and lungs. Insert of alveolar duct and alveoli.

Lungs

Occupying most of the space within the thoracic cavity, the two lungs contain all the components of the bronchial tree beyond the primary bronchi. Because they are mostly air spaces surrounded by the alveolar cells and elastic connective tissue, the lungs are soft and spongy in consistency. They are separated from each other by the mediastinum, which contains the heart, trachea, and esophagus. The only point of attachment for each lung is at the hilum (or root) on their medial sides. The hilum is where the bronchi, blood vessels, lymphatics, and nerves enter the lungs.

The right lung is divided into three lobes, and each lobe is supplied by one of the secondary bronchi. It is shorter, broader, and has a greater volume than the left lung. The left lung has two lobes and is longer and narrower than the right lung. The cardiac notch is an indentation on the medial surface of the left lung to accommodate for the apex of the heart.

The *pleura* is a double-layered serous membrane which encloses each lung. The visceral pleura is securely attached to the surface of the lung. At the hilum, the visceral pleura is continuous with the parietal pleura that lines the inner wall of the thorax. The pleural cavity is the small space between the visceral and parietal pleurae. It contains a thin layer of serous fluid that is produced by the pleura. The pleural fluid acts as a lubricant to reduce friction as the two layers slide against each other. It also helps to hold the two layers together as the lungs inflate and deflate.

Chapter 9

Introduction to the Cardiovascular System

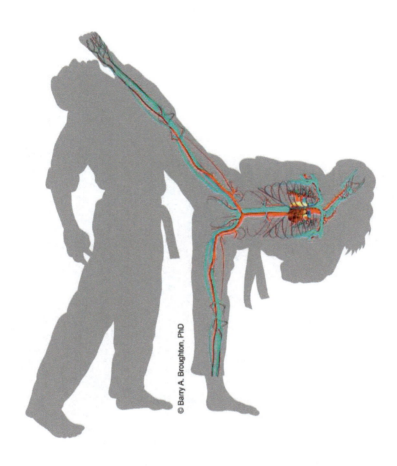

Fig. 9.1 - Introduction to the cardiovascular system.

The cardiovascular, or circulatory, system consists of the heart, blood, and blood vessels called arteries, capillaries, and veins. As the name implies, blood is pumped by the heart throughout the closed circuit of vessels as it passes continuously through the tissues of the body.

The cardiovascular system plays a vital role in maintaining homeostasis. Nutrient rich blood passes through the thousands of miles of vessels and capillaries to permeate every tissue and reach every cell within the human body. It is in the microscopic capillaries that blood performs its ultimate transport function. Nutrients and other essential materials pass from blood within the capillaries, into fluids surrounding the cells as waste products are removed.

Heart

The heart is a muscular pump that that is situated in the thoracic cavity between the lungs, posterior to the sternum and anterior to the vertebral column. The contracting heart provides the force necessary to circulate the blood throughout the cardiovascular system to all the tissues in the body. The circulatory system is vital to survival because it provides the tissues with a continuous supply of oxygen and nutrients, and aids in the removal of metabolic waste products. While blood is the transport medium, the heart is the organ that keeps the blood moving throughout the complex of vessels. The normal adult heart pumps about 5 liters (1.2 gallons) of blood every minute. If it loses its pumping effectiveness for even a few minutes, the irreversible changes can lead to death.

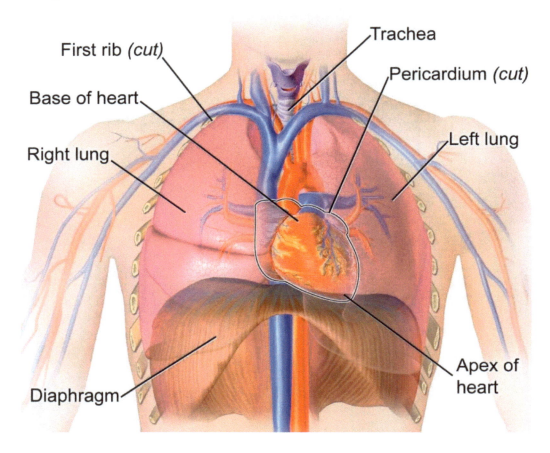

Fig. 9.2 - Location of the heart within the thoracic cavity. Image Credit: biologydictionary.net/thoracic-cavity

The heart is enclosed in a fibroelastic pericardial sac, or pericardium, which separates it from other structures with the mediastinum. The double-walled pericardium protects and lubricates the heart while keeping it in place within the thorax. The visceral layer of the serous membrane forms the epicardium.

Three layers of tissue form the heart wall. The outer layer of the heart wall is called the epicardium, the middle layer is the myocardium, and the inner layer is called the endocardium.

Chambers of the Heart

The internal cavity of the heart is divided into four chambers: the right atrium, right ventricle, left atrium, and the left ventricle.

The atria are the two thin-walled upper chambers of the heart that receive blood from the veins, while the two ventricles are the larger lower chambers. The ventricles are thick-walled chambers that forcefully pump blood out of the heart. The difference in thickness of the walls of each heart chamber are due to the amount of myocardium that is present. More myocardium is required in the chambers that need to produce more force in moving blood further distances.

The right atrium receives deoxygenated blood from the body via the systemic veins. The left atrium receives oxygenated blood from the lungs via the pulmonary veins. The right ventricle receives blood from the right atrium and pumps it to the lungs for oxygenation. The left ventricle receives blood from left atrium and pumps it throughout the body.

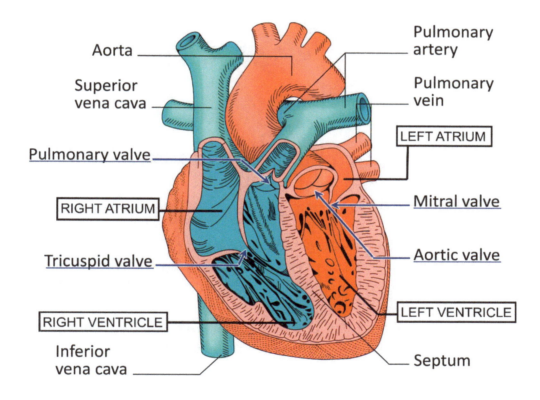

Fig. 9.3 - Cross section of human heart demonstrating the chambers and valves.

Valves of the Heart

The heart has two types of valves that prevents the backflow of blood and keeps it flowing in the correct direction. The valves between the atria and ventricles are called atrioventricular valves (or cuspid valves). The valves at the bases of the large vessels leaving the ventricles are called semilunar valves.

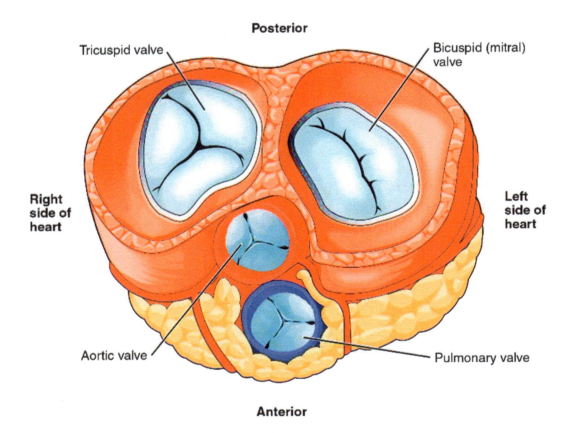

*Fig. 9.4 - Cuspid and semilunar valves of the heart.
Image Credit: OpenStax College, [CC BY 3.0], via Wikimedia Commons*

The right atrioventricular valve is called the *tricuspid valve*. The left atrioventricular valve is the *bicuspid* (or *mitral*) valve. The valve between the right ventricle and the trunk of the pulmonary arteries is the *pulmonary* valve. The valve between the left ventricle and the aorta is the *aortic* valve.

When the ventricles contract the atrioventricular valves close to prevent blood from flowing back into the atria. When the ventricles relax, the semilunar valves close to prevent blood from flowing back into the ventricles.

Blood Flow through the Heart

The heart functions as two separate pumps working simultaneously, one on the right and one on the left. Although it is easier to describe the flow of blood through the right side of the heart and then through the left side, it is important to realize that both atria and ventricles contract at the same time.

Blood flows from the right atrium to the right ventricle and is then pumped to the lungs to receive oxygen. From the lungs, the oxygenated blood flows to the left atrium, then to the left ventricle where it is pumped throughout the body via the systemic circulation.

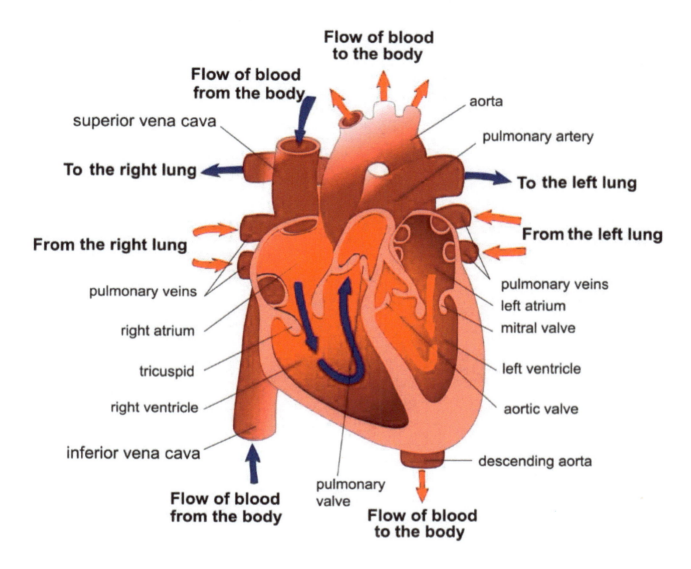

Fig. 9.5 - Blood flow through the heart.

Blood Supply to the Myocardium

The myocardium of the heart wall is a continuously working muscle, therefore it needs a continuous supply of oxygen and nutrients to function efficiently. An extensive network of blood vessels delivers oxygen to the cardiac tissue and cells while removing the waste products. Blood is supplied to the walls of the myocardium via the right and left coronary arteries, which branch off the ascending aorta. After blood passes through the capillaries in the myocardium, it enters the coronary (cardiac) veins which drain into the coronary sinus and into the right atrium.

Cardiac Conduction System

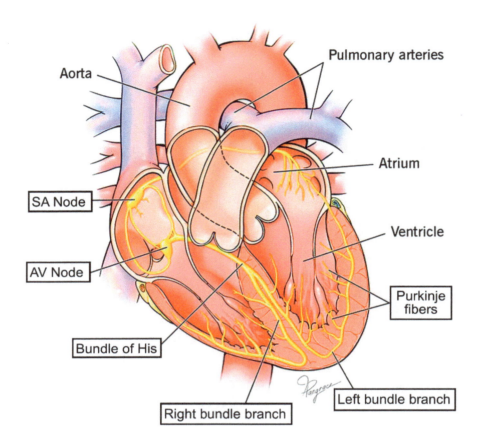

Fig. 9.6 - Cardiac conduction system. Image Credit: Modified by Barry A. Broughton, PhD. Original: Cleveland Clinic 2021, clevelandclinic.org

The electrical conduction system of the heart is a network of nodes, cells, and signals that controls the heartbeat. For each heartbeat, electrical signals travel through the conduction pathway within the cardiac muscle.

Known as the pacemaker of the heart, the sinoatrial (SA) node rhythmically initiates impulses 70 to 80 times per minute. The cells within the SA node contain electrolytes both inside and outside of the cells. The most common electrolytes within the human body include calcium, sodium, potassium, magnesium, phosphorus, and chloride. Sodium and calcium generally reside outside the cells of the SA node, while potassium generally lies within them. The cell membrane acts as a barrier between these electrolytes. Pressure within the bloodstream allows sodium to pass through the membrane and enter the cell, causing potassium to leave it — with less potassium leaving the cell than sodium entering it. The result is a continually growing positive charge. When the charge reaches a certain point, calcium channels in the cell membrane open and allows for calcium to enter. This makes the interior of the cell extremely positive compared to the outside of the cell, causing what is known as an *action potential*. Once that potential reaches a certain point it has enough power to create an excitation signal and discharge down the nerves of the heart. This bioelectricity causes the muscles to contract and the heart to beat.

- The conduction cycle begins when the sinoatrial (SA) node creates an excitation signal.
- The excitation signal travels to the atria causing them to contract.
- The signal continues to the atrioventricular (AV) node which delays the signal until the atria are empty of blood.
- The impulse moves through the Bundle of His (the center bundle of nerve fibers between the ventricles), carrying the signal to the Purkinje fibers (around the ventricles).
- The Purkinje fibers in turn cause the ventricles to contract pumping blood from the ventricles.

Blood

Blood is the circulating fluid within the cardiovascular system that provides the body with nutrients, oxygen, and waste removal. Blood is mostly liquid, with numerous cells and proteins suspended within it. The average person has about 5 liters (1.32 gallons) of blood.

Plasma is a liquid that makes up about half of the content of blood. It contains proteins that help blood to clot and transport substances through the blood. Blood plasma also contains glucose and other dissolved nutrients.

About half of blood volume is composed of blood cells:

- Red blood cells (RBC), which carry oxygen to the tissues.
- White blood cells (WBC), which fight infections.
- Platelets, smaller cells that help blood to clot.

Blood Vessels

Blood vessels are the elastic tubes through which blood is distributed to body tissues. The vessels form two separate closed systems that each begin and end at the heart. One system includes the pulmonary vessels which transports blood from the right ventricle to the lungs and back to the left atrium. The other system includes the systemic vessels which carries blood from the left ventricle to the remaining tissues of the body, and then returns the blood back to the right atrium. Based on the blood vessels' structure and function, they are classified as: arteries, capillaries, or veins.

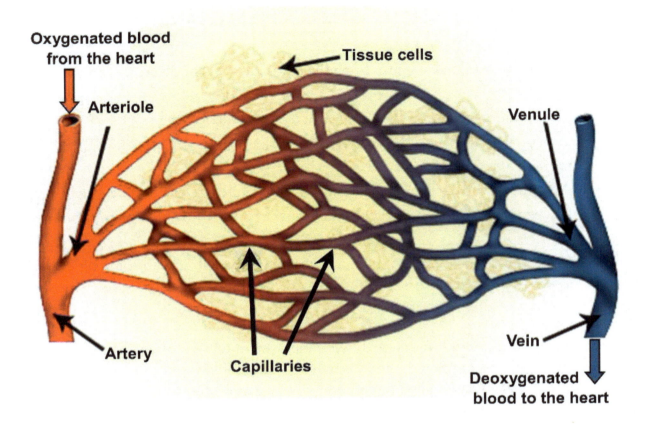

Fig. 9.7 - Vessels transport blood from the heart to the body tissues, and back to the heart via a complex of arteries, capillaries, and veins.

By understanding the specific location of major blood vessels, the knowledgeable martial artist has an advantage when defending against, or when using, an edged weapon.

Arteries

Arteries transport blood away from the heart. Pulmonary arteries carry deoxygenated blood from the right ventricle to the lungs. Systemic arteries carry oxygenated blood from the left ventricle to the body tissues. Blood is pumped from the ventricles into large arteries that branch repeatedly into smaller arteries until the branching results in microscopic arteries called arterioles.

Capillaries

Capillaries, the smallest and most numerous of the blood vessels, form the connection between the arteries that carry blood away from the heart, and the veins that return blood to the heart. The primary function of capillaries is the exchange of oxygen, carbon dioxide, other nutrients, and waste products between the blood and tissue cells.

Smooth muscle cells in the arterioles where they branch to form capillaries regulate blood flow from the arterioles into the capillaries.

Veins

Veins transport blood toward the heart. After blood passes through the capillaries, it enters the smallest veins, called venules. From the venules, the blood flows into progressively larger veins until it reaches the heart. The pulmonary veins transport oxygenated blood from the lungs to the left atrium of the heart. Systemic veins transport deoxygenated blood from the body tissue to the right atrium of the heart. This blood has a reduced oxygen content because the oxygen has been used for metabolic activities in the tissue cells.

Medium and large veins have one-way valves that help keep the blood flowing toward the heart. Venous valves are crucial in the extremities, where they prevent the backflow of blood in response to the pull of gravity.

Major Systemic Arteries

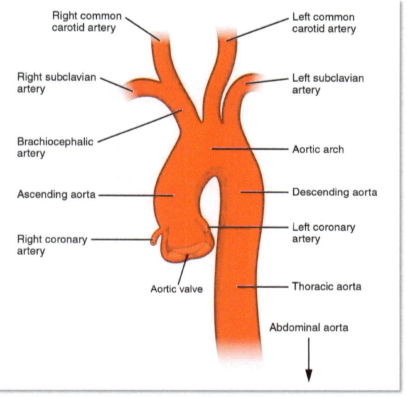

Fig. 9.8 - The aortic artery. Image Credit: OpenStax College, [CC BY 3.0], via Wikimedia Commons

- **Aorta**

The systemic arteries all branch, either directly or indirectly, from the aorta. The aorta ascends from the base of the left ventricle, and then curves posteriorly and to the left before descending through the thorax and abdomen. The aorta is divided into three sections: the ascending aorta, the aortic arch, and the descending aorta. The descending aorta is further subdivided into the thoracic aorta and abdominal aorta.

- **Common Carotid Arteries**

The common carotid arteries are present in the neck bilaterally supplying the head and neck with oxygenated blood. They originate from different arteries but follow symmetrical courses. The right common carotid originates from the brachiocephalic trunk, while the left common carotid originates from the aortic arch. Both common carotids divide into the external and internal carotid arteries at the upper border of the thyroid cartilage.

Carotid and Vertebral Arteries

The main arteries that provide blood to the brain are the internal carotid arteries and the vertebral arteries. The internal carotid arteries supply approximately 80% of the oxygenated blood to the brain, while the vertebral arteries contribute the remaining 20%. The carotid and vertebral arteries begin in the neck and travel superiorly into the cranium. Within the cranial vault the terminal branches join to form a circle, commonly known as the *Circle of Willis*. This interconnection allows collateral blood circulation to continue if a major vessel is blocked on one side of the brain. Cerebral artery branches arise from the circle to supply blood to most of the cerebrum.

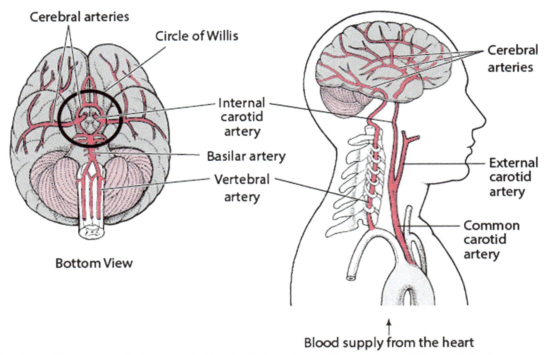

Fig. 9.9 - Blood supply to the brain is provided by the internal carotid arteries and the vertebral arteries. Collateral blood supply is provided by arteries with the Circle of Willis. Image Credit: merckmanuals.com/home/brain,-spinal-cord,-and-nerve-disorders/stroke-cva/ischemic-stroke

The internal carotid arteries originate from the bifurcation of left and right common carotid arteries in the neck at the level of the C4 vertebrae. The arteries travel superiorly within the carotid sheath and into the brain; branching off into other arteries that perfuse different portions of the brain.

The right and left vertebral arteries branch off from the subclavian arteries just inferior to the clavicles. They travel superiorly to the posterior portion of the neck and then pass through a bony canal within the cervical vertebrae. Upon entering the cranial cavity, they branch off to form other arteries before converging to form the basilar artery.

Cerebral blood flow (CBF) refers to the blood supply to the brain at any given period. In an adult, CBF is typically 15 - 20% of the cardiac output. Because the brain is extremely sensitive to oxygen starvation, cerebral blood flow is vital to its proper function. When an area of the brain is cut off from adequate blood flow for an extended period of time, loss of consciousness or a stroke can occur.

Clinical Significance and Martial Arts Relevance:

• Carotid Triangle

The carotid triangle of the anterior neck is formed by the following borders:
- Superior: by the posterior belly of the digastric muscle.
- Lateral: by the medial border of the sternocleidomastoid muscle.
- Inferior: by superior belly of the omohyoid muscle.

Many of the vessels and nerves in the carotid triangle are relatively superficial, which makes them vulnerable to the knowledgeable practitioner. The common carotid arteries bifurcate into the internal and external carotid arteries in the carotid triangle. The internal jugular vein, the vagus and hypoglossal nerves, the carotid sinus, and special sensory cells called baroreceptors are also located within its borders.

The baroreceptors detect stretch within the blood vessel walls, and helps to regulate the blood pressure within the cardiovascular system. The glossopharyngeal nerve relays this information to the brain to help regulate blood pressure.

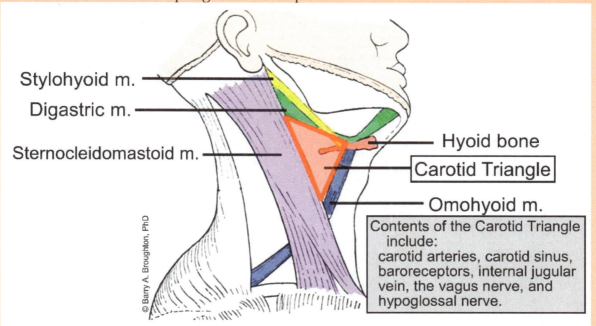

Fig. 9.10 - Structures within the carotid triangle include the common carotid, external, and internal carotid arteries, carotid sinus, baroreceptors, internal jugular vein, and the vagus and hypoglossal nerves.

In some people the baroreceptors are hypersensitive to stretch, and external pressure on their carotid sinus can cause slowing of the heart rate and a decrease in blood pressure. In response, the brain becomes under perfused, and syncope (fainting) results.

▪ **Vascular Neck Restraints**

Note: Please see a more detailed discussions on Vascular Neck Restraints and Strangulations in *Section Four- Physiology of Specific Techniques*.

One of the most powerful tools in the arsenal of jujitsu and combatives grappling art practitioners is the ability to render an assailant unconscious without striking. This most often occurs by encircling the neck and decreasing the cerebral blood flow by occluding the carotid arteries. These vascular neck restraints (VNR), often referred to as a "rear choke", are actually strangulations.

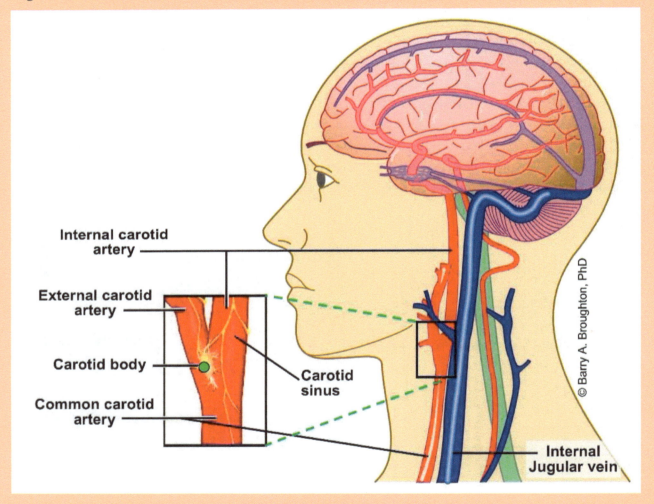

Fig. 9.11 - The carotid sinus is located in the internal carotid artery just superior to the bifurcation. It contains a baroreceptor that senses changes in systemic blood pressure.

The internal carotid arteries supply the brain with about 80% of its oxygenated blood, while the vertebral arteries contribute the remaining 20%. Cerebral hypoxia, which contributes to loss of consciousness, occurs when the cerebral blood flow velocity drops below 50% in both the right and left carotid arteries. The compression force required to effectively compress the carotid arteries must be at least 100 mmHg. However, applying a greater amount of pressure *does not* result in a faster response of unconsciousness. The average time for unconsciousness following the application of the vascular neck restraint is approximately 9.5 seconds (+/- 0.4 sec.).

With the proximity of other structures to the carotid arteries within the carotid triangle; subsequent compression of the jugular veins causes an increase in intracranial pressure, thereby also contributing to the loss of consciousness during VNR. Applying only 4.4 pounds of pressure to the jugular veins causes venous outflow obstruction from the brain and subsequent stagnant hypoxia, while eleven pounds of pressure to the carotid arteries can cause loss of consciousness.

Even though the application of "chokes" in sporting environments have been demonstrated to be relatively safe, bear in mind that research studies are most often performed on young healthy individuals attempting to isolate the vasculature while avoiding the airway. Additionally, VNR that are applied in a martial arts training are infrequently held for a period long enough to induce unconsciousness. Executing vascular neck restraints on an older, less healthy person can have dire consequences. There is the potential for plaque within the carotid arteries to dislodge, occlude the blood flow to the brain and cause a stroke. Neck compression in individuals who have a hypersensitive carotid sinus can cause a significant drop in blood pressure and heart rate, causing a dangerously irregular heartbeat (arrhythmia) resulting in a heart attack.

▪ Injury to the External Jugular Vein

The external jugular vein is situated relatively superficially in the neck, leaving it vulnerable to injury. If it becomes severed, in an injury such as a knife wound, the lumen of the vessel is held open due to the thick layer of investing fascia in the neck. Air is subsequently drawn into the vein, producing cyanosis, and can stop blood flow through the right atrium. This is a true medical emergency, managed by the application of pressure to the wound to stop the bleeding and the entry of air.

Major Systemic Arteries

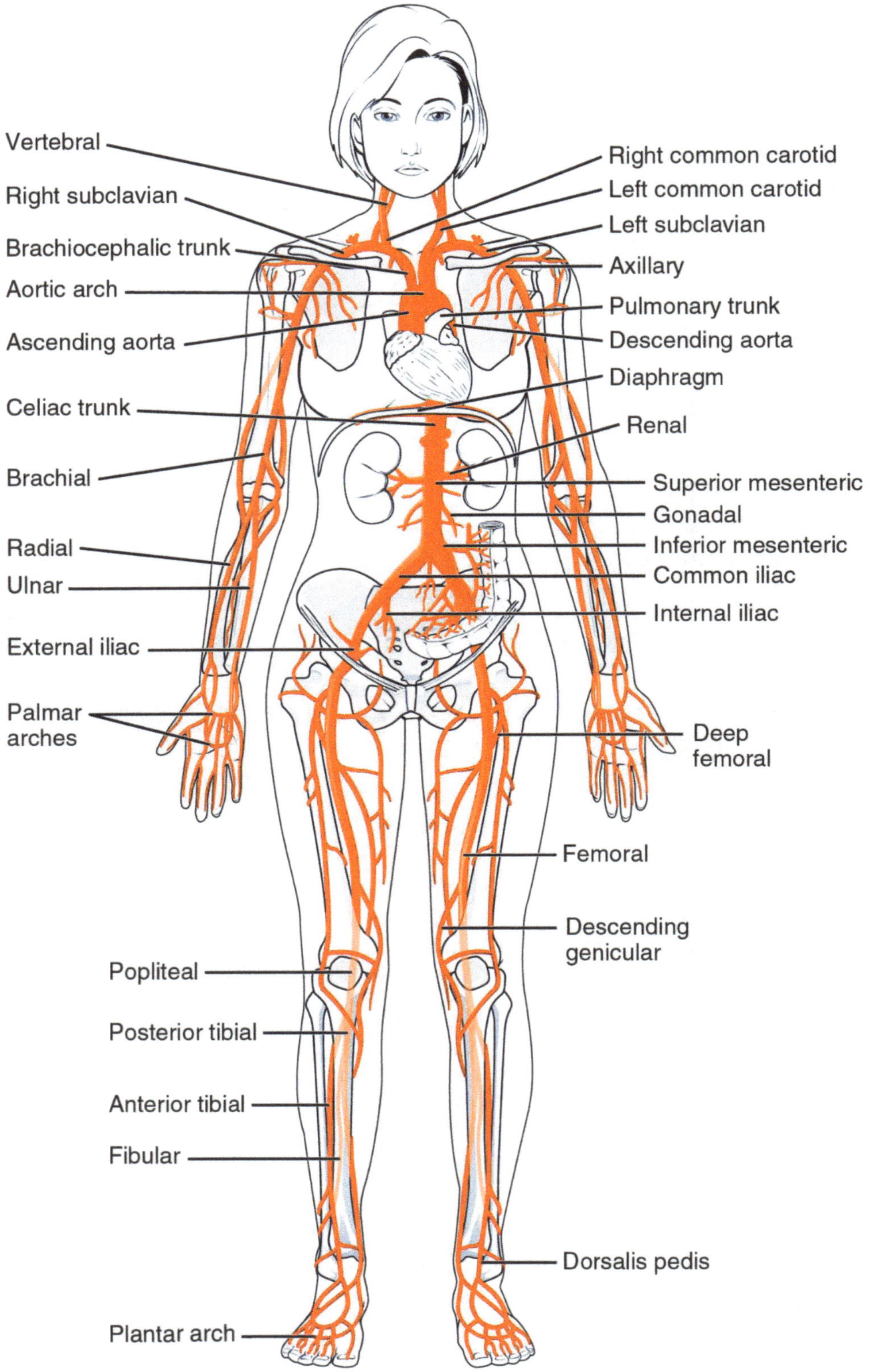

Fig. 9.12 - Major systemic arteries. Image Credit: OpenStax College, [CC BY 3.0], via Wikimedia Commons

Major Systemic Veins

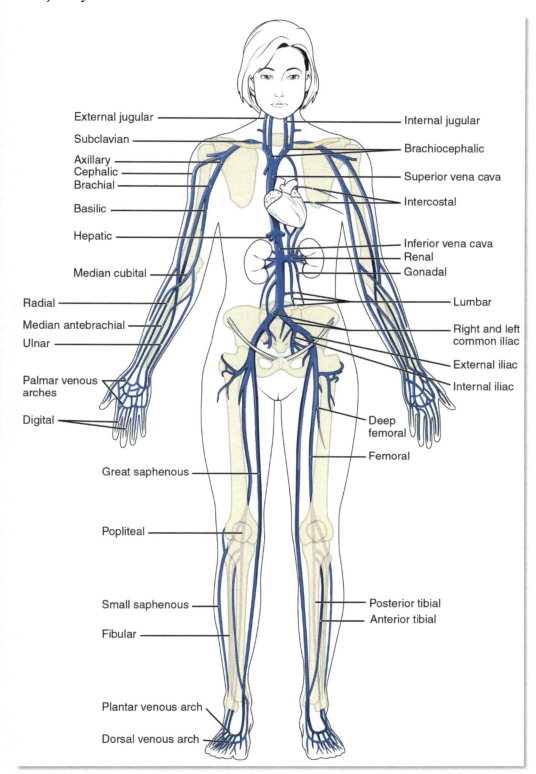

After blood delivers oxygen and nutrients to the tissues, and picks up carbon dioxide and other waste products, it returns to the heart through the systemic veins. Gaseous exchange occurs at the capillaries which merge into venules, and then converge to form larger veins until the blood reaches either the inferior vena cava or the superior vena cava, which drain into the right atrium.

Fig. 9.13 - Major systemic veins. Image Credit: OpenStax College, [CC BY 3.0], via Wikimedia Commons

Chapter 10

Introduction to the Lymphatic System

The lymphatic system has three primary functions: 1) to remove excess fluid from body tissue, 2) absorption of fats and transporting them to the circulatory system, and 3) the production of immune cells.

The lymphatic system removes excess interstitial fluid from body tissues and returns it back to the blood. Of all the fluid that crosses the capillary walls into tissue, about 90% is returned. The remaining 10% that does not return becomes part of the interstitial fluid that surrounds the tissue cells. Small protein molecules may pass through the capillary wall and increase the osmotic pressure of the interstitial fluid; inhibiting the return of fluid into the capillaries, causing fluid to accumulate in the tissue spaces. If this process continues, blood volume and blood pressure decrease and the volume of tissue fluid increases, resulting in tissue swelling (edema). Lymph capillaries pick up the excess interstitial fluid and proteins and return them to the circulatory system via venous blood.

The lymphatic system is responsible for the absorption of fats and fat-soluble vitamins from the digestive system, and their subsequent transportation back to the venous circulation. The mucosal lining of the small intestine is covered with fingerlike projections called villi. In the center of each villus there are blood capillaries and special lymph capillaries, called lacteals. The fats and fat-soluble vitamins are absorbed by the lacteals, while the blood capillaries absorb most of the other nutrients. The lymph in the lacteals, called chyle, has a milky appearance because of its high fat content.

The third and probably most well-known function of the lymphatic system is its defense against invading microorganisms and disease. The lymph nodes and other lymphatic organs filter the lymph to remove microorganisms and other foreign substances. Lymphatic organs contain lymphocytes (a type of white blood cell) that destroy invading organisms.

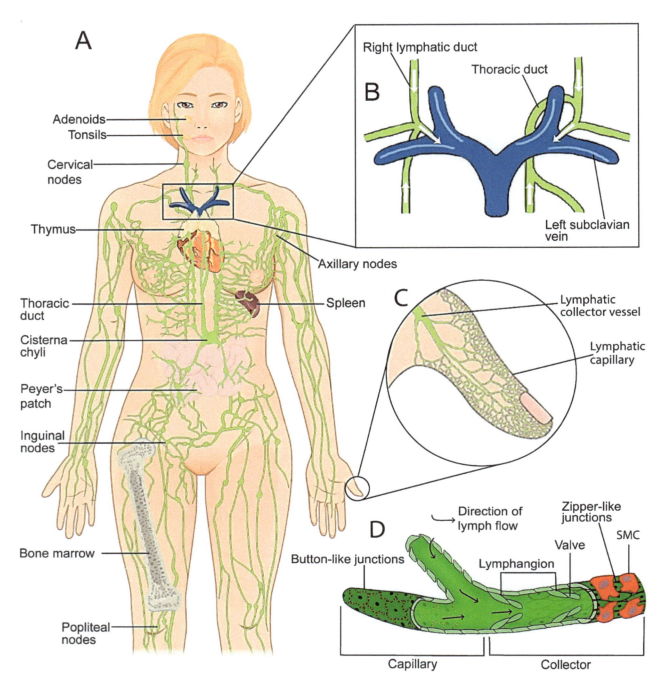

Fig. 10.1 - Mechanics of the lymphatic system. Image Credit: in (A) modified from OpenStax College under a CC BY 3.0 license. (C) modified from OpenLearn Create under a CC BY-NC-SA 4.0 license. SGUL lymers, [CC BY-SA 4.0], via Wikimedia Commons

See full descriptions on next page.

(**A**) The lymphatic system includes the primary and secondary lymphoid organs and a series of lymphatic vessels, providing a one-way drainage route from all tissues back to the blood circulation via the great veins in the neck. In the primary lymphoid organs (bone marrow and thymus) immune cell production and maturation takes place, whereas secondary lymphoid organs (lymph nodes, spleen, and mucosa associated lymphoid organs such as Peyer's patch, tonsils and adenoids) are the sites for lymphocyte activation. The initial dermal lymphatic capillaries absorb interstitial material and fluid to make lymph which drains into lymphatic collectors. Lymph is pumped from the gut and lower half of the body to the cisterna chyli, a sac-like structure situated below the diaphragm, and then on to the thoracic duct.

(**B**) The thoracic duct is responsible for the lymph drainage coming from most of the body except for the right sides of the head and neck, the right side of the thorax and the right upper extremity that drain primarily into the right lymphatic duct. Both ducts drain into the great veins of the neck.

(**C**) The intricate dermal lymphatic capillary network drains downstream into the lymphatic collector vessels on route to the lymph nodes.

(**D**) Oak leaf-shaped initial lymphatic capillary cells are connected via discontinuous junctions or buttons allowing the fluid to enter the system passively, the lymphatic collector endothelial cells, on the other hand, present with continuous junctions or zippers. Collectors differ from initial lymphatics by possessing intraluminal valves, smooth muscle cells (SMC) and a continuous basement membrane. Contractions of the lymphangions, the vessel segment between two valves, generate the pressure gradient ensuring the unidirectional flow of lymph.

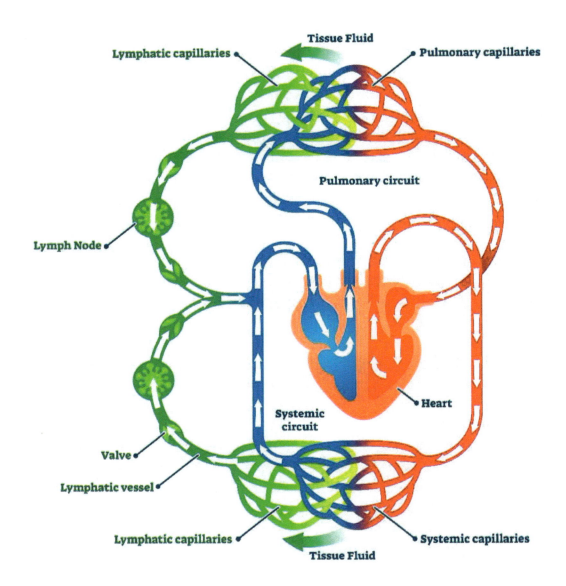

Fig. 10.2 - Lymphatic circulation.

Components of the Lymphatic System

The lymphatic system consists of lymph fluid, lymph vessels that transport the lymph, and organs that contain lymphoid tissue.

- **Lymph**

Lymph is a fluid that is derived from blood plasma as fluids pass through capillary walls. As the interstitial fluid begins to accumulate, it is picked up and removed by tiny lymphatic vessels and returned to the venous blood. Once the interstitial fluid enters the lymph capillaries, it is called lymph. Returning lymph to the blood prevents edema and helps to maintain normal blood volume and blood pressure.

Lymphatic Vessels

Unlike blood vessels, lymphatic vessels only carry fluid away from the tissues. The smallest of lymphatic vessels are the lymph capillaries, which begin in the tissue spaces as projection-like sacs. Lymph capillaries are found in all regions of the body except for bone marrow, the central nervous system, and tissues that lack blood vessels, such as the epidermis. The interior walls of lymph capillaries contain one-way valves that are composed of overlapping squamous cells. This permits fluid to enter the lymph capillary but prevents the lymph from leaving the vessel.

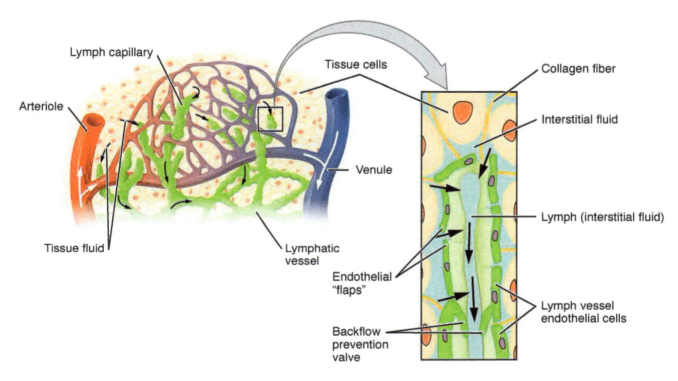

Fig. 10.3 - Lymph capillaries in the tissue spaces. Image Credit: OpenStax College, [CC BY 3.0] via Wikimedia Commons

The microscopic lymph capillaries merge forming lymphatic vessels. The small lymphatic vessels join together forming larger tributaries (lymphatic trunks) which drain large regions of tissue. Lymphatic trunks merge until the lymph enters into two lymphatic ducts. The *right lymphatic duct* drains lymph from the upper right quadrant of the body, while the *left thoracic duct* drains the rest of the body.

Like veins, the lymphatic tributaries have thin walls and one-way valves that prevent the backflow of lymph. Unlike the cardiovascular system, there is no pump in the lymphatic system. The action of skeletal muscles, respiratory movement, and the contraction of smooth muscle in vessel walls provide the pressure gradients required to move lymph through the lymphatic vessels.

Lymphatic Organs

Lymphatic organs are characterized by clusters of lymphocytes, macrophages, and other cells, intertwined in a framework of short, branching connective tissue fibers. Lymphocytes originate in the red bone marrow of long bones and are carried in the blood to the lymphatic organs. When the human body is exposed to invading microorganisms and other foreign substances, the lymphocytes proliferate within the lymphatic organs. As part of the immune response, lymphocytes are then sent via the blood to the site of the invasion and attempts to destroy the invading agent.

Organs of the lymphatic system include: the lymph nodes, tonsils, spleen, and the thymus gland.

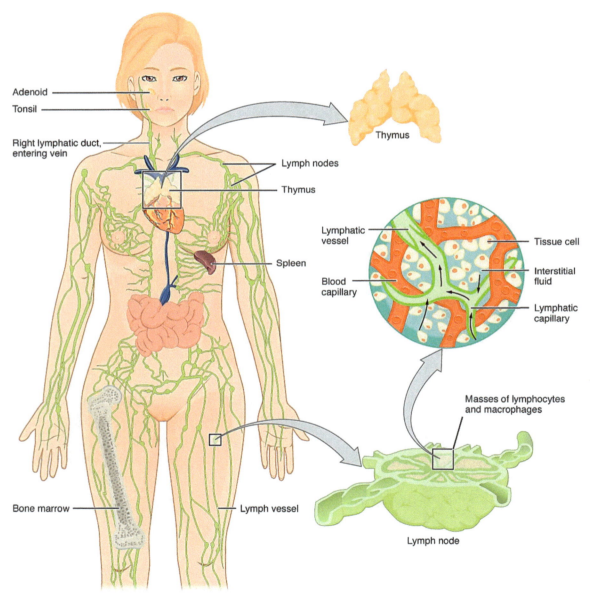

Fig. 10.4 - Anatomy of the lymphatic system. Image Credit: OpenStax College, [CC BY 3.0], via Wikimedia Commons

Lymph Nodes

Lymph nodes are small bean-shaped structures, usually measuring less than 2.5 cm (< 1 inch) in length, which are distributed throughout the body along the lymphatic pathways. The lymph nodes filter the lymph from tissues before it is returned into the bloodstream. There are predominately three regions on each side of the body where lymph nodes tend to cluster superficially. These areas include: the cervical nodes in the neck, the axillary nodes in the armpit, and the inguinal nodes in the groin.

Lymph nodes are surrounded by a connective tissue capsule and are divided into compartments called lymph nodules. The lymph nodules are dense masses of lymphocytes and macrophages that are separated by spaces called lymph sinuses. Entering on the convex side, the afferent lymphatic vessels carry lymph into the node. The lymph moves through the lymph sinuses and enters the efferent lymphatic vessel located at an indented region called the hilum. The efferent lymphatic vessels then carry the lymph away from the lymph node.

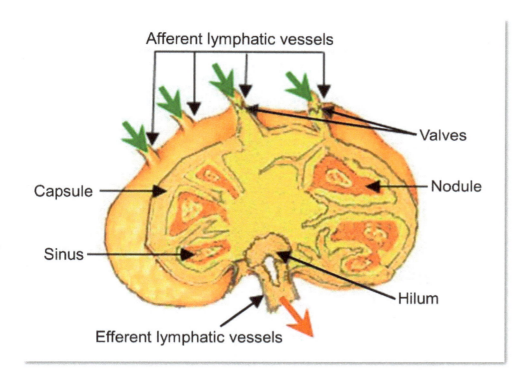

Fig. 10.5 - Lymph node structure.

Tonsils

The tonsils are clusters of lymphatic tissue situated just under the mucous membranes of the nose, mouth, and pharynx. There are primarily three groups of tonsils: the pharyngeal, palatine, and lingual tonsils.

The pharyngeal tonsils are located in the pharynx near the opening of the nasal cavity. The palatine tonsils are located near the opening of the oral cavity into the pharynx. The lingual tonsils are located on the posterior surface of the tongue, which also places them near the opening of the oral cavity into the pharynx.

The tonsils contain lymphocytes and macrophages that provide protection against pathogens and harmful substances that may enter the body through the nose or mouth.

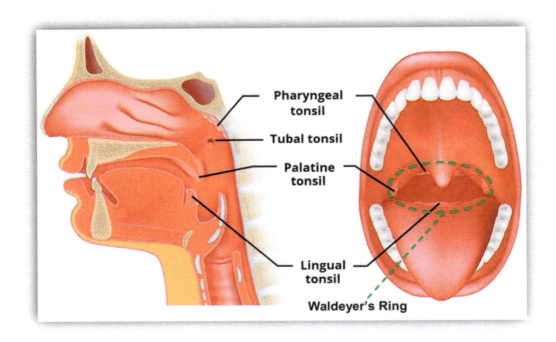

Fig. 10.6 - The pharyngeal, palatine, tubal, and lingual tonsils (called Waldeyer's Ring) are located in the pharynx. The ring of tonsils acts as a first line of defense against microbes that enters the body through the nasal and oral routes.

- **Spleen**

The spleen is the largest lymphatic organ in the human body. It is located in the upper left abdominal cavity, just inferior to the diaphragm, and posterior to the stomach. The spleen is surrounded by a connective tissue capsule which extends inward, dividing the spleen into lobules. The spleen contains two main types of tissue called white pulp and red pulp. The white pulp is lymphatic tissue consisting mainly of lymphocytes (white blood cells) around arteries. The red pulp consists of venous sinuses filled with blood and cords of lymphatic cells, such as lymphocytes and macrophages. The venous sinuses also act as a reservoir for blood. Blood enters the spleen through the splenic artery, passes through the sinuses where it is filtered, then exits via the splenic vein.

The spleen filters blood in much the way that the lymph nodes filter lymph. Like other lymphatic tissue, the spleen produces lymphocytes, especially in response to invading pathogens. Lymphocytes then react to microorganism and pathogens in the blood and act to destroy them. The macrophages then engulf the resulting debris, the damaged cells, and the other large particles and removes them. The spleen, along with the liver, removes old and damaged erythrocytes (red blood cells) from the circulating blood.

In emergencies such as hemorrhage (significant blood loss), smooth muscle in the vessel walls and in the capsule of the spleen contracts and release blood out of the spleen and into the general circulation.

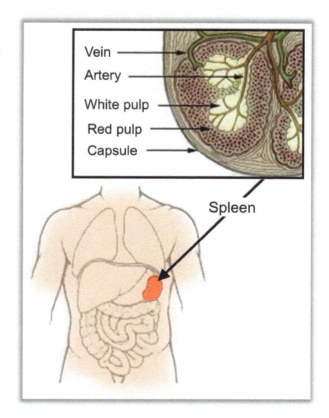

Fig. 10.7 - Structure of the spleen.

Clinical Significance and Martial Arts Relevance:

- **Rupture of the Spleen**

The abdominal organ with the highest incidence of injury is the spleen, accounting for 49% of blunt abdominal injuries. A splenic rupture occurs when there is a break in its fibroelastic capsule, disrupting the underlying tissue. Splenic rupture is most often caused by penetrating or blunt force trauma, such as knee strikes or kicks to the abdomen or forceful throws; and is often associated with left rib fractures.

Because the spleen is highly vascularized, a splenic rupture results in profuse bleeding into the peritoneal (abdominal) cavity. Surgical removal of the spleen (splenectomy) is indicated when injury to the spleen, and the subsequent hemorrhage, are life threatening.

In the case of splenectomy, the liver and bone marrow take over some of the functions provided by the spleen. However, an individual who has had a splenectomy are more susceptible to some bacterial infections and may require lifelong antibiotics.

Thymus Gland

The thymus gland is a two-lobed soft lymphatic organ that is located in the upper chest, anterior to the ascending aorta and directly posterior to the sternum between the lungs. The thymus increases in size throughout infancy and childhood until puberty, at which point it decreases in size so that in older adults it is quite small.

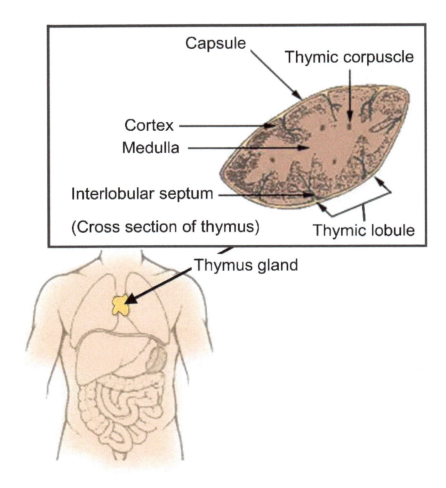

Fig. 10.8 - Thymus gland structure.

The primary function of the thymus gland is the maturation of special lymphocytes called T-lymphocytes (or T-cells). While in the thymus, the lymphocytes do not respond to foreign microorganism and pathogens. After the lymphocytes have matured, they are released into the blood and go to other lymphatic organs where they help provide defense against disease. The thymus also produces thymosin, a hormone which stimulates the maturation of lymphocytes in other lymphatic organs.

Chapter 11

Introduction to the Digestive System

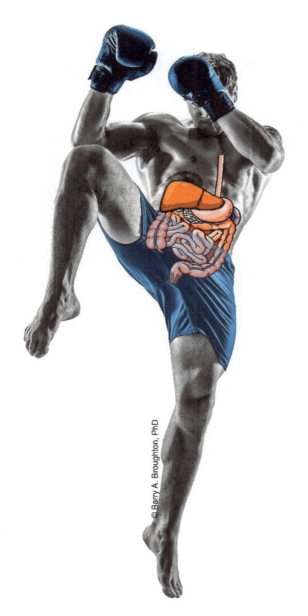

Fig. 11.1 - The digestives system provides nutrients to aid in the demands of daily activities.

The digestive system includes the digestive tract, also called the gastrointestinal (GI) tract or alimentary canal, and its accessory organs. This specialized system of organs processes food into molecules that can be absorbed and utilized by the cells of the body and eliminates the waste products. The digestive tract consists of a long continuous tube that extends from the mouth to the anus. It includes the mouth, pharynx, esophagus, stomach, small intestine, and large intestine. The teeth and tongue are accessory structures located in the mouth. The salivary glands, liver, gallbladder, and pancreas are accessory organs that secrete fluids into the digestive tract to aid in digestion.

Upon entering the digestive tract food undergoes three types of processes in the body: digestion, absorption, and elimination. The digestive system prepares nutrients for utilization by body cells through six activities: ingestion, mechanical digestion, chemical digestion, movements, absorption, and elimination.

- *Ingestion* occurs when food is taken into the mouth in preparation for digestion.

- *Mechanical Digestion* begins in the mouth with chewing (mastication). Large pieces of food that are ingested are broken into smaller particles that can be acted upon by various enzymes. Mechanical digestion continues with the mixing and churning actions in the stomach.

- *Chemical Digestion* is the process in which digestive enzymes and water break down the complex molecules of proteins, fats, and carbohydrates into smaller molecules that can be absorbed and utilized by the cells.

- *Movement* within the digestive system propels food particles from the mouth throughout the gastrointestinal tract. After ingestion and mastication, the food bolus moves from the mouth into the pharynx and esophagus via deglutition (swallowing). Mixing movements within the stomach occur as a result of smooth muscle contraction. Food particles mix with enzymes and other fluids as it is propelled through the digestive tract via movements called peristalsis. These rhythmic waves of contractions move the food particles through the various regions of the gastrointestinal tract in which mechanical and chemical digestion occurs.

- *Absorption* is the process in which simple molecules that result from chemical digestion pass through cell membranes of the lining in the small intestine into the blood and lymph capillaries.

- *Elimination* is the process of removing food molecules that cannot be digested (or absorbed) from the body. The removal of indigestible wastes (feces) through the anus is referred to as defecation or elimination.

Organs of the Digestive System

The organs that comprise the digestive system (in order of their function) are the mouth, esophagus, stomach, small intestine, large intestine, rectum, and anus. Accessory organs that aid in digestion includes the salivary glands, pancreas, gallbladder, and liver.

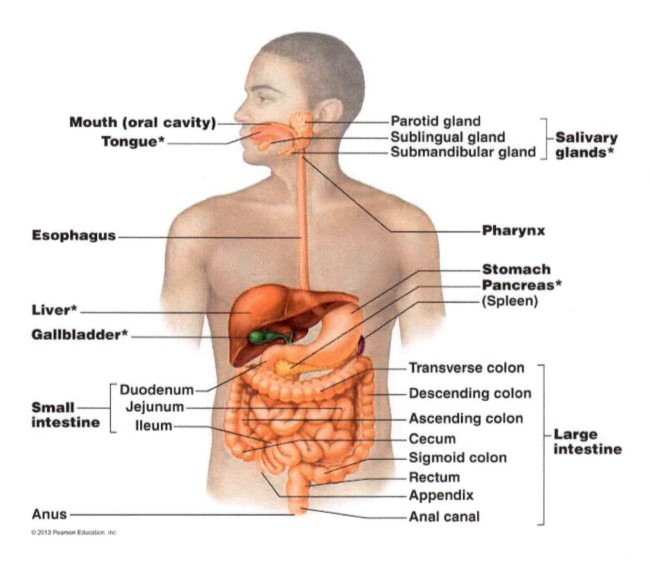

Fig. 11.2 - The digestive tract and accessory organs (*) of the digestive system. Image Credit: Pearson Education, Inc. 2013.

- **Mouth**

The mouth, or oral cavity, is the beginning of the digestive tract. Digestion begins before food enters the oral cavity. The salivary glands in the mouth become active upon seeing or smelling food. The process of chewing (mastication) mechanically breaks down food into pieces that are more easily digested. Saliva mixes with the food to begin chemically breaking it down into a form the body can absorb and use. Upon swallowing, the tongue passes the food into the pharynx and into the esophagus.

- **Esophagus**

Located in the throat near the trachea, the esophagus receives food from the oral cavity. The epiglottis is a small flap of tissue that folds over the trachea preventing food from entering and causing choking. Peristalsis, a series of muscular contractions, within the esophagus moves food towards the stomach.

The lower esophageal sphincter, a ring-like muscle at the distal esophagus relaxes to allow food to enter the stomach. The sphincter then contracts preventing stomach contents from flowing back into the esophagus. When the esophageal sphincter does not close the contents flow back into the esophagus causing acid reflux or heartburn.

- **Stomach**

The stomach is a hollow organ that contains the masticated food while it is being mixed with stomach enzymes. These enzymes continue the chemical digestion process of breaking down food into a usable form. Cells in the lining of the stomach secrete the powerful enzymes and strong acid responsible for the digestion process. When the contents of the stomach are processed, they are passed into the small intestine.

- **Small intestine**

The small intestine is divided into three segments: the duodenum, jejunum, and ileum. Peristalsis moves the food mixture through the seven meter (22 feet) long muscular tube that breaks it down using enzymes released by the pancreas, and bile from the liver.

The duodenum, the most proximal segment of the small intestine is primarily responsible for the continuous breaking-down process of food. The jejunum and ileum (middle and distal portions) are responsible for the absorption of nutrients into the bloodstream.

Contents within the small intestine start out semi-solid and end in a liquid form after passing through the entire organ. Water, enzymes, bile, and mucus contribute to the liquid consistency. Once the nutrients have been absorbed, and the nondigested food residue liquid has passed through the small intestine, it then passes along into the large intestine (colon).

- **Pancreas**

The pancreas secretes digestive enzymes into the duodenum that breaks down protein, fats, and carbohydrates. The pancreas also produces insulin, secreting it directly into the bloodstream. Insulin is the chief hormone for metabolizing sugars.

- **Liver**

The liver has multiple functions, but its primary job within the digestive system is to process the nutrients absorbed from the small intestine. It produces bile that plays a key role in the digestion of fat and some vitamins.

The liver takes the raw materials absorbed by the intestine and performs over 500 different chemical functions within the body. The liver detoxifies potentially harmful chemicals and also breaks down and secretes many drugs that could be potentially toxic.

- **Gallbladder**

The gallbladder stores and concentrates the bile produced from the liver; and then releases it into the duodenum to help absorb and digest fats.

- **Colon**

The colon or large intestine is a long muscular tube that connects the small intestine to the rectum. Measuring approximately five feet (1.5 meters) in length, the colon is divided into the cecum, the ascending colon, the transverse colon, the descending colon, and the sigmoid colon which connects to the rectum.

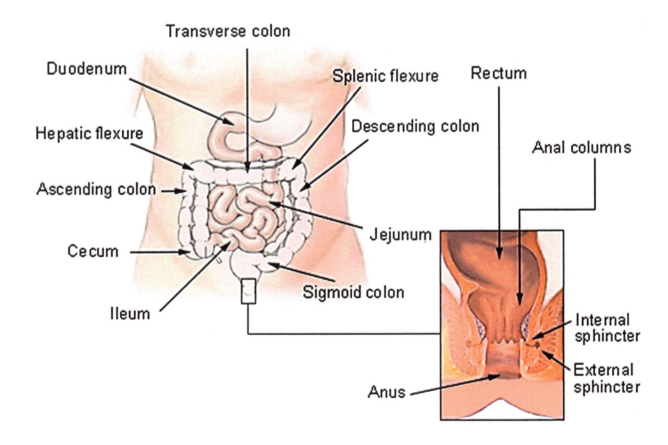

Fig. 11.3 - Structures of the small and large intestines.

Stool, or feces, is the waste product that remains after the digestive process. As stool passes through the colon by peristalsis, where water is removed, it enters the colon in a liquid state and ultimately is eliminated in a semi-solid form. Stool is stored in the sigmoid (S-shaped) colon until it empties into the rectum once or twice a day.

It normally takes approximately 36 hours for stool to get through the colon. The stool itself is mostly undigested food debris and bacteria. These "good" bacteria perform numerous useful functions, such as synthesizing various vitamins, processing waste products and food particles, and protecting against harmful bacteria. As the descending colon becomes full, it empties the fecal contents into the rectum to begin the process of elimination (bowel movement).

- **Rectum**

The rectum is a straight chamber that connects the colon to the anus. When stool (or gas) enters the rectum, nerve sensors relay a message to the brain. The brain then decides if the rectal contents can be released or not. If the contents cannot be excreted, the sphincter contracts and the rectum relaxes so that the sensation temporarily goes away. If the contents can be eliminated, the sphincters relax and the rectum contracts, disposing its contents.

- **Anus**

The anus is the most distal portion of the digestive tract. It consists of pelvic floor muscles and the internal and external anal sphincters. The lining of the upper anus detects rectal contents and signals whether the contents are liquid, gas, or solid.

The sphincter muscles surrounding the anus are important in allowing control of stool within the rectum. The pelvic floor muscle creates an angle between the rectum and the anus that prevents stool from exiting. Except when stool enters the rectum, the internal sphincter is always tight which maintains continence while sleeping or otherwise unaware of the presence of stool. Upon receiving an urge to have a bowel movement, the external sphincter remains tight to retain the stool. Once it is safe to eliminate the feces, the external sphincter relaxes to release the contents.

Clinical Significance and Martial Arts Relevance:

- **Liver Shot**

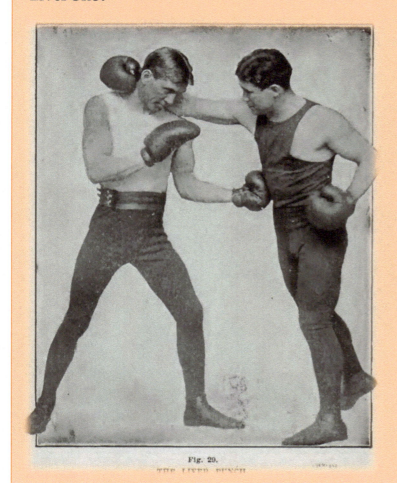

Many experienced practitioners of martial arts and combat sports are aware that a well-placed liver shot can be as effective at incapacitating an opponent as a knockout strike to the head. Most, however, are not aware of the cascade of events involved that cause it to happen.

While the ribcage does provide some protection to the liver, it remains partially exposed and vulnerable to attack. Direct blows to the liver from knee strikes, kicks, or punches can be extremely painful and debilitating, at least temporarily. To the uninitiated, these strikes can appear somewhat innocuous. Those who have been on the receiving end, however, are fully aware of the effectiveness of the liver shot.

Fig. 11.4 - Vintage image of a boxing liver punch. Image Credit: Boxing: A Guide to the Manly Art of Self Defense. American Sports Publishing Company, 1917.

The liver receives sympathetic nerve fibers from the celiac (solar) plexus, and parasympathetic nerve fibers from branches of the vagus nerve. The vagus nerve innervates many vital organs of the cardiovascular, respiratory, and digestive systems; and is part of the parasympathetic nervous system, known for its "rest and digest" response (*Note:* Please see the *Introduction to the Nervous System* chapter).

When the liver gets compressed and stretched from an impact force, it causes a series of events to unfold: the heart rate slows down, blood vessels dilate, and the blood pressure drops, all causing reduced blood flow to the brain which can cause fainting (vasovagal syncope). There can also be confusion and/or temporary paralysis as the legs give out. To overcome this cascade of events, the body tries to overcome the lack of brain perfusion by forcing itself into a horizontal position. Some people can also feel breathless and often describe a feeling like their body was momentarily turned off. Because the capsule surrounding the liver is highly innervated, a direct liver shot can also cause excruciating pain.

Understanding the physiology of a liver shot not only informs the practitioner of more viable targets, but it also allows them to exploit the vulnerabilities and potential weaknesses of the human body in order to overcome an opponent or assailant. Note: Please see a more detailed discussions on the *Physiology of the Liver Shot in Section Four- Physiology of Specific Techniques*.

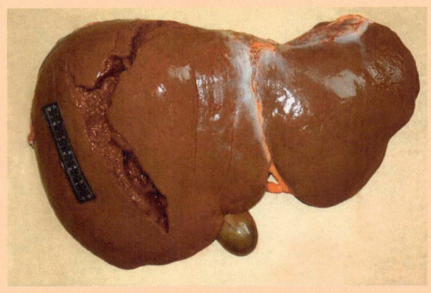

Fig. 11.5 - Liver rupture from blunt force abdominal trauma. Image Credit: Yu Shao, et. al., doi: https://doi.org/10.1371/journal.pone.0052366.g005

Chapter 12

Introduction to the Genitourinary System

The genitourinary system includes all the organs of the reproductive and the urinary systems. Although their functions are unrelated, they are grouped together because of their proximity to each other and the structures involved in reproduction and excretion use of common ducts, i.e., the male urethra. The urinary system is the body's primary excretory system, allowing it to regulate its fluid and electrolyte levels. The urinary system has both abdominal and pelvic structures that allow it to produce, store, and eliminate urine.

Organs and structures of the genitourinary systems include the kidneys, ureters, urinary bladder, and urethra. In males it also includes the testes, sperm ducts, and penis; in females, the genitourinary system also includes ovaries, fallopian tubes, uterus, and vagina.

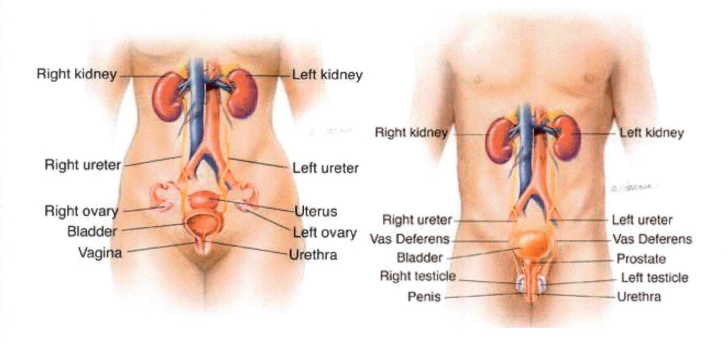

Fig. 12.1 - The female and male genitourinary system.

Components of the Urinary System

The urinary system consists of the kidneys, ureters, urinary bladder, and urethra. The bilateral kidneys form the urine. The ureters carry urine from kidneys to the urinary bladder. The bladder is emptied via the urethra; a tubular structure that carries urine from the urinary bladder to outside the body.

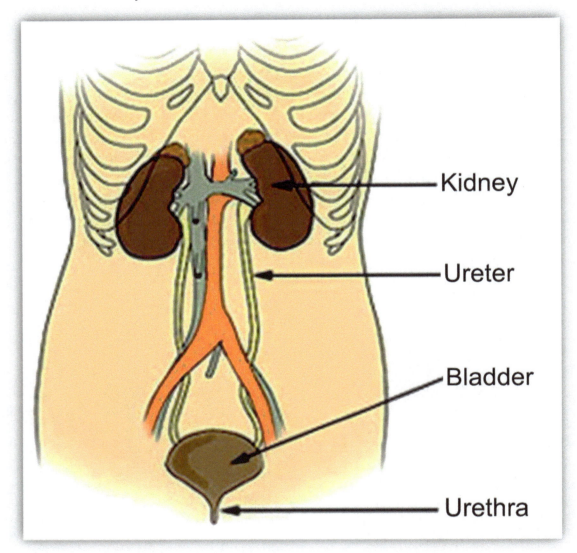

Fig. 12.2 - Components of the Urinary system.

Kidneys

As the primary organs of the urinary system, the kidneys filter the blood, remove the wastes, and excrete the wastes in the urine. Lying against the posterior abdominal wall, on either side of the vertebral column, the kidneys are partially protected by the 11th and 12th ribs bilaterally.

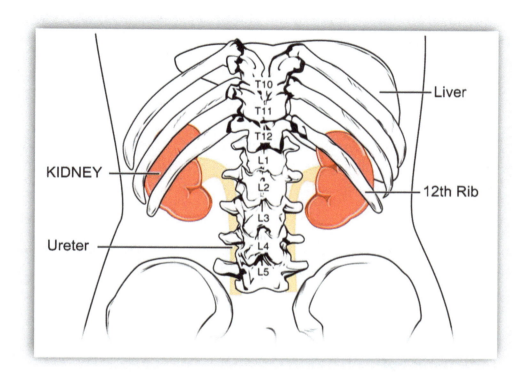

The right kidney is usually slightly lower than the left because the liver displaces it inferiorly.

Fig. 12.3 - The kidneys are partial protected by the ribcage.

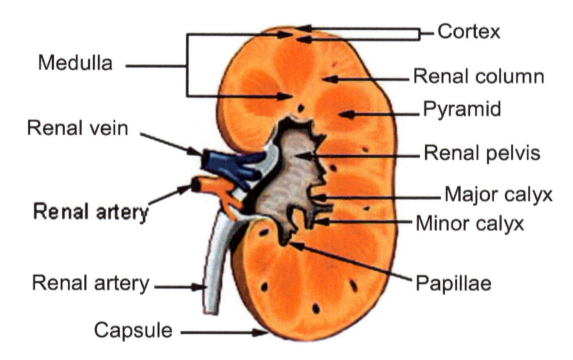

Fig. 12.4 - Sagittal section of the kidney.

The kidneys are extremely vascular and are divided into three main regions: the cortex, medulla, and pelvis. The renal cortex is the outer region, containing approximately 1.25 million renal tubules. The renal medulla is the middle region of the kidney that filters the blood and acts as a collecting chamber. The renal pelvis, the inner region of the kidney, receives urine through the major calyces.

Ureters

The ureter are small tubes that carries urine from the renal pelvis of each kidney to the urinary bladder. They descend from the renal pelvis along the posterior abdominal wall and enter the posterior surface of the urinary bladder.

Urinary Bladder

Located in the pelvic cavity, posterior to the symphysis pubis, the urinary bladder functions as a temporary storage reservoir for urine. The size of the urinary bladder changes based on the volume of urine it contains.

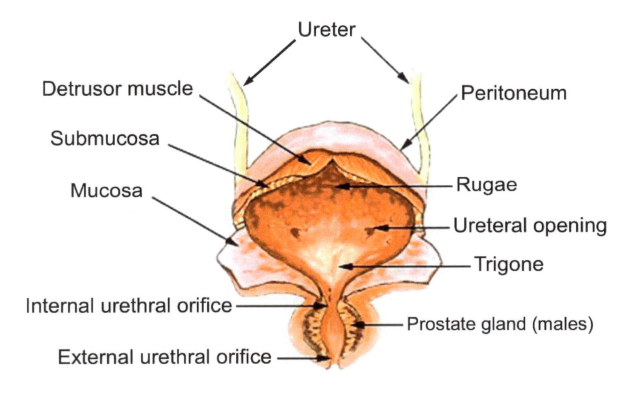

Fig. 12.5 - Structure of urinary bladder.

The trigone is a triangular area in floor of the urinary bladder formed by the openings of the two ureters into the bladder and the urethra. Small flaps of mucosa cover the openings from the ureters and function as one-way valves, allowing urine to enter the bladder but prevent it from backing up into the ureters.

Urethra

The thin-walled tube that allows urine to flow from the floor of the urinary bladder to outside the body is the urethra.

Two sphincters control the flow of urine through the urethra. A small band of smooth (involuntary) muscle encircles the urethra where it leaves the urinary bladder, forming the internal urethral sphincter. The external urethral sphincter is formed by skeletal (voluntary) muscle where the urethra exits through the pelvic floor.

In males, the urethra is about 20 cm (7 to 8 inches) in length, and transports both urine and semen. Upon exiting the urinary bladder, the urethra passes through the prostate gland, penetrates the pelvic floor and enters the penis. The urethra extends the length of the penis and opens to the outside at its tip.

In females, the urethra is much shorter measuring only 3 to 4 cm (about 1.5 inches) long. The external urethral orifice opens to the outside just anterior to the opening for the vagina.

Components of the Reproductive System

While organ systems such as the urinary and endocrine systems, continuously function to maintain homeostasis for survival of the individual, the major function of the reproductive system is to ensure the survival of the species. An individual may live a long, healthy and happy life without producing offspring; however, for the continuation of the species, some of the individuals must produce offspring.

The primary reproductive organs in females are the ovaries, and the testes in males. These organs are responsible for producing the gamete (egg and sperm cells), as well as hormones. The secondary organs, ducts, and glands of the reproductive system transport and sustain the gametes and nurture the developing offspring.

Male Reproductive System

The male reproductive system consists of a pair of testes and a network of ducts, seminal vesicles, the prostate, the bulbourethral glands, and the penis.

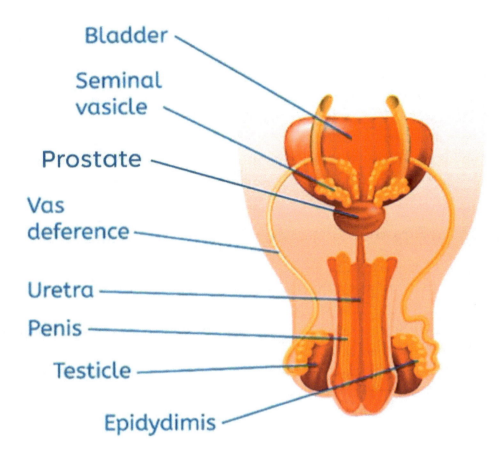

Fig. 12.6 - Components of male reproductive system.

Testes

The testes, or testicles, begin to form during fetal development high in the abdominal cavity, near the kidneys. During the last two months of gestation, or shortly after birth, they descend through the inguinal canal and into the scrotum. The scrotal sac consists of skin and subcutaneous tissue that extends below the abdomen and is posterior to the penis. Although the location of the testes, outside the abdominal cavity may make them vulnerable to injury, it provides a lower temperature to produce viable sperm.

Each testis contains interstitial cells (cells of Leydig) located between the seminiferous tubules within a lobule, which produces testosterone. Sperm are produced within the seminiferous tubules.

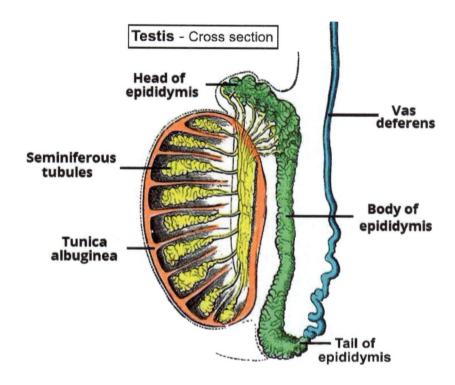

Fig. 12.7 – Cross section of testis.

Urethra

The urethra extends from the urinary bladder to the external urethral orifice at the tip of the penis. It is a passageway for sperm and fluids from the reproductive system, and urine from the urinary system. While reproductive fluids are passing through the urethra, sphincters contract tightly to keep urine from entering the urethra.

Accessory Glands

The accessory glands of the male reproductive system are the seminal vesicles, prostate gland, and the bulbourethral glands. Each of these glands secrete fluids that enter the urethra.

Seminal Vesicles

The seminal vesicles are two small glands posterior to the urinary bladder that store and produce the majority of the fluid that makes up semen.

Prostate

The prostate is a firm dense walnut-sized gland located just inferior the bladder, and anterior to the rectum. The prostate secretes fluid that nourishes and protects sperm cells. The urethra runs from the bladder through the center of the prostate where numerous short ducts empty secretions into the prostatic urethra.

Bulbourethral Glands

The paired bulbourethral (Cowper's) glands are pea-shaped glands located beneath the prostate gland at the beginning of the internal portion of the penis. The bulbourethral glands add fluids to semen and neutralizes the acidity of urine residue in the urethra.

Penis

Located anterior to the scrotum the penis is a cylindrical pendant organ formed by three columns of erectile tissue wrapped in connective tissue and covered with skin. The two dorsal columns are the corpora cavernosa. The single ventral midline column surrounds the urethra and is called the corpus spongiosum.

The root of the penis attaches to the pubic arch, while the body (shaft) is the visible pendant portion. The corpus spongiosum expands at the distal end to form the glans penis. The urethra extends throughout the length of the corpus spongiosum and opens at the tip of the glans penis. The loose fold of skin called the prepuce (or foreskin), covers the glans penis.

Clinical Significance and Martial Arts Relevance:

Injuries to the Genitalia

Trauma to the testes or scrotum can cause harm to any of its contents. When the tough cover of the testicle is shattered or torn, blood leaks from the injured area. A hematoma may develop in the scrotum as a result of the trauma. This causes swelling and discoloration of the scrotal skin. Occasionally the origin of bleeding may not arise from the scrotal contents (i.e., spermatic cord and testis) but from the basal part of the penile urethra as in "straddle injuries" – direct perineal trauma such as falling onto a bicycle crossbar or being kicked in the groin area. The pooling of blood stretches the scrotum until it is tense and can lead to an infection.

Blunt force trauma can cause injury to female external genitalia as well. In women, this includes the highly innervated vulva. Injuries to the labia may cause bruising, bleeding, and significant pain. A straddle injury may also injure the area between the genitals and the anus called the perineum. Severe trauma can also cause a fracture of bones in the pelvis.

Female Reproductive System

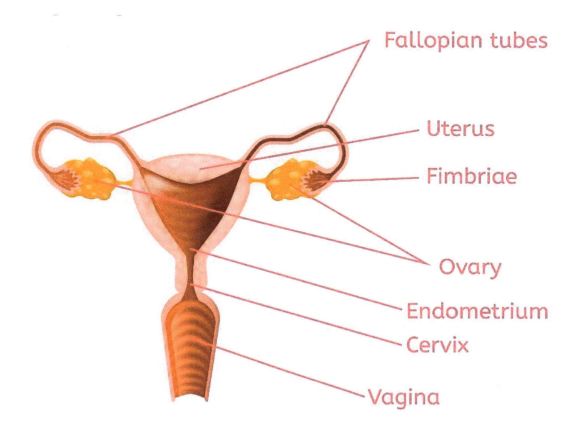

Fig. 12.8 - Coronal view of components of the female reproductive system.

In addition to producing female sex hormones, the female reproductive system organs produce and sustain the female gamete (egg cells or ova) and transports them to where they may be fertilized by sperm. Should an egg become fertilized, it provides an environment for the developing fetus through the end of gestation.

The female reproductive system includes the ovaries, fallopian tubes, uterus, vagina, accessory glands, and the external genital organs.

Ovaries

The primary female reproductive organs are the two ovaries in which the eggs form and the female hormones estrogen and progesterone are made. The ovaries are located in shallow depressions on each side of the uterus in the pelvic cavity. The ovaries are held loosely in place by peritoneal ligaments.

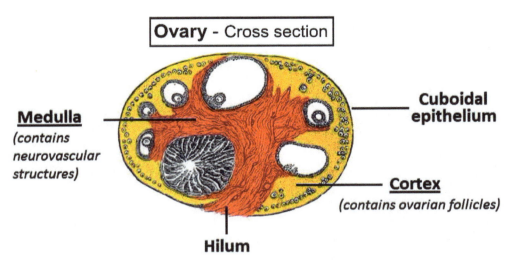

Fig. 12.9 – Cross section of ovary.

The ovaries are divided into an outer cortex and an inner medulla. The cortex appears denser and more granular due to the presence of numerous ovarian follicles in various stages of development. Each of the follicles contains an oocyte, a female germ cell. The medulla is a loose connective tissue containing blood vessels, lymphatic vessels, and nerve fibers.

Fallopian Tubes

The fallopian tubes are muscular J shape tubes extending from both sides of the uterus. There is one fallopian (uterine) tube associated with each ovary. Their main function is to transmit the ovum to the uterus. There is no direct connection between the end of the tube and the ovary, therefore the oocyte enters the peritoneal cavity before it enters the fallopian tube.

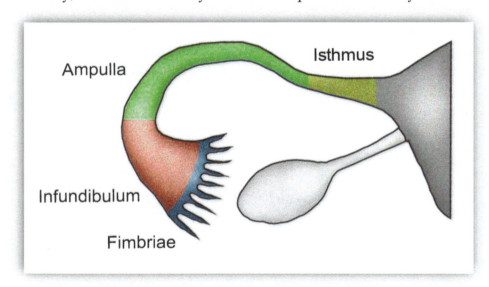

Fig. 12.10 - Fallopian tubes.

The fimbriae (finger-like projections) are the entry point of the ovum into the infundibulum, a funnel shaped opening to the fallopian tube. Fertilization of the ovum with the sperm may occur in the ampulla, the widest section of the tube. The ovum travels down the isthmus, the narrowest part of the fallopian tube which connects the tube with the uterine wall.

Uterus

The uterus is a pear-shaped relatively mobile muscular organ that receives the fertilized oocyte and provides a supporting environment for the developing fetus.

The lower end of the uterus is located at the level of the ischial spine and is supported by pelvic floor muscles and cervical ligaments. During pregnancy, it reaches the epigastric area due to growth of the fetus.

Vagina

The vagina is a fibromuscular tube extending from the vulva to the uterus. Located anterior to the rectum and posterior to the urethra and urinary bladder, the vagina is tilted posteriorly as it ascends. Due to its obliquity, its posterior wall is larger than the anterior wall.

The vagina serves as the outlet for the menstrual blood flow, and acts as a birth canal.

External Genitalia

The area containing the external genitalia of the female reproductive system is called the vulva. The vulva includes the labia majora, mons pubis, labia minora, clitoris, and the glands within the vestibule. The vestibule is the area between the labia minora which contain the urethral opening and the vaginal opening.

Chapter 13

Introduction to the Endocrine System

The endocrine system, along with the nervous system, is responsible for the regulation of bodily activities. While the nervous system acts through electrical impulses and neurotransmitters, the endocrine system acts through chemical messengers called hormones. The short-term (i.e., seconds) localized effect of stimuli from the nervous system cause muscle contraction and glandular secretion. Hormones regulate many biological processes such as metabolic activities, influencing growth and development, and is therefore longer acting (i.e., minutes, hours, or weeks) and is more generalized than the actions of the nervous system.

The ductless glands of the endocrine system secrete hormones directly into the bloodstream, which is then carried throughout the body. The hormones influence only those cells that have receptor sites equipped to respond to that specific hormone.

Chemical Nature of Hormones

Hormones are classified chemically as either proteins or steroids. Of the over fifty hormones in the human body, all (except the sex hormones and those from the adrenal cortex) are proteins or protein derivatives.

Mechanism of Hormone

Hormones are carried via the circulatory system throughout the entire body yet only target certain cells. Target cells that have receptor sites for a given hormone act in a quasi-lock-and-key fashion activating the target tissue.

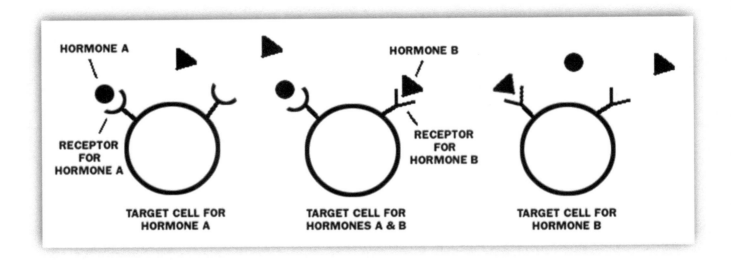

Fig. 13.1 - Hormone target cells.

Some hormonal responses affect localized tissue in a single gland or organ; while in others the target tissue is diffuse and affects many areas of the body. Hormones bring about their specific characteristic effects on target cells by modifying cellular activities.

Protein hormones react with receptors on the surface of the target cell, and the sequence of events that results during the hormone action is relatively rapid. Steroid hormones typically react with receptor sites inside a cell. Because this method of action involves synthesis of proteins, it is relatively slow in comparison.

Control of Hormone Action

Because of their potency, very small amounts of a hormone may have profound effects on metabolic processes. Therefore, hormone secretion must be regulated within very narrow limits in order to maintain a state of stability, or homeostasis, in the body.

To aid in maintaining these narrow parameters, many hormones are controlled by a negative feedback loop. In negative feedback systems, a stimulus causes the release of a substance whose effects then inhibits further release of hormones — thereby allowing the concentration of hormones in blood to be maintained within a narrow range.

Some endocrine glands secrete hormones in response to hormones secreted by another gland. While a third mechanism of regulating hormone secretion is by direct nervous stimulation which causes a gland to secrete its hormone.

Endocrine Glands & Their Hormones

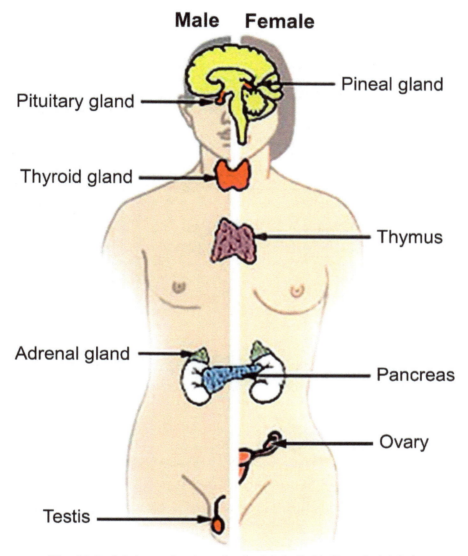

Fig. 13.2 - Major endocrine glands. Male (left), Female (right).

Although there are eight major endocrine glands scattered throughout the body, because they have similar functions, mechanisms of influence, and interrelationships, they are considered to be one system.

    Some glands also have non-endocrine regions that have functions other than hormone secretion. For example, the pancreas has a major exocrine (duct containing) portion that secretes digestive enzymes, and an endocrine (ductless) portion that secretes hormones. Some organs, such as the stomach, intestines, and heart, produce hormones, but it is not their primary function. The testes and ovaries secrete hormones and produce the ova and sperm.

Pituitary & Pineal Glands

Pituitary Gland

The pituitary gland is often called the "master gland" because it produces many hormones that control different processes in the body. The pituitary is a small gland measuring about 1 centimeter in diameter, the size of a kidney bean, resting in a bony depression in the sphenoid bone. The pituitary gland is connected to the hypothalamus of the brain by a slender stalk called the infundibulum.

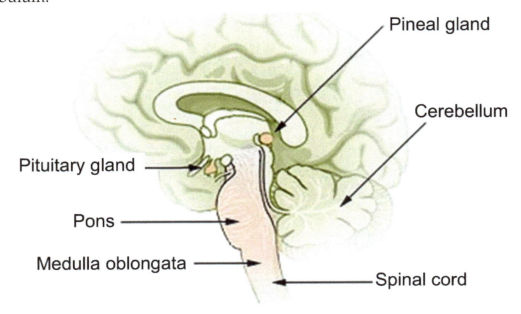

Fig. 13.3 - Sagittal of the brain showing pituitary and pineal glands.

There are two distinct regions in the gland: the anterior lobe and the posterior lobe. The activity of the anterior lobe is controlled by releasing hormones from the hypothalamus. The posterior lobe is controlled by nerve stimulation.

Hormones of the Anterior Lobe

The pituitary gland secretes a variety of hormones into the bloodstream which transmits information to distant cells, regulating their activity. For example, the pituitary gland controls metabolism, growth, sexual maturation, reproduction, blood pressure and many other vital physical functions and processes. The pituitary gland also secretes hormones that act on the thyroid gland, adrenal glands, ovaries and testes, which in turn produce other hormones.

Hormones of the Posterior Lobe

The hormones of the posterior pituitary that are synthesized by the hypothalamus include oxytocin and antidiuretic hormone. Oxytocin causes contraction of the smooth muscle wall of the uterus and stimulates the ejection of lactating breast milk.

Antidiuretic hormone helps regulate the amount of water in the body by controlling the amount of water the kidneys reabsorb.

Pineal Gland

The pineal gland is a small cone-shaped structure that extends posteriorly from the third ventricle of the brain. The pineal gland synthesizes the hormone melatonin, secreting it directly into the cerebrospinal fluid which takes it into the blood. Melatonin affects reproductive development and is best known for the role it plays in regulating sleep patterns.

Thyroid & Parathyroid Glands

Thyroid Gland

Lying just under the skin in the anterior neck, the thyroid gland secretes hormones that control the body's metabolic rate. It consists of two lobes, one on each side of the trachea, which are connected by a narrow band of tissue (called the isthmus) giving it the shape of a bow tie.

Thyroid hormones affect many vital functions such as growth, skin maintenance, heart rate, heat production, digestion, the rate at which calories are burned, and fertility.

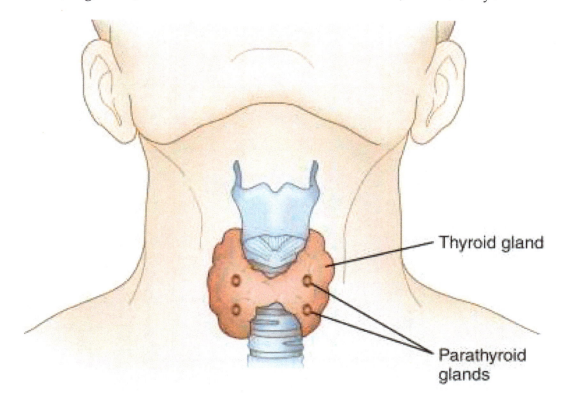

Fig. 13.4 - Thyroid and parathyroid glands.

Parathyroid Glands

The parathyroid glands are two pairs of small, oval-shaped glands located on the posterior surface of two thyroid gland lobes.

The parathyroid glands produce parathyroid hormone, which plays a key role in the regulation of calcium levels in the blood. Insufficient secretion of parathyroid hormone leads to low blood calcium levels, causing increased nerve excitability that stimulates muscle contraction.

Adrenal Glands

The paired adrenal glands are located near the superior portion of each kidney. Each gland is divided into the inner medulla and the outer cortex. The medulla and cortex of the adrenal gland secrete different hormones. The adrenal cortex is essential to life, while the medulla may be removed with no long-term life-threatening effects.

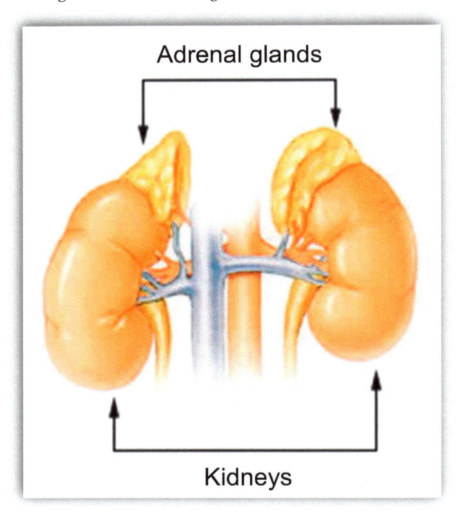

Fig. 13.5 - Adrenal glands.

Hormones of the Adrenal Cortex

The adrenal cortex produces several hormones. The most important are cortisol, aldosterone, and estrogen and androgens (sex hormones).

Cortisol is released during times of stress, providing an energy boost to help handle an emergency situation. It suppresses inflammation, regulates blood pressure, and increases blood sugar. Cortisol helps manage the body's use of fats, proteins, and carbohydrates, and also controls the sleep/wake cycle.

Aldosterone plays a key role in regulating blood pressure by helping the kidneys control certain electrolytes in the bloodstream and tissues of the body. Aldosterone sends signals resulting in the kidneys absorbing more sodium into the bloodstream and releasing potassium into the urine

DHEA (Dehydroepiandrosterone) and androgenic steroids are precursor hormones that are converted in the ovaries into female hormones (estrogens) and in the testes into male hormones (androgens). However, estrogens and androgens are produced in much larger amounts by the ovaries and testes. Androgens, male sex hormones, are produced in the adrenal glands of both men and women, but in different amounts.

Hormones of the Adrenal Medulla

Produced in the adrenal medulla, epinephrine and norepinephrine have similar functions in initiating the flight or fight response. Together they increase the heart rate and the force of heart contractions, increasing blood flow to the muscles and brain, while relaxing smooth muscles of the airway. They also control vasoconstriction (the squeezing of the blood vessels), helping maintain blood pressure, and assist in glucose (sugar) metabolism.

Epinephrine and norepinephrine are activated when the body needs additional resources and energy to endure unusual physical and emotionally stressful events.

Clinical Significance and Martial Arts Relevance:

- **Fight, Flight, or Freeze**

During a stressful situation — whether something psychological, such as persistently worrying about losing a job; or something environmental such as a physical assault — a cascade of stress hormones that produce well-orchestrated physiological changes occur. A stressful incident can cause an increased heart rate and pound with more force while causing more rapid breathing. Muscles tense along with an increase in perspiration.
Because it evolved as a survival mechanism, this combination of reactions to stress is often referred to as the "fight-or-flight" response, enabling people and other mammals to react

quickly to potentially life-threatening situations. These nearly instantaneous physiological responses and sequence of hormonal changes helps a person to fight the threat or flee to safety.

This same adrenal response that allows a person to run faster and jump higher in potentially dangerous situations, also causes tunnel vision and loss of fine motor control during that time. Therefore, intricate, and complicated martial arts techniques may be ineffective during times of great stress and danger. These involuntary physiological responses can be severe enough to cause the unexpecting and/or inexperienced practitioner to even become momentarily immobilized, thereby freezing in place.

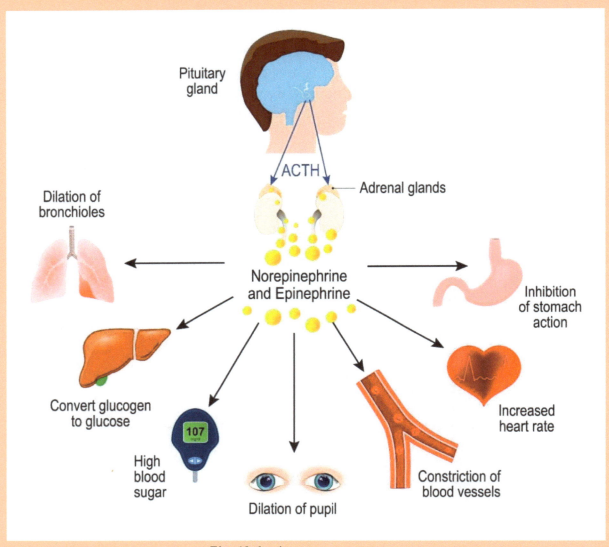

Fig. 13.6 - Acute stress response.

Pancreas — Islets of Langerhans

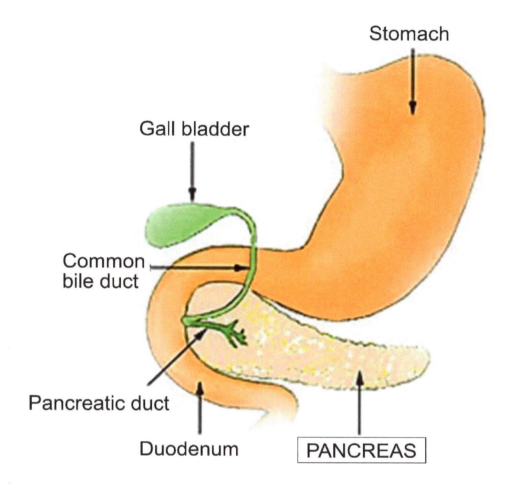

Fig. 13.7 - Pancreas.

The pancreas is a long organ that lies transversely along the posterior abdominal wall, posterior to the stomach, and extends from the region of the duodenum to the spleen. The pancreas serves two functions, as a digestive exocrine gland and a hormone-producing endocrine gland. Functioning as an endocrine gland, the pancreatic islets secrete the hormones glucagon and insulin to control blood sugar levels throughout the day.

Gonads

The primary reproductive organs (the gonads) are the testes in the male and the ovaries in the female. Along with producing the sperm and ova, they also secrete hormones and are therefore considered to be endocrine glands.

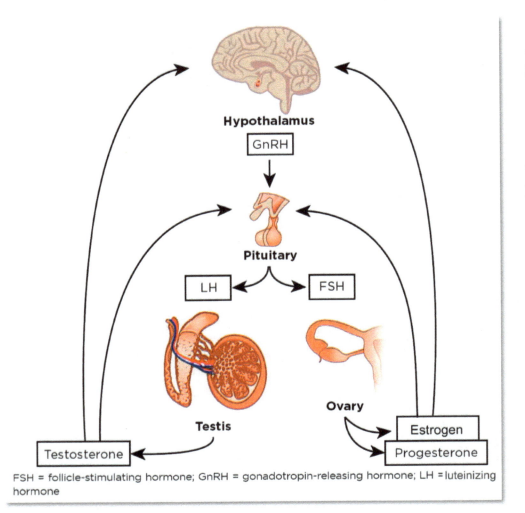

Fig. 13.8 - Hypothalamic-pituitary-gonadal axis

The release of sex hormones from the testes and ovaries is governed by the *hypothalamic-pituitary-gonadal axis* (Fig. 13.8). The levels of testosterone and estrogen are continually monitored by the hypothalamus gland. When sex hormone levels begin to fall, gonadotropin-releasing hormone (GnRH) is released by the hypothalamus signaling the pituitary gland. The anterior pituitary then secretes luteinizing hormone (LH) and follicle-stimulating hormone (FSH) into the systemic circulation.

Testes

Testosterone is the principal androgen, male sex hormone, secreted by the testes. Production of testosterone begins during fetal development and continues for a short time after birth; then nearly ceases during childhood but resumes at puberty.

Testosterone is vital in the development of male physical characteristics such as:

- The development and growth of the male reproductive organs.
- Enlargement of the larynx accompanied by voice changes.
- Increased skeletal and muscular growth.
- Distribution and growth of body hair.
- Increased male sexual drive.

Testosterone secretion is regulated by a negative feedback loop that involves releasing hormones from the hypothalamus and gonadotropins from the anterior pituitary. In addition to producing testosterone, the testes also produce estrogen, a female sex hormone, to a lesser degree.

Ovaries

There are two groups of female sex hormones that are produced in the ovaries, the estrogens and progesterone. Both groups of steroid hormones contribute to the development and function of female sex characteristics of the reproductive organs.

During puberty estrogen plays a role in the development of female sex characteristics such as:

- The development of the breasts.
- Wider hips.
- Distribution of fat in the hips, legs, and breasts.
- Pubic hair and armpit hair.
- Maturation of reproductive organs such as the uterus and vagina

Progesterone causes the uterine lining to thicken in preparation for pregnancy. Together with progesterone, the estrogens are responsible for the changes that occur in the uterus during the female menstrual cycle.

Other Endocrine Glands

In addition to the major endocrine glands, the thymus, stomach, small intestines, heart, and placenta have some hormonal activity as part of their function.

Thymosin, produced by the thymus gland, plays a vital role in the development of the body's immune system.

The gastric mucosa (the stomach lining) produces the hormone gastrin, in response to the presence of food in the stomach. Gastrin then stimulates the production of hydrochloric acid and the enzyme pepsin, which are used in the digestion of food.

Secretin and cholecystokinin are secreted by the mucosa of the small intestine. In response to acid in the small intestine, secretin is release and stimulates the pancreas to release a flood of bicarbonate-rich fluid, which neutralizes the stomach acid. Cholecystokinin stimulates the contraction of the gallbladder, which releases stored bile into the intestine. It also stimulates the pancreas to secrete digestive enzyme.

In addition to its major role of pumping blood, the heart also acts as an endocrine organ. Special cells in the wall of the atria, the upper chambers of the heart, produce atriopeptin, a cardiac hormone involved in fluid, electrolyte, and blood-pressure balance.

Human chorionic gonadotropin (HCG) is secreted by the placenta of pregnant females. HCG signals the mother's ovaries to secrete hormones to maintain the uterine lining so that it does not shed off during menstruation.

SECTION FOUR

Physiology of Specific Techniques

Chapter 14

Physiology of Specific Techniques

Because of their complex nature, the cascade of events that occur, and the potential for significant injury, the three topics presented in this section are discussed in greater detail than in the previous chapters of this text.

Vascular Neck Restraints

One of the most powerful tools in the arsenal of jujitsu and combatives grappling art practitioners is the ability to render an assailant unconscious without striking. This most often occurs by encircling the neck, thereby decreasing cerebral blood flow via occluding the carotid arteries. Commonly referred to by the misnomer of "choke", these types of techniques, are actually strangulations. Even though the terms "rear naked *choke*", "baseball *choke*", "side *choke*", etc. are widely used in martial arts vernacular, the verbiage is wrong. According to Dorland's Medical Dictionary a *strangulation is the impairment of blood supply*. Whereas a *choke is the mechanical obstruction of the glottis, larynx, or trachea*. Therefore, a strangle affects blood flow, while chokes affect breathing. Complicating the picture somewhat, is that oftentimes when attempting to apply a technique that isolates the carotid artery bilaterally, the trachea and larynx may also be obstructed (incidentally or intentionally). For those of us who practice the combatives application of these techniques; in what can initially begin as a somewhat innocuous technique, by simply changing the direction of force, the technique can transition to a neck crank and also affect the cervical spine.

Therefore, to be more precise with our terminology, rather than use the broad stroke term of "choke", when applying techniques that occlude blood flow to the brain, the term *vascular neck restraint* (VNR) is a more accurate term, i.e., *rear naked VNR*. Additionally, when applying a technique that disrupts cerebral blood flow *and* the airway (or possibly the cervical spine), the term *neck restraint* may be more accurate, i.e., *guillotine neck restraint*.

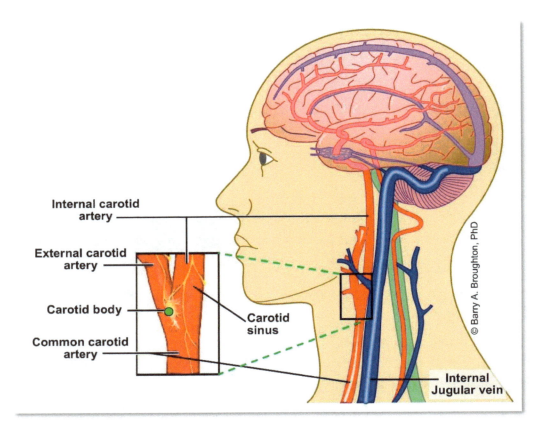

Fig. 14.1 - The carotid sinus is located in the internal carotid artery just superior to the bifurcation. It contains a baroreceptor that senses changes in systemic blood pressure.

In order to apply these techniques more safely and effectively, an understanding of the physiology of a vascular neck restraint is beneficial. The internal carotid arteries supply the brain with about 80% of its oxygenated blood, while the vertebral arteries contribute the remaining 20%. A study by Mitchell, et al. published in the *Journal of Applied Physiology* in 2012 evaluated the "Mechanism of loss of consciousness during vascular neck restraint". By applying a VNR (commonly referred to as a "rear naked choke") on compliant volunteers, their findings reveal that the most important mechanism resulting in loss of consciousness was bilateral carotid artery compression causing decreased cerebral flow. Carotid sinus baroreceptor reflex appears to have little effect of the efficacy of VNR. Also of importance is the finding that cerebral hypoxia, contributing to loss of consciousness, occurs when the cerebral blood flow velocity drops below 50% in both the right and left carotid arteries. Of significance, the compression force required to effectively compress the carotid arteries must be at least 100 mmHg. However, applying a greater amount of pressure *did not* result in a faster response in which the subject was rendered unconscious. The average time for unconsciousness following the application of the vascular neck restraint was 9.5 seconds (+/- 0.4 sec.).

A 2020 study published in the *International Journal of Performance Analysis in Sport* by Stellpflug, et al. confirmed similar times for loss of consciousness (LOC) in fully resisting highly trained competitors. In evaluating 81 Ultimate Fighting Championship bouts that ended in stoppage due to LOC via "choke", the average time for LOC was 9 seconds. There was no discernible statistical difference when comparing 11 different "chokes" (five neck-only chokes, and six arm-in chokes).

In addition to the above finding, some studies suggest that due to their proximity to the carotid arteries, jugular vein compression causing increased intracranial pressure combined with the carotid sinus baroreceptor reflex, may potentially be contributing mechanisms to LOC during VNR to a lesser degree. Applying only 4.4 pounds of pressure to the jugular veins causes venous outflow obstruction from the brain and subsequent stagnant hypoxia, while eleven pounds of pressure to the carotid arteries can cause loss of consciousness.

The data presented in these studies reveals that when applying a vascular neck restraint; ensure that gradual pressure is applied to the bilateral carotid arteries so that force can be held for greater than 10 seconds. Squeezing harder does not necessarily provide greater results, demonstrating that the application of proper technique is more effective than brute force.

Even though the application of "chokes" in sporting environments have been demonstrated to be relatively safe, bear in mind that all these studies were performed on young healthy individuals attempting to isolate the vasculature while avoiding the airway. Additionally, VNR that are applied in a martial arts training are infrequently held for a period long enough to induce unconsciousness. When applied in the context of sport, the chokehold is typically managed in a controlled setting by trained referees, instructors, and participants who consent in advance. Executing these same techniques on an older, less healthy person can have dire consequences. There is the potential for plaque within the carotid arteries to dislodge, occlude the blood flow to the brain and cause a stroke. Some individuals have a hypersensitive carotid sinus which when compressed, or stimulated, can cause a vast drop in blood pressure and heart rate, causing a dangerously irregular heartbeat (arrhythmia) resulting in a heart attack.

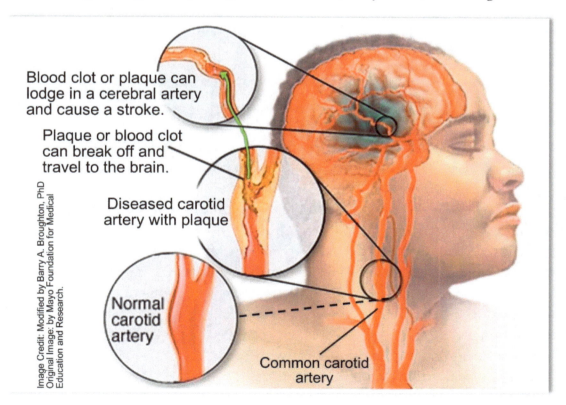

Fig. 14.2 - A vascular neck restraint could cause disastrous results in the presence of a diseased carotid artery. Image Credit: Modified by Barry A. Broughton, PhD; Original: Mayo Foundation for Medical Education and Research.

Airway Chokes

It is important to understand that not all chokes are "blood chokes" (or more accurately-strangulations). Arguably, the most used choke in combat sports is some variation of a rear choke or rear naked choke. Although most rear naked choke variations are indeed "blood chokes"; in reality *not all* rear choke variations are "blood chokes". In medicine, a *choke* is the interruption, or prevention, of *respiration* by *obstruction or compression of the airway*.

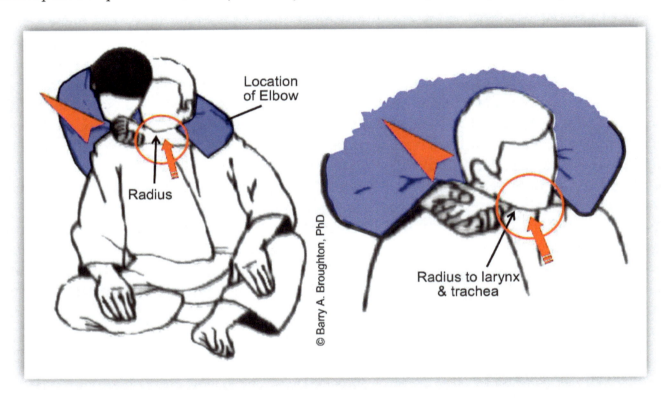

Fig. 14.3 - Rear choke attacking the airway.

There are a host of chokes that directly attack the larynx and trachea (windpipe) that can disrupt the opponent's ability to breathe. In grappling related martial arts, these are often referred to as "airway chokes" or "air chokes". Because of the potential for severe injury, or even death associated with "airway chokes", they are often illegal in combat sport competition; and therefore, are often neglected and frequently are not taught.

There is often confusion regarding the difference between an "airway choke" and a "blood choke". This may be perpetuated because oftentimes in traditional Japanese Jiu-jitsu systems and Judo (and BJJ to a lesser degree), both airway and blood choke variations of the rear choke share the same Japanese name - *Hadaka Jime*.

The lack of distinction regarding "air" and "blood" choke variations is unfortunate because the physiology between the two variations is dramatically different; therefore, there are different concerns for injury and safety precaution in their application.

Airway chokes, either intentionally or inadvertently, directly attack the soft tissue, cartilaginous, and bony structures of the airway. Numerous anatomical structures within the neck can be severely injured during the application of airway chokes. This can be accomplished by using innumerable objects to include: the attacker's hand, arm, forearm, leg, clothing, or other inanimate objects.

During the conventional application of the rear (*airway*) choke, the elbow of the choking arm is far lateral from the anterior midline of the opponent; unlike the "blood choke" variation of *rear naked choke*. In the airway choke there is no intentional pressure over the area the carotid arteries or carotid sinus. Instead, the pressure is placed directly over the laryngotracheal area.

Airway chokes can directly injure the hyoid bone, thyroid cartilage, cricoid cartilage, trachea, and surrounding membranes. Injury to any of these structures can be severe and require immediate medical intervention.

Research by Travis, et. al., evaluated static and dynamic impact trauma of the human larynx. Their findings revealed that fracture of the cricoid and thyroid cartilages occurred at 20.8 kg (45.85 lbs.) and 15.8 kg (34.8 lbs.) of force, respectively. Structural collapse of the larynx occurs at 55 kg (121.25 lbs.) of force. Occlusion of the trachea requires 33 pounds of force, and just 35 pounds to fracture the tracheal cartilage. All relatively easily achieved when it has been reported that trained practitioners can apply chokes in excess of 100 pounds of force.

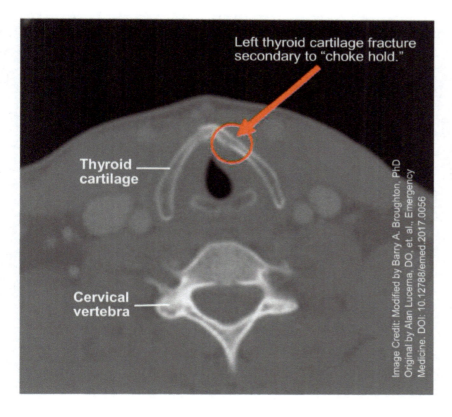

Fig. 14.4 - Computed tomography image showing a minimally displaced fracture of the left thyroid cartilage with soft-tissue swelling and minimal narrowing of the subglottic trachea. Case History: A 38-year-old man presented with a complaint of throat pain after his 15-year-old son applied a "choke hold" while wrestling. He reported that he felt a "crack" in his anterior neck, and soon afterwards felt throat pain with swallowing, along with discomfort with breathing.

Image Credit: Modified by Barry A. Broughton, PhD Original by Alan Lucerna, DO, et. al., Emergency Medicine. DOI: 10.12788/emed.2017.0056

When employing any variation of airway chokes (and vascular neck restraints), in addition to the local trauma that occurs from the direct pressure, underlying medical conditions can also be exacerbated. Much like carotid plaques breaking off and causing strokes after the application of "blood chokes"; airway chokes applied to those with comorbidities such as asthma can also have a deleterious effect.

▪ Physiology of the Liver Shot

Many experienced practitioners of martial arts and combat sports are aware that a well-placed liver shot can be as effective at incapacitating an opponent as a knockout strike to the head. Most, however, are not aware of the cascade of events involved that cause it to happen.

While the ribcage does provide some protection to the liver, it remains partially exposed and vulnerable to attack. Direct blows to the liver from knee strikes, kicks, or punches can be extremely painful and debilitating, at least temporarily. To the uninitiated, these strikes can appear somewhat innocuous. Those who have been on the receiving end, however, are fully aware of the effectiveness of the liver shot.

A research study published in 2013 evaluated simulated liver injuries sustained by blunt force abdominal trauma. The study measured five different impact velocities (4, 5, 6, 7, 8 meters per second) of a punch to the right hypochondrium (overlying the area of the liver) delivered from three different directions (anterior, lateral, and posterior) of impact. Their findings revealed that a direct punch laterally to the side of the abdomen with a minimum punch speed of five meters per second, is enough to cause liver injury. Subsequent fractures of the right ribs were not needed to cause liver injury.

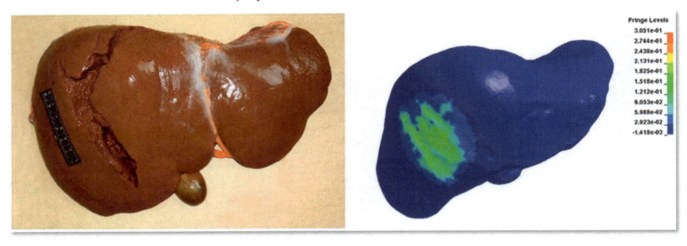

Fig. 14.5 - The comparison between the liver rupture of the victim and the simulated results. Results of lateral punch simulations with an impact velocity of 6 m/s were illustrated. High gradients of color indicate region of greatest strain and location of injuries. Image Credit: Yu Shao, et. al., doi: https://doi.org/10.1371/journal.pone.0052366.g005

For perspective on the amount of impact velocity that can be delivered by a punch; a 2007 study by engineers at the University of Manchester in England measured the punching velocity of a professional boxer. They found that the average punching velocity was 11 m/s, while his fastest velocity was 15.3 m/s. The punching velocity of an average untrained person was estimated to be 6.7 m/s, certainly enough to cause liver injury.

A well-placed strike to the liver, even with moderate power and speed, could result in injuring the liver without fracturing the ribs. When a strike initially lands on the ribcage overlying the liver, there are dynamic pressure changes within the organ itself. The 2013 study demonstrated that the impact force and energy to the overlying ribs is transferred to the liver. Because the liver is flexible and malleable, when one side of the liver gets compressed with a strike, the other side will stretch. Envision holding an air-filled balloon in your hand; as you squeeze the balloon, the displaced air causes the balloon to bulge on the opposite side of the squeeze.

The liver receives sympathetic nerve fibers from the celiac (solar) plexus, and parasympathetic nerve fibers from branches of the vagus nerve. The vagus nerve innervates many vital organs of the cardiovascular, respiratory, and digestive systems; and is part of the parasympathetic nervous system, known for its "rest and digest" response (*Note:* Please see the *Introduction to the Nervous System* chapter).

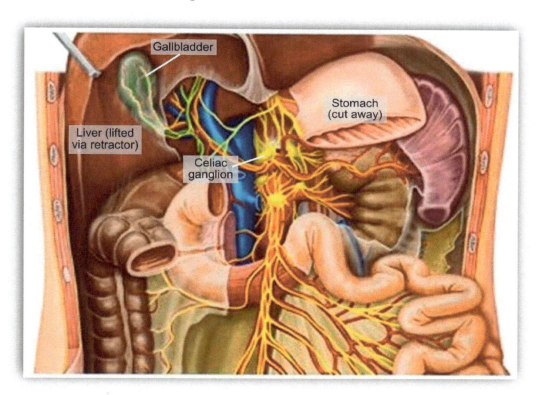

Fig. 14.6 - The liver is innervated by sympathetic and parasympathetic nerve fibers.

When the liver gets compressed and stretched from an impact force, it causes a series of events to unfold: the heart rate slows down, blood vessels dilate, and the blood pressure drops, all causing reduced blood flow to the brain which can cause fainting (vasovagal syncope). There can also be confusion and/or temporary paralysis as the legs give out. To overcome this cascade of events, the body tries to overcome the lack of brain perfusion by forcing itself into a horizontal position. Some people can also feel breathless and often describe a feeling like their body was momentarily turned off. Because the capsule surrounding the liver is highly innervated, a direct liver shot can also cause excruciating pain.

Understanding the physiology of a liver shot not only informs the practitioner of more viable targets, but it also allows them to exploit the vulnerabilities and potential weaknesses of the human body in order to overcome an opponent or assailant.

SECTION FIVE

Pseudoscience In Martial Arts

Chapter 15

Pseudoscience In Martial Arts

Numerous times throughout the course of writing *Comprehensive Anatomy for Martial Arts*, I was asked by fellow martial artists if I would include sections on pressure points, nerve points, meridians, and similar notions. Not surprisingly, I was never asked that same type of question by non-martial artists, physicians, advanced healthcare providers, or those who are scientifically literate. I have struggled with the idea of including anything in this text that is not based on empirical evidence, or that could potentially provide credibility to outdated erroneous concepts. However, because of the prevalence of martial arts lore and those perpetuating misinformation, however unintentional, I felt it necessary to include a section on Pseudoscience in Martial Arts. My goal is not to belittle or offend anyone but rather to advance the level of education and professionalism within the martial arts community. To this end, I strongly encourage you to read the Introduction, and the chapters on Biomechanics, and Skeletal, Muscular, and Neuroanatomy of this textbook before you continue this section.

As mentioned in the *Introduction* of this text, we cannot gain a full appreciation of human anatomy and biomechanics by just memorizing two-dimensional basic anatomy wall charts. Furthermore, to truly understand how each of the anatomy systems function and interact with each other requires a more in-depth study than what can be presented in this one reference text. Yet, in numerous sections throughout each of these chapters I have attempted to briefly present the physiology of how certain techniques work, or how injures occur. Physiology is the study of how cells, individual organs, organ systems, and organisms carry out chemical and physical functions. Therefore, a basic understanding of biology and chemistry are truly required to fully appreciate what is at play during physical human movement. An advanced knowledge of human anatomy is not possible without also knowing the physiology.

Having a vague or superficial understanding of the human body oftentimes leads to erroneous assumptions. That is why biology, physics, chemistry, organic chemistry, and biochemistry are all required courses prior to obtaining a degree in the medical sciences. Not having that knowledge stifles the comprehension of how the human organism truly works. Historically, in an attempt to explain certain health and martial arts related phenomena; specific concepts and practices have been developed over multiple centuries that have been proved inaccurate. I was first introduced to the concept of chi (qi or ki) and meridians in the early 1970s during the height of the kung-fu craze in the United States. The television series *Kung-Fu* and the movie *Billy Jack* that both came out in the early 1970s inspired me to pursue martial arts training. I was initially taught that chi was a "life force" or "life energy" that was present in all living things. It was something that could be "focused and channeled", providing almost supernatural abilities to those who could harness its power. I was taught that if you focus your chi, you will have devastating knockout techniques and can even break cinder blocks! I did learn how to break boards and cement patio blocks, but I never honestly sensed the power of chi that many others professed to experience. I questioned my technique and myself. *Was I doing it wrong? If so, how much more powerful would I be once I learned how to focus my chi?*

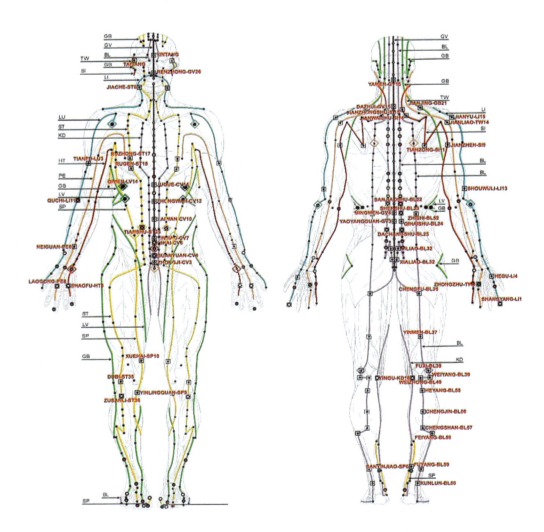

Fig. 15.1 - A schematic of the "human body meridians".
Image Credit: KVDP, Public domain, via Wikimedia Commons.

Not long after learning how to break cinder blocks, I stumbled across an article in *Scientific American* magazine at the local library. That serendipitous finding ignited a thirst for applying science to my martial arts training. I carried a Xerox copy of the article around with me in my instructor briefcase for years. "The Physics of Karate" by Feld, McNair, and Wilk published in the April 1979 issue of *Scientific American* demonstrated that boards and bricks are strong under compression, however, they are susceptible to breaking when bent, even microscopically.

Boards and bricks are indeed strong under compression, making them ideal for the construction of houses and buildings. While performing martial arts breaks, *compression* does occur on the *striking* surface side of the board or brick. However, the *expansion* on the opposite side cannot resist the stretching force of the microscopic bend, thereby causing the material to break. No chi power or mystical force required — only kinetic energy and physics.

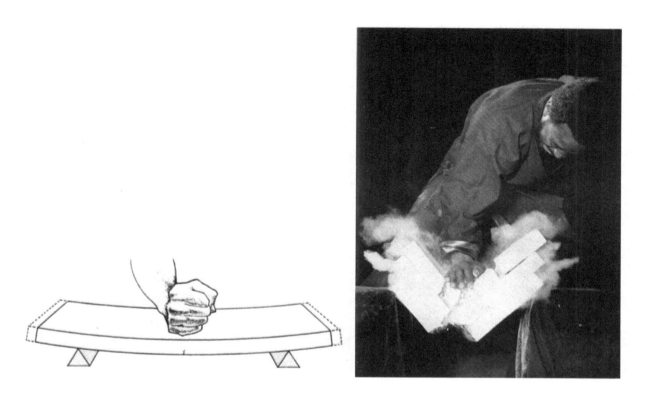

Fig. 15.2 – Left Image: Hammer-fist strike breaking a wooden board is shown in a schematic diagram. The top of the board is compressed; the bottom is stretched. Because wood is weaker under tension than it is under compression the board cracks first on the bottom surface (near the center). The crack propagates rapidly upward as the board continues to be forced downward.

Fig. 15.3 – Right Image: Three concrete patio blocks are broken by one of the authors (Ronald E. McNair, PhD) of The Physics of Karate with a right vertical downward palm strike. Bone can resist 40 times more stress, or force per unit area, than concrete. Image Credit: The Physics of Karate. Scientific American. Volume 240, Issue 4 (April 1979): 150-58.

▪ Where did the term chi (qi, ki) come from and why is it still being used today?

The use of chi was developed in a pre-scientific era steeped in superstition. The original proponents existed in a time of *philosophy-based* health practices, prior to the advent of *scientific-based* medicine. Chi is much like *astrology* (a pseudoscience), or the *medieval* idea of *bodily humors* for maintaining health and wellbeing. They were both our first awkward attempts to describe real-world phenomena that were eventually proven to have incorrect foundations. As is now widely accepted, the planets do not move the way in which astrology described, and the theory of the four humors (yellow bile, black bile, blood, and phlegm) were just speculation that turned out to be wrong. Similarly, chi was just a way to vaguely describe perceived medical processes and martial phenomena that people did not fully understand at that time. As is often the case, our first attempts to explain something is usually our worst attempt.

The human brain has powerful control of the body that is not yet fully understood at this time. For example, a connection between the nervous system and the immune system *does* exist, but until recently has not been well studied. The emergence of neuroimmunology as a medical specialty in the early 1980s is attempting to address that area. However, until it is fully understood, we do not need to attribute external forces or supernatural powers to try to explain such things.

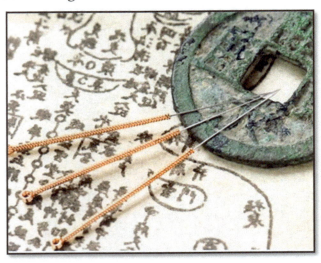

Fig. 15.4 - Example of stainless-steel acupuncture needles.

In an effort to validate the use of chi in the martial arts, proponents will frequently cite the use of acupuncture and the presumed manipulation of chi by penetrating the skin with thin, solid, metallic needles into specific points along certain meridians. Some proudly proclaim that acupuncture is even being used *instead* of general anesthesia for open heart surgery. These misinformed comments are usually referencing (often unwittingly because these types of tales customarily circulate unchecked) a television show titled *Alternative Medicine: The Evidence?* (Notice the question mark!) that was aired by the BBC in January of 2006. The narrator of the series misleadingly implied that acupuncture was used *instead* of anesthetics during open heart surgery in China. Shortly after the TV show aired, the scientists involved with the study publicly complained that elements of the program were misleading and that the findings were sensationalized. They also revealed that intravenous anesthetic agents and narcotic drugs, such as fentanyl and midazolam, were indeed used; as well as large doses of local anesthetic injected at the surgical incision site. Therefore, even though acupuncture was being used during the surgical procedures, it was *not* being used *instead* of modern anesthetic agents. It was being used as an *adjunct* secondary to the primary anesthetics.

My point is that many chi proponents seem to believe acupuncture somehow validates the use of chi in martial arts. Therefore, I would like to present an abbreviated description of different approaches to acupuncture. It is not my goal to debunk or debate the use of acupuncture as a medical practice.

There are several types and styles of acupuncture that are practiced with varying degrees of efficacy and usefulness. Most types of acupuncture fall into the categories of either Traditional

Chinese Acupuncture or Western Medical Acupuncture. Traditional Chinese Acupuncture (TCA) is a *philosophy-based* practice dating back a few hundred centuries BCE. It was built on the premise of regulating the flow of energy to aid in improving health by incorporating the concept of yin and yang. By stimulating points along 12-14 meridian pathways, the TCA practitioner's objective is to improve the body's flow of vital energy, or chi. The meridians are presumed to represent major organs and functions within the body; however, they do not follow the pathways of blood vessels or nerves. The belief is that when there are disruptions in the flow of chi, it causes imbalances, ill health, and pain. TCA is therefore used to purportedly restore the balance of energy and reduce blockages or barriers.

There is a distinct difference in the basis for Western Medical Acupuncture. The western model of acupuncture uses a more targeted evidence-based approach employing a modern understanding of anatomy and physiology. Western Medical Acupuncture is only administered after a full diagnosis is made and is most often associated with managing specific symptoms (not the overall restoration of "energy flow"). Dry needling in western acupuncture is frequently used in treating pain. The needle is inserted directly into a muscle trigger point, *not* a meridian acupuncture point. The objective of western medical dry needling is to release the tight area, thereby diminishing muscle restriction and reducing pain. Some scientists assert that the needle insertion causes the hypothalamus and pituitary glands to release endorphins, natural painkillers, and may increase blood flow while stimulating biochemical changes in the brain. These biochemicals are thought to stimulate the body's natural healing properties while promoting mental and physical well-being.

The reason *traditional* acupuncture, a chi-based practice, still exists today, and medieval bloodletting does not, is the historical happenstance that scientific medicine was developed first in the West and not in the East. This text is not designed to provide a full context of the historical and geopolitical isolationist environments that allowed for the significant divergence of ideas at that point in time — and even exists today to a certain degree.

Those advancing the idea of the use of chi in martial arts often teach that chi flows along unseen meridians throughout the body. They suggest that in striking or manipulating these meridians or pressure points, the practitioner can somehow control or disrupt the flow of the opponent's chi, or life-force, and in doing so, potentially render the person unconscious.

Having performed thousands of surgeries, I have never seen a meridian, never inadvertently cut an unseen meridian, or have had to repair a meridian that was injured from trauma.

Pseudoscientific practices are often highly developed, backed by a subculture of believers, and frequently have an evolved and sophisticated doctrine. But if a certain practice requires a person to *believe* it works for it to *actually* work, what happens when they attempt a technique against a nonbeliever? *Nothing* happens — or they learn a painfully hard and possibly deadly lesson.

In the case of martial arts and self-defense: to depend on the use of chi power (and the need to believe in chi for it to work) while trying to protect oneself is a recipe for getting hurt, or worse. This has been demonstrated now countless times when self-professed "chi-masters" fight a *non*-believing martial artist who uses real techniques to attack anatomical vulnerabilities. The video from National Geographic's "Is it Real?" series, vigorously demonstrates the ineffective use of chi on the "non-believer".

Some people, including myself, have been told that chi is *intended* to be an "unexplainable phenomenon". Many people use the term *chi* as a catch-all because they don't know or can't explain the biomechanics or physiology of certain techniques. But because someone personally may not understand how something works does not mean that those more scientifically literate cannot explain it.

And yet, the *appeal to antiquity* (or tradition), an argument in which an idea or concept is deemed correct on the basis of correlation with past or present tradition, doggedly persists. The appeal takes the form of "this is right because it has *always* been done this way". In an attempt to modernize the concept of chi in martial arts, some martial arts instructors claim that chi is now understood to be neurological pathways. This is a gross misunderstanding of human anatomy and neurology. Chi is *not* neuroscience!

What old school martial arts practitioners understood as chi, or spirit energy, is actually just good old biomechanics and physics. When a chi practitioner is "building up chi", what they are really doing is relaxing their muscles which provides more "snap" in their technique. When they "use chi to root into the ground", they are simply dropping their weight down (like dead weight) to get centered. This is easily demonstrated by attempting to pick up a person when their muscles are tense and rigid, and then again when their muscles are limp and relaxed (dead weight). Using proper form in delivering martial arts techniques does not open meridians and allow for chi to flow better; it does, however, improve the *biomechanics* that provide for more power and more efficiency in their execution.

If you happen to subscribe to the concept of pressure point fighting, and you assert that it is about *energy* (meaning *chi* and *not kinetic energy*) transfer; and that pressure point techniques can stun, disorient or "loosen joints", etc., and that they *can* work in the "*right* scenario" against a "believer"... remember that we are talking about MARTIAL arts, Combat, and Personal <u>Protection</u>. Techniques *must* be effective against a *non*compliant adversary who is intent on hurting you; not someone who is standing still in a coffee line.

I am not saying that pushing, manipulating, or striking a specific area on the body will not produce a certain response. I am asserting that the response is a result of biomechanics and physical dysfunction, not a mystical force that must be believed in for it to work.

Although some have attempted to migrate away from overtly using the terms meridian, chi, or even pressure points, and have begun using terms they believe to be more acceptable such as nerve points, nerve motor points, or nerve pressure points; they still imply there is some hidden secret (i.e., "revealing the 10 most deadly nerve points", etc.). Please stop using terms and phrases like "this will shut down the body", "disconnect from the brain", or "create total dysfunction", when exaggerating the purported effectiveness of pressure point techniques. Moreover, please avoid making elaborate excuses for why these mystical techniques don't work against a noncompliant, non-believing aggressor. Especially when the explanation for "nullifying" their effectiveness — *it didn't work because they didn't believe in it* — is even more illogical and irrational than the intended technique itself. In every other area of scholarly research and the hard sciences, fantastical claims demand real evidence to support their proposition. Outside of the martial arts there are very few topics in our society that we allow for such loose "evidence", or that you must "believe" for it to work. Unfortunately for us, as martial artists, in our arena such claims can cost the unwitting their lives.

Similarly, although there are *bio*electrical impulses that run throughout the nervous system between the origin of the nerve stimuli and the spinal cord and brain, you can't "shut down the body" like pulling an electric cord from a wall socket. Also, using pseudoscientific sounding phrases such as "we are electrical-magnetic beings that can generate chi and move energy through our bodies" does not add validity to such claims. That is a HUGE oversimplification that may have worked as in explanation in the early 1970s; but it is idiotic to the well-informed populous of the 21st century.

In addressing the often-presented notion that this mysterious "electrical-magnetic current" in the human body is indeed chi, *and* that *it* cannot be explained is… well, erroneous and *it* can be explained. An understanding of biochemistry and neurology demonstrates that an "electrical" nerve impulse is actually the movement of an *action potential* along a neuron, as a series of sodium and potassium ion channels open and close. It is not chi, nor is it like the conventional *alternating* electric current in your house. A nerve impulse is much slower than an electrical current, and the strength of a nerve impulse is always the same. There is either an impulse to the stimuli or there is not. For a more thorough explanation please see the "*How does the human body create electricity?*" section of the *Introduction to the Nervous System* chapter, and the *Cardiac Conduction System* section of the *Introduction to the Cardiovascular System* chapter.

Additionally, regarding humans being "magnetic", that is not completely accurate either. When discussing magnets, we usually think of ferromagnetism — the type of magnet that *attracts* metallic alloys such as iron. The human body is actually diamagnetic; a type of magnetism that *weakly repels* a magnetic field. *How does this magnetism occur?* The human body is comprised of approximately 60% water. Water is diamagnetic. Each of the billions of water molecules in the body consists of one oxygen atom and two hydrogen atoms. Electrons spin around the nucleus of each atom on a randomly aligned axis. The orbiting electrons *act like* tiny electromagnets. When exposed to a very strong magnetic field (such as an MRI) it forces all the proton axes to align with that field. This understanding allows for the development and use of Magnetic Resonance Imaging (MRI). During an MRI a radiofrequency pulse is introduced that disrupts the proton axis and forces it into either a 90-degree or 180-degree realignment with the static magnetic field. Because the radiofrequency pulse pushed the proton against its natural axis, once this pulse is turned off, the protons realign with the magnetic field, releasing electromagnetic energy along the way. The MRI is then able to detect this energy and can differentiate various body tissues based on how quickly they release energy after the pulse is removed.

The electromagnetic properties of the human body *can* be explained; however, these properties do not create a mystical force field that can be manipulated or used to counter or direct techniques.

There are indeed tender points on the human body where nerves lie in close proximity to the skin, along a bony prominence, or that are not well protected. But a nerve is distinctly different than what is implied by the notion of meridians.

Vital points *do* exist — in a way. They exist in a framework of:

- if you poke someone in the eye, their hands come up to protect their eyes.
- if you slap someone in the ear or to the side of their head, they may stumble sideways away from the strike as they cover the affected target.
- if you kick someone in the groin, their hands drop down, knees come together, and their hips move posteriorly.
- if someone grabs your lapel and you strike down forcefully in the crook of their elbow, their head will move forward and down.
- if you kick someone in the back of the knee or lower leg, their knee will buckle.

All predictable kinesthetic responses... Biomechanics!

If you strike someone unexpectedly in a highly innervated sensitive area — mistakenly called a "pressure point" — it is going to hurt. The human body is not designed to be hit, and there are multiple places where it causes harm when that occurs. Strikes to the solar plexus, or liver shots, are responsible for many body-shot "knockouts". The jawline, temples, bony orbit of the eye, and the medial and lateral thigh, are all painful places to get hit. That does not mean "chi" has been disrupted. It simply means that the recipient of the strikes is responding to the predictable physiological event that transpired in the midst of physical and psychological trauma.

Unfortunately, for those who focus on hitting pressure points in specific directions to activate them, it is going to be difficult to achieve against an assailant with their guard up, and even more difficult when the opponent begins to fight back. Any combination that requires striking two pressure points as a set-up, prior to rubbing a third "knockout" pressure point is not going to work against a noncompliant moving target.

Similarly, a *kiai*, (vocalization, or "spirit yell") is not a release of "internal energy". It is a forceful contraction of the diaphragm that increases core stability, in turn improving perceived power — much like the short exhale used when lifting weights, or while punching in boxing. Have you ever noticed that no one uses a kiai during boxing or MMA bouts, or while playing football, rugby, baseball, or golf? The kiai might, however, distract or intimidate an assailant — *IF* it is not used as a *SCREAM* on every-single-technique!

Let me express again, this section is not intended to be offensive or hurtful to anyone. As I mentioned in the Introduction of this reference text, which I encouraged you to read before this section, the *scientific method* is the inquiry and testing of a hypothesis through achieving empirical and measurable data as evidence. Sometimes while testing and examining the question at hand, it is found that the conclusion is *correct*, despite the presumed *cause* being *wrong*. In other words, even though a technique works, it does not mean the traditional explanation of how or why it works is correct. Direct physical pressure over certain points on the body may temporarily control an opponent, such as jamming your fingers into the hollow of the throat just over the suprasternal notch. Pushing straight-in, in an anterior to posterior direction, is indeed uncomfortable; but directing the force inferiorly and posterior to the sternum is miserable for the one on the receiving end. It is not because of the redirection of presumed chi that makes it miserable but rather because of the compression of vulnerable physical anatomical structures and nerves that were not intended to be traumatized.

As *martial scientists,* it is our moral obligation to evaluate the efficacy of what we teach our students. Understanding the anatomical, physiological, and biomechanical principles governing individual techniques allows each of us to not only learn the individual *mechanics* of physical techniques, but also the *intellectual* mastery of the much larger concepts in their application.

From a science-based center, we need to frequently rethink and reevaluate what we teach based on new evidence. That is often hard to do in a traditional environment, where honoring tradition is valued above evolving and integrating new information. This can be dangerous and even deadly when personal safety is at stake.

Letting go of outdated traditions and concepts one believes to be true is not easy. I understand how some martial artists are strongly vested in their worldview and find it hard to integrate new information into their curriculum, but in the arena of real-world self-defense, holding onto to falsehoods can be fatal.

This book is not intended to be a biochemistry or physics text; however, such topics must be touched upon to demonstrate that certain claims thought to be mysterious and beyond our understanding are indeed explicable and not supernatural.

BIBLIOGRAPHY

Adderson, E. E., & Bohnsack, J. F. (1996). Traumatic myositis ossificans simulating soft tissue infection. *The Pediatric Infectious Disease Journal, 15*(6), 551–553. https://doi.org/10.1097/00006454-199606000-00020

Ahmad, C. S., Redler, L. H., Ciccotti, M. G., Maffulli, N., Longo, U. G., & Bradley, J. (2013). Evaluation and management of hamstring injuries. *The American Journal of Sports Medicine, 41*(12), 2933–2947. https://doi.org/10.1177/0363546513487063

Almeida, T. B., Dobashi, E. T., Nishimi, A. Y., Almeida, E. B., Pascarelli, L., & Rodrigues, L. M. (2017). Analysis of the pattern and mechanism of elbow injuries related to armbar-type armlocks in jiu-jitsu fighters. *Acta Ortopédica Brasileira, 25*(5), 209–211. https://doi.org/10.1590/1413-785220172505171198

Boriskie, L. (2009). Muscle Origin Insertion Actions, PDF file. Public Domain, Colorado.edu

Brewer, J. (2017). *Pocket anatomy of the moving body: The compact guide to the science of human locomotion.* Barron's.

Broughton, B.A. (2016). *Beyond Self-Defense: AKT Combatives Reality-Based Personal Protection.* New York, Rustic Studio Publishing.

Bryce, C. D., & Armstrong, A. D. (2008). Anatomy and biomechanics of the elbow. *Orthopedic Clinics of North America, 39*(2), 141–154. https://doi.org/10.1016/j.ocl.2007.12.001

Buckwalter, J. A. (2003). Sports, joint injury, and posttraumatic osteoarthritis. *Journal of Orthopaedic & Sports Physical Therapy, 33*(10), 578–588. https://doi.org/10.2519/jospt.2003.33.10.578

Dashnaw, M. L., Petraglia, A. L., & Bailes, J. E. (2012). An overview of the basic science of concussion and subconcussion: Where we are and where we are going. *Neurosurgical Focus, 33*(6). https://doi.org/10.3171/2012.10.focus12284

de Haan, J. (2011). Stability of the elbow joint: Relevant anatomy and clinical implications of in vitro biomechanical studies. *The Open Orthopaedics Journal, 5*(1), 168–176. https://doi.org/10.2174/1874325001105010168

Doyle-Baker, P. K., Mitchell, T., & Hayden, K. A. (2021). Stroke and athletes: A scoping review. *International Journal of Environmental Research and Public Health, 18*(19), 10047. https://doi.org/10.3390/ijerph181910047

El-Menyar, A., Parchani, A., Peralta, R., Zarour, A., Al-Thani, H., Al-Hassani, A., Abdelrahman, H., & Arumugam, S. (2015). Frequency, causes and pattern of abdominal trauma: A 4-year descriptive analysis. *Journal of Emergencies, Trauma, and Shock, 8*(4), 193. https://doi.org/10.4103/0974-2700.166590

Estevan, I., & Falco, C. (2013). Mechanical analysis of the roundhouse kick according to height and distance in taekwondo. *Biology of sport, 30*(4), 275–279. https://doi.org/10.5604/20831862.1077553

Farke, A. A. (2008). Frontal sinuses and head-butting in goats: A finite element analysis. *Journal of Experimental Biology, 211*(19), 3085–3094. https://doi.org/10.1242/jeb.019042

Feld, M. S., McNair, R. E., & Wilk, S. R. (1979). The physics of karate. *Scientific American, 240*(4), 150–158. https://doi.org/10.1038/scientificamerican0479-150

Fitzsimons, M. G., Peralta, R., & Hurford, W. (2005). Cricoid fracture after physical assault. *The Journal of Trauma: Injury, Infection, and Critical Care*, 1237–1238. https://doi.org/10.1097/01.ta.0000197557.16613.a4

Gavagan, C.J., & Sayers, M.G.L. (2017). A biomechanical analysis of the roundhouse kicking technique of expert practitioners: A comparison between the martial arts disciplines of Muay Thai, Karate, and Taekwondo. *PLoS ONE* 12(8): e0182645. https://doi.org/10.1371/journal.pone.0182645

Glick, Y. (2022, January 18). *Myositis ossificans: Radiology reference article*. Radiopaedia Blog RSS. Retrieved March 26, 2022, from https://radiopaedia.org/articles/myositis-ossificans-1

Grieve, G.P., & Worth, D.R. (1986). Motion of the cervical spine. Modern Manual Therapy of the Vertebral Column London: Churchill Livingstone, 77-78.

Guardian News and Media. (2006, March 25). *A groundbreaking experiment ... or a sensationalised TV stunt?* The Guardian. Retrieved May 10, 2022, from https://www.theguardian.com/media/2006/mar/25/science.broadcasting

Hassmann, M., Buchegger, M., Stollberg, K.-P., Sever, A., & Sabo, A. (2010). Motion analysis of performance tests using a pulling force device (PFD) simulating a judo throw. *Procedia Engineering, 2*(2), 3329–3334. https://doi.org/10.1016/j.proeng.2010.04.153

Hodges, B. H., Meagher, B. R., Norton, D. J., McBain, R., & Sroubek, A. (2014). Speaking from ignorance: Not agreeing with others we believe are correct. *Journal of Personality and Social Psychology, 106*(2), 218–234. https://doi.org/10.1037/a0034662

Hoppenfeld S, Deboer P, Buckle R. (2009) *Surgical Exposures in Orthopedics: The anatomic approach*, 4th Edition. Philadelphia, Lippincott Williams and Wilkins

https://medical-dictionary.thefreedictionary.com

Imamura, R. T., Hreljac, A., Escamilla, R. F., & Edwards, W. B. (2006). A three-dimensional analysis of the center of mass for three different judo throwing techniques. Journal of sports science & medicine, 5(CSSI), 122–131.

Jabbari Ali, et al., (2019). Western medical acupuncture is an alternative medicine or a conventional classic medical manipulation, Caspian Journal of Internal Medicine. 10(2): 239–240

Kato, S., & Yamagiwa, S. (2021). Statistical extraction method for revealing key factors from posture before initiating successful throwing technique in Judo. *Sensors, 21*(17), 5884. https://doi.org/10.3390/s21175884

Keerthi, R., & Quadri, A. (2015). Hyoid bone fracture: Associated with head and neck trauma—a rare case report. *Journal of Maxillofacial and Oral Surgery, 15*(S2), 249–252. https://doi.org/10.1007/s12663-015-0761-x

Kinoshita, M., Fujii, N. The Analysis of Kinematical Characteristics in Taekwondo Roundhouse Kick. Retrieved May 1, 2022, from https://ojs.ub.uni-konstanz.de/cpa/article/view/5737

Koga, H., Muneta, T., Bahr, R., Engebretsen, L., & Krosshaug, T. (2015). Video analysis of ACL injury mechanisms using a model-based image-matching technique. *Sports Injuries and Prevention*, 109–120. https://doi.org/10.1007/978-4-431-55318-2_9

Kokabi, N., Shuaib, W., Xing, M., Harmouche, E., Wilson, K., Johnson, J.-O., & Khosa, F. (2014). Intra-abdominal solid organ injuries: An enhanced management algorithm. *Canadian Association of Radiologists Journal, 65*(4), 301–309. https://doi.org/10.1016/j.carj.2013.12.003

Kragha, K. O. (2015). Acute traumatic injury of the larynx. *Case Reports in Otolaryngology, 2015*, 1–3. https://doi.org/10.1155/2015/393978

Kreighbaum, E. F., & Barthels, K. M. (1996). *Biomechanics: A qualitative approach for studying human movement*. Allyn and Bacon.

Krogmann, R.J., Jamal, Z., & King, K.C., Auricular Hematoma. (Updated 2022 Jan 24). In: StatPearls [Internet]. Treasure Island (FL): StatPearls Publishing; 2022 Jan-. https://www.ncbi.nlm.nih.gov/books/NBK531499/

Lawson, K. A., Ayala, A. E., Morin, M. L., Latt, L. D., & Wild, J. R. (2018). Ankle fracture-dislocations. *Foot & Ankle Orthopaedics, 3*(3), 247301141876512. https://doi.org/10.1177/2473011418765122

Levine, W. N., & Flatow, E. L. (2000). The pathophysiology of shoulder instability. *The American Journal of Sports Medicine, 28*(6), 910–917. https://doi.org/10.1177/03635465000280062501

Liu, H., Zhang, Y., Rang, M., Li, Q., Jiang, Z., Xia, J., Zhang, M., Gu, X., & Zhao, C. (2018). Avulsion fractures of the ischial tuberosity: Progress of injury, mechanism, clinical manifestations, imaging examination, diagnosis and differential diagnosis and treatment. *Medical Science Monitor, 24*, 9406–9412. https://doi.org/10.12659/msm.913799

Lucerna, A., Espinosa, J., & Hertz, R. (2017). Thyroid cartilage fracture in context of noncompetitive "Horseplay" wrestling. *Emergency Medicine, 49*(9). https://doi.org/10.12788/emed.2017.0056

Magee, D. J., & Manske, R. C. (2021). *Orthopedic physical assessment*. Saunders.

Mandal, A. (2019, June 19). *Acupuncture history*. News. Retrieved February 10, 2021, from https://www.news-medical.net/health/Acupuncture-History.aspx

McCance, K.L., & Heuther, S.E., (2010). *Pathophysiology*. 6th ed. Maryland Heights, Mo: Mosby Elsevier

Meaney, D. F., & Smith, D. H. (2011). Biomechanics of concussion. *Clinics in Sports Medicine, 30*(1), 19–31. https://doi.org/10.1016/j.csm.2010.08.009

Mercier, L. R. (2008). *Practical orthopedics*. Mosby Elsevier.

Mitchell, J. R., Roach, D. E., Tyberg, J. V., Belenkie, I., & Sheldon, R. S. (2012). Mechanism of loss of consciousness during Vascular neck restraint. *Journal of Applied Physiology, 112*(3), 396–402. https://doi.org/10.1152/japplphysiol.00592.2011

Neidecker, J., Sethi, N. K., Taylor, R., Monsell, R., Muzzi, D., Spizler, B., Lovelace, L., Ayoub, E., Weinstein, R., Estwanik, J., Reyes, P., Cantu, R. C., Jordan, B., Goodman, M., Stiller, J. W., Gelber, J., Boltuch, R., Coletta, D., Gagliardi, A., ... Inalsingh, C. (2018). Concussion management in combat sports: Consensus statement from the Association of Ringside Physicians. *British Journal of Sports Medicine, 53*(6), 328–333. https://doi.org/10.1136/bjsports-2017-098799

Neligan, P. C. (2013). *Plastic surgery. vol 6: Hand and upper extremity.* Elsevier Saunders.

Neumann, D. A. (2010). *Kinesiology of the Musculoskeletal System Foundations for physical rehabilitation.* Mosby/Elsevier.

O'Driscoll, S.W., Jupiter, J.B., King, J., Hotchkiss, R.N., & Morrey, B.F. (2001). The unstable elbow. Instructional Course Lecture 2001;50:89–102.

Parnes, Lorne & Agrawal, Sumit & Atlas, Jason. (2003). Diagnosis and management of benign paroxysmal positional vertigo (BPPV). CMAJ: Canadian Medical Association journal = journal de l'Association medicale canadienne. 169. 681-93.

Patella dislocation - statpearls - NCBI bookshelf. (n.d.). Retrieved May 10, 2022, from https://www.ncbi.nlm.nih.gov/books/NBK538288/

Rodriguez, G., Vitali, P., Nobili, F., & Nobili, F. (1998). Long-term effects of boxing and judo-choking techniques on brain function. *The Italian Journal of Neurological Sciences, 19*(6), 367–372. https://doi.org/10.1007/bf02341784

Rozzi, H.V., & Riviello, R. (2019, April 17). How to Evaluate Strangulation. *ACEP Now.* American College of Emergency Physicians.

Shao, Y., Zou, D., Li, Z., Wan, L., Qin, Z., Liu, N., Zhang, J., Zhong, L., Huang, P., & Chen, Y. (2013). Blunt liver injury with intact ribs under impacts on the abdomen: A biomechanical investigation. *PLoS ONE, 8*(1). https://doi.org/10.1371/journal.pone.0052366

Standring, S., & Standring, S. (2016). *Gray's anatomy: The anatomical basis of Clinical Practice.* Elsevier Limited.

Stellpflug, S. J., Menton, T. R., Corry, J. J., & Schneir, A. B. (2019). There is more to the mechanism of unconsciousness from vascular neck restraint than simply carotid compression. *International Journal of Neuroscience, 130*(1), 103–106. https://doi.org/10.1080/00207454.2019.1664520

Stellpflug, S. J., Menton, W. H., Dummer, M. F., Menton, T., Corry, J., & LeFevere, R. (2020). Time to unconsciousness from sportive chokes in fully resisting highly trained combatants. *International Journal of Performance Analysis in Sport, 20*(4), 720–728. https://doi.org/10.1080/24748668.2020.1780873

Stellpflug, S. J., Schindler, B. R., Corry, J. J., Menton, T. R., & LeFevere, R. C. (2020). The safety of Sportive Chokes: A cross-sectional survey-based study. *The Physician and Sportsmedicine, 48*(4), 473–479. https://doi.org/10.1080/00913847.2020.1754734

Takakura, Y., Yamaguchi, S., Akagi, R., Kamegaya, M., Kimura, S., Tanaka, H., & Yasui, T. (2020). Diagnosis of avulsion fractures of the distal fibula after lateral ankle sprain in children: A diagnostic accuracy study comparing ultrasonography with radiography. *BMC Musculoskeletal Disorders, 21*(1). https://doi.org/10.1186/s12891-020-03287-1

Thalken, J. (2015). *Fight like a physicist - the incredible science behind Martial Arts*. Ymaa Publication Center.

Tran, D. Q., Salinas, F. V., Benzon, H. T., & Neal, J. M. (2019). Lower Extremity Regional Anesthesia: Essentials of Our Current Understanding. *Regional Anesthesia & Pain Medicine, 44*(2), 143–180. https://doi.org/10.1136/rapm-2018-000019

Travis, L. W., Snyder, R. G., Melvin, J. W., & Olson, N. R. (1975). *Static and dynamic impact trauma of the human larynx* (Pt 1, Vol. 80, Ser. 382-90). American Academy of Ophthalmology and Otolaryngology.

University of Manchester. (2007, June). *Engineers Prove That Boxer, 'Hitman' Hatton, Packs a Mighty Punch*. Science Daily

Weintraub, C. M. (1961). Fractures of the Hyoed Bone. *Medico-Legal Journal, 29*(4), 209–216. https://doi.org/10.1177/002581726102900405

White, A. (2009). Western Medical acupuncture: A definition. *Acupuncture in Medicine, 27*(1), 33–35. https://doi.org/10.1136/aim.2008.000372

Wright, S. (n.d.). *Concussion: Symptoms, causes, diagnosis, treatments, & recovery*. WebMD. Retrieved March 10, 2022, from https://www.webmd.com/brain/concussion-traumatic-brain-injury-symptoms-causes-treatments

Zhang, L., Yang, K. H., & King, A. I. (2004). A proposed injury threshold for mild traumatic brain injury. *Journal of Biomechanical Engineering, 126*(2), 226–236. https://doi.org/10.1115/1.1691446

Zhou, J., Chi, H., Cheng, T. O., Chen, T.-yu, Wu, Y.-yao, Zhou, W.-xiong, Shen, W.-dong, & Yuan, L. (2011). Acupuncture anesthesia for open heart surgery in contemporary China. *International Journal of Cardiology, 150*(1), 12–16. https://doi.org/10.1016/j.ijcard.2011.04.002

GLOSSARY

abdominal – referring to the abdomen (commonly called the belly) is the body space between the thorax (chest) and pelvis.

abdominopelvic – cavity is a body cavity that consists of the abdominal cavity and the pelvic cavity.

abduction – to move something laterally away from the midline.

acetabulofemoral – referring to the hip joint.

acetabulum – the cup-shaped cavity at the base of the pelvis into which the ball-shaped head of the femur fits.

Achilles tendon – heel cord, also known as the calcaneal tendon, is a tendon at the back of the lower leg and is the thickest in the human body.

acute – sudden or short term.

adduction – movement that brings something towards the midline.

adductor – a muscle whose contraction moves an extremity or other part of the body toward the midline of the body.

agonist – a muscle that on contracting is automatically checked and controlled by the opposing simultaneous contraction of another muscle.

anatomical snuffbox – (also known as the radial fossa), is a triangular depression found on the lateral aspect of the dorsum of the hand, overlying the scaphoid bone of the wrist.

anatomy – the branch of biology concerned with the study of the structure of organisms and their parts.

anterior – situated to the front.

anterior cruciate ligament (ACL) – one of a pair of structures (the other being the posterior cruciate ligament) in the middle of the knee joint that provides forward and rotational stability by preventing the tibia from sliding forward on the distal femur.

anteroinferiorly – situated in front and below.

anterolateral – situated or occurring in front and to the side.

appendicular skeleton – the portion of the skeleton that support the extremities.

arm – referring to the anatomical structures between the shoulder and the elbow.

articular – relating to a joint.

articulating – to unite by forming a joint.

auditory – relating to the sense of hearing.

axial skeleton – includes the bones that form the skull, vertebral column, and thoracic cage.

baroreceptors –sensors that are sensitive to pressure changes located in the carotid sinus (at the bifurcation of external and internal carotids) and in the aortic arch.

bilateral – refers to something occurring on both sides of the body.

bimalleolar – referring to the bones on the inside and outside of the ankle.

biomechanics – the study of the structure, function, and motion of the human body.

blood – fluid in the circulatory system that transports oxygen and nutrients to the cells and carries away carbon dioxide and other waste products.

boxer's fracture – a break (fracture) of the neck of the 5th metacarpal.

brachii – a Latin word meaning "of the arm".

brevis – a Latin word meaning short or brief.

bronchus – a airway in the lower respiratory tract that conducts air into the lungs.

bursa – a small, fluid-filled sac that lies near bony prominences and joints.

calcaneus – also known as the heel bone, it is the largest and strongest bone of the foot.

cancellous bone – the sponge-like tissue inside bones.

capitis – a Latin word meaning "of the head".

capsuloligamentous – referring to capsule and ligaments around a joint.

cardiac – relating the heart.

carpals – the eight small bones of the wrist.

carpi – referring to the carpal bones of the wrist.

cauda equina – a Latin term that literally means "horse's tail"; the roots of the lumbar and sacral spinal nerves, which form a bundle within the lowest part of the spinal column.

cervical – refers to the neck region that consists of seven vertebrae.

chronic – persisting for a long time or constantly recurring.

clavicle – also known as the collar bone, that acts as a strut from the sternum to the acromion of the scapula/shoulder blade. the only long bones of the body that lie horizontal.

coccyx – also known as the tailbone. The distal tip of the spine inferior to the sacrum.

collateral ligament – a band of tissue that connects a bone to another bone, providing side-to-side stability.

common peroneal nerve – a branch of the sciatic nerve that travels around the lateral knee to the foot, innervating the skin of the lateral knee and leg and the musculature of the anterior leg and foot.

comorbidities – the presence of one or more additional conditions often co-occurring with a primary condition.

concussion – a traumatic brain injury that affects brain function.

contralateral – refers to something on the other side of the body.

coronal plane – a vertical plane at right angles to a sagittal plane, dividing the body into anterior and posterior portions.

cortical bone – the harder, outer tissue of bones.

cranial – relating to the skull or cranium.

cruris – a Latin word referring to the leg.

deltoid – meaning triangular: the muscle forming the rounded contour of the shoulder.

dermatome – an area of skin that is primarily supplied by a single nerve root: communicating sensation from this skin region to the brain.

digiti – referring to the finger.

distal – anatomical term of location relative to something else: meaning further away.

dorsal – relating to the back or upper side.

dorsiflexion – refers to flexion at the ankle towards the dorsum (superior surface).

endorphins – a group of hormones in the brain and nervous system that act as the body's natural pain relievers.

epicondyles – a protuberance above or on the condyle of a long bone.

epididymis – a long, coiled tube that transports sperm from the testes to the vas deferens.

epistaxis – nosebleed.

extension – refers to a movement that increases the angle between two body segments.

external – the outer surface.

externus – a Latin word meaning "of, on, or from the outside".

extremity – referring to the limbs of the human body, i.e., arms and legs.

extrinsic – not forming part of or belonging to a thing, i.e., the extrinsic muscles of the hand are in the forearm (not in the hand).

fasciitis – inflammation of the fascia.

femoral head – the rounded proximal end of the femur that articulates with the pelvis forming the hip joint.

femoral neck – connects the femoral head to the proximal end of the shaft of the femur.

femoris – a Latin word referring to the femur.

femur – long bone of the thigh that runs from the hip to the knee.

fibrosus – the thickening and scarring of connective tissue, usually as a result of injury.

fibula – the smaller of the two bones of the lower leg and is located lateral to the tibia.

fight bite – a laceration to the metacarpophalangeal joint capsule caused by a tooth puncture that occurs when one person punches another person in the mouth with a clenched fist.

flexion – refers to a movement that decreases the angle between two body segments.

floating ribs – the two most inferior ribs of the rib cage that only attaches to the thoracic spine, and do not have a ventral attachment to the sternum, either directly or via cartilage.

force – strength or energy as an attribute of physical action or movement.

forearm – referring to the anatomical structures between the elbow and the wrist.

forefoot – the anterior aspect of the foot comprised of the phalanges and the metatarsals.

fossa – a shallow depression in the bone surface or formed by anatomical structures.

fracture – a break in a bone or cartilaginous structure.

glands – an organ that secretes a substance.

glenoid – a shallow surface on the lateral scapula providing an articulating surface for the humerus. Referring to the shoulder.

gonadotropins – hormones secreted by the pituitary which stimulate the activity of the gonads.

greater trochanter – the irregular lateral prominence at the proximal end of the femur.

groin – the hallow at the junction of the truck and the inner portion of each thigh, containing the pubic region.

hallucis – a Latin word referring "of the big toe".

hematoma – localized bleeding outside of blood vessels, often due to trauma.

hindfoot – the posterior aspect of the foot that is formed by four of the tarsal bones including the calcaneus, talus, navicular, and cuboid.

homeostasis – a relatively stable state of equilibrium or balance.

hormone – the chemicals secreted by glands that are responsible for controlling and regulating the activities of certain cells and organs.

humerus – the arm bone. The long bone of the upper extremity that runs from the shoulder to the elbow.

hyoid – a u-shaped bone in the neck which supports the tongue.

hypothenar – referring to a group of three muscles of the palm of the hand that control the motion of the little finger.

iliac – relating to or situated near the ilium.

iliotibial band – a thick strip of connective tissue connecting several muscles in the lateral thigh.

ilium – the uppermost and largest region of the pelvis.

inferior – lower, below.

inferolaterally – situated both inferior and lateral.

inferomedial – situated both below and toward the middle.

intercostal – several groups of muscles that run between the ribs and help form and move the chest wall.

intermedius – a Latin word meaning "intermediate", or between.

intervertebral – situated between vertebrae.

intrinsic – being a part of; within; built-in.

ipsilateral – the opposite of contralateral and occurs on the same side of the body.

kinetic energy – energy which a body possesses by virtue of being in motion.

lateral – away from the midline.

lateral collateral ligament (LCL) – the structure on the outer aspect of the knee that provides side-to-side stability.

lateral femoral cutaneous nerve – the nerve that innervates the skin on the lateral aspect of the thigh.

leg – referring to the anatomical structures between the knee and the ankle.

ligament – a short band of tough, flexible fibrous connective tissue which connects two bones.

linea aspera – a Latin term for rough lines, referring to longitudinal ridges of the femoral shaft.

linear – arranged in or extending along a straight or nearly straight line.

long bone – a bone that has greater length than width. a long bone has a shaft and two distinct ends.

lower extremity – referring to the anatomical structures between the hip and the toes.

lumbar – refers to the lower back that consists of five vertebrae.

lymph – the fluid that flows through the lymphatic system.

macrophages – a type of white blood cell of the immune system that engulfs and digests pathogens.

magnus – a Latin word meaning great.

major – referring to something being more than something else.

mandible – the lower jawbone.

maximus – a Latin word referring to greatest or largest.

mechanoreceptors – a sense organ or cell that responds to mechanical stimuli such as touch or sound.

medial – towards the midline.

medial collateral ligament (MCL) – the structure on the inner aspect of the knee that provides side-to-side stability.

medioinferior – situated medial and inferior to something.

medius – an anatomic structure that is situated between two other similar structures or that is midway in position.

melanocytes – specialized skin cell that produces the protective skin-darkening pigment melanin.

meninges – the three membranes that envelop the brain and spinal cord.

meniscus – crescent shaped cartilaginous structure in the knee – both medial and lateral.

metatarsals – the five long bones of the foot.

midfoot – refers to the bones and joints that make up the arch of the foot and connect the forefoot to the hindfoot.

minimus – refers to being the smallest.

myotomes – refers to the group of muscles that are innervated by a specific spinal nerve root.

nerve – a cordlike structure within the body that conducts impulses that relay information from one part of the body to another.

neuroimmunology – medical specialty combining neuroscience, the study of the nervous system, and immunology, the study of the immune system.

neuromusculoskeletal – a connection and interaction between the neurological, muscular, and skeletal systems.

nondisplaced – a fracture (broken bone) that remains aligned after the injury.

oblique – slanting; neither parallel nor at a right angle to a specified or implied line.

odynophagia – painful swallowing.

oligodendrocytes – a type of nerve cell whose main functions are to provide support and insulation to axons in the central nervous system.

orbit of the eye – refers to the bony socket in the skull that contains the eye and its associated structures.

origin – the point or place where structure begins or is derived.

osteitis – inflammation of bone.

osteoarthritis – a degenerative joint process than can affect bone and surrounding tissues.

patella – also known as the kneecap; the small circular-triangular shaped bone imbedded in the quadriceps tendon and articulates with the distal femur.

pedis – a Latin wording referring to the foot.

pelvic ilium – the largest and uppermost bone of the pelvis.

pelvis – refers to the bony structures that form the cavity of the lower torso.

peroneal nerve – a branch of the sciatic nerve, which supplies movement and sensation to the lower leg, foot, and toes.

phalanges – the small bones that form the fingers and toes.

phalanx – singular of the term phalanges.

philtrum – the vertical groove from the base of the nose to the border of the upper lip overlying the teeth and gums.

photoreceptors – specialized cells in the eye's retina that are responsible for converting light into signals that are sent to the brain.

plantar flexion – refers extension at the ankle towards the plantar surface (the sole), so that the foot points inferiorly.

platelets – or thrombocytes, are small, colorless cell fragments in the blood that form clots and stop or prevent bleeding.

pollicis – the thumb.

popliteal fossa – the shallow depression located at the back of the knee joint.

posterior – refers to the back of, behind of, or to the rear of something.

posterior cruciate ligament (PCL) – one of a pair of structures (the other being the anterior cruciate ligament) in the middle of the knee joint that provides knee stability by preventing excessive posterior translation of the tibia relative to the distal femur.

posterolateral – situated on the side and toward the posterior aspect.

profundus – Latin word referring to "deeper" in relation to other more superficial structures.

pronate – to rotate (the hand or forearm) so that the surface of the palm is downward or toward the back; to turn (the sole of the foot) outward so that the inner edge of the foot bears the weight when standing.

prone – lying flat, face downward.

proximal – situated nearer to the center of the body or the point of attachment. The opposite of distal.

pubic ramus – inferior most part of the pelvis.

pubic symphysis – the midline cartilaginous joint formed by the right and left superior rami of pubic bones.

quadratus – referring to any of several roughly square or rectangular muscles.

radial – referring to the radius bone.

radiograph – an image produced on a sensitive plate or film by x-rays.

radioulnar – referring to the articulations or anatomical structures related to the radius and ulna bones.

radius – one of the two bones of the forearm that runs from the lateral side of the elbow to the thumb side of the wrist.

rheumatism – a chronic disease which is characterized by inflammation, muscle weaknesses, and muscle pains.

rhinorrhea – excess drainage from the nose and nasal passages.

ribs – twelve pairs of long curved bones that form the rib cage.

rotator cuff – a group of muscles and their tendons that act to stabilize the shoulder and allow for its extensive range of motion.

sacrum – the wedge-shaped bone at the inferior end of the spine that intersects with the pelvis.

sagittal – longitudinal plane which divides the body into right and left parts.

scapula – also known as the shoulder blade.

sciatic nerve – the longest and widest single nerve in the human body, runs from the lumbar spine through the buttock down the posterior thigh and leg to the foot. The sciatic nerve provides innervations to the majority of the skin and musculature of the thigh and lower leg.

sequalae – an abnormal condition or complication resulting from a previous injury or disease.

skeletal muscles – voluntary muscles that are attached to bones and are involved with the movement of different parts of the body.

skeleton – composed of bones which provides an internal framework and structure for the body.

skull – also known as cranium, comprises the bony structures that form the head and houses the brain.

spinal cord – a long, thin, tubular structure made up of nervous tissue extending from the medulla oblongata in the brainstem to the lumbar region of the vertebral column.

spine – also known as the backbone; the series of vertebrae extending from the skull to the lower back, enclosing the spinal cord and providing support for the thorax and abdomen.

staphylococcus – a group of bacteria that cause a multitude of diseases, especially in the skin and mucous membranes.

static – pertaining to or characterized by a fixed or stationary condition.

sternum – the long flat bone in the center of the chest to which the ribs connect via cartilage, also known as the breastbone.

streptococcus – a group of round gram-positive bacteria that occur in pairs or chains and can cause various infections in humans, including strep throat, erysipelas, and scarlet fever.

subglottis – the region in the lower portion of the larynx, extending from just beneath the vocal cords down to the top of the trachea.

sublimis – referring to "on top" or more superficial in relation to other deeper structures.

subtalar – below the talus bone.

superficial – located near the surface.

superior – upper; above; toward the head end of the body.

supinate – to turn or hold (a hand, foot, or limb) so that the palm or sole is facing upward or outward.

supine – lying on the back or having the face upward.

supraglottis – The upper part of the larynx, from just above the vocal cord to the tip of the epiglottis.

synovium – a specialized connective tissue that lines the inner surface of capsules of synovial joints and tendon sheath.

tarsals – seven irregular shaped bones of the foot and ankle.

T-cells – (T-lymphocytes) one of the important white blood cells of the immune system and play a role in the adaptive immune response.

testis – a testicle (plural testes) is the male reproductive gland or gonad.

thenar – referring to the rounded fleshy part in the palm of the hand at the base of the thumb

thigh – referring to the anatomical structures between the hip and the knee.

thoracic – refers to the mid back region that consists of twelve vertebrae.

tibia – also known as the shin bone it is the larger and stronger of the two bones of the lower leg.

T-lymphocytes – one of the important white blood cells of the immune system and play a role in the adaptive immune response.

transverse – lying or extending across or in a cross direction.

triangular fibrocartilage complex – (TFCC) a structure formed by the triangular fibrocartilage discus, the radioulnar ligaments and the ulnocarpal ligaments in the wrist.

trochanter – a bony protuberances to which muscles are attached to the upper part of the thigh bone.

ulna – one of the two bones of the forearm that runs from the elbow to the small finger side of the wrist.

ulnar – referring to the ulna bone.

upper extremity – referring to the anatomical structures between the shoulder and the fingers.

valgus stress – stress or pressure applied to a joint in the lateral to medial direction.

varus stress – stress or pressure applied to a joint in the medial to lateral direction.

vertebrae – the bony segments of the spine.

vertebral column – also known as the backbone or spine; part of the axial skeleton.

Printed in Poland
by Amazon Fulfillment
Poland Sp. z o.o., Wrocław